3D-Printed Prosthesis in Orthopedic Oncology

Zheng Guo • Ling Wang • Bin Liu
Editors

3D-Printed Prosthesis in Orthopedic Oncology

Springer

Editors
Zheng Guo
Orthopedics
Tangdu Hospital, Air Force Medical University
Xian, China

Ling Wang
Mechanical Engineering
School of Mechanical Engineering, Xi'an Jiaotong University
Xi'an, China

Bin Liu
GBA Center for Medical Device Evaluation and Inspection
National Medical Products Administration
Shenzhen, China

ISBN 978-981-95-1453-3 ISBN 978-981-95-1454-0 (eBook)
https://doi.org/10.1007/978-981-95-1454-0

Jointly published with Science Press

The print edition is not for sale in China (Mainland). Customers from China (Mainland) please order the print book from: Science Press.

This Springer imprint is published by the registered company Springer Nature Singapore Pte Ltd.
The registered company address is: 152 Beach Road, #21-01/04 Gateway East, Singapore 189721, Singapore

Preface

The use of 3D printing technology in the design and manufacture of prosthetics has been rapidly developing and applied to bone defect repair after bone tumor resection due to its abilities to promote efficient preparation and customization of prostheses as well as to create porous structures that meet specific needs. The use of this technique allows surgeons to plan the boundaries for surgical tumor removal based on the extent of bone tumor invasion and then propose customized prosthetic designs. Prosthetics that are fabricated by customized 3D printing precisely match the bone defects during surgery, ensuring alignment between surgical planning and execution. Moreover, the porous structures of personalized 3D-printed prosthetics facilitates bone integration at the interface, enhancing the long-term stability of these prosthetics and significantly improving the outcomes of bone repair and reconstruction.

Professor Guo is a pioneer and leader in the clinical application of customized 3D-printed orthopedic implants for the treatment of bone tumors in China. He led the team that was first in the world to implant a 3D-printed titanium clavicle and scapula prosthesis as well as the first in the world to treat necrosis of the femoral head with a 3D-printed biomimetic porous support rod, among other innovative techniques. These accomplishments have provided a foundation for the clinical application of personalized 3D-printed prostheses. Additionally, Professor Guo proposed the principle of "applying technology with control of standards" and played a leading role in drafting several standards and consensus documents, including "Specific Requirements for the Quality System of Customized Medical Devices," "Additive Manufacturing of Metal Intercalary Prostheses for Limbs," "Additive Manufacturing of Tantalum Spinal Prostheses," and "Consensus on the Design and Clinical Application of Customized 3D-Printed Pelvic Tumor Prostheses." These documents provide crucial guidelines for the product standards and clinical application of customized 3D-printed prostheses, ensuring the standardized and rational use of the technology.

Even when standards are established to guide and regulate the use of new technologies and products, their clinical application remains an iterative process of discovering and solving problems. Professor Guo's team has spent years exploring various aspects, such as the design and preparation of customized prostheses for bone tumors, clinical application, product certification, regulations, and interactions between medicine and engineering as well as between medicine and enterprises, accumulating a wealth of experience. This book summarizes these valuable experiences, aiming not only to help beginners quickly understand and begin using customized prostheses by resolving doubts but also to serve as a reference for experienced engineers, doctors, and managers by increasing their understanding of related issues.

The development of technology should benefit the public. This book hopes to provide knowledge to answer readers' questions and allow more patients to benefit from 3D-printed prostheses.

Xi'an, China Zheng Guo
Xi'an, China Ling Wang
Shenzhen, China Bin Liu

Contents

Editors and Contributors

About the Editors

Zheng Guo Department of Orthopedics, Tangdu Hospital, Air Force Medical University, Xi'an, China

Ling Wang State Key Laboratory for Manufacturing System Engineering, School of Mechanical Engineering, Xi'an Jiaotong University, Xi'an, China

Bin Liu GBA Center for Medical Device Evaluation and Inspection, National Medical Products Administration, Shenzhen, China

Associate Editors

Xiaokang Li Department of Orthopedics, Tangdu Hospital, Xi'an, China

Yongquan Zhang Wedo (Xian) Bio-Medical Technology Co., Ltd, Xi'an, China

Suhua Wu Wedo (Xian) Bio-Medical Technology Co., Ltd, Xi'an, China

Lei Shi Department of Orthopedics, Xijing Hospital, Xi'an, Shaanxi, China

Qiong Ma Department of Orthopedics, Tangdu Hospital, Xi'an, China

Jintao Gao GBA Center for Medical Device Evaluation and Inspection, NMPA, Shenzhen, China

Dan Han GBA Center for Medical Device Evaluation and Inspection, NMPA, Shenzhen, China

Contributors

Shusen Bao Department of Orthopedics, Tangdu Hospital, Xi'an, China

Changcheng Chen Department of Orthopedics, Tangdu Hospital, Xi'an, China

Yibei Chen GBA Center for Medical Device Evaluation and Inspection, NMPA, Shenzhen, China

Jinju Ding GBA Center for Medical Device Evaluation and Inspection, NMPA, Shenzhen, China

Enchun Dong State Key Laboratory for Manufacturing System Engineering, School of Mechanical Engineering, Xi'an Jiaotong University, Xi'an, China

National Medical Products Administration (NMPA) Key Laboratory for Research and Evaluation of Additive Manufacturing Medical Devices, Xi'an Jiaotong University, Xi'an, China

National Innovation Platform (Center) for Industry-Education Integration of Medical Technology, Xi'an Jiaotong University, Xi'an, China

Jun Fu Department of Orthopedics, Xijing Hospital, Xi'an, China

Shuo Guo Department of Orthopedics, Tangdu Hospital, Xi'an, China

Department of Radiology, Functional and Molecular Imaging Key Lab of Shaanxi Province, Tangdu Hospital, Xi'an, China

Hai Huang Department of Orthopedics, Tangdu Hospital, Xi'an, China

Jianfeng Kang School of Mechatronic Engineering and Automation, Foshan University, Foshan, China

Xiaoqi Lian GBA Center for Medical Device Evaluation and Inspection, NMPA, Shenzhen, China

Niya Li GBA Center for Medical Device Evaluation and Inspection, NMPA, Shenzhen, China

Jiayin Liu State Key Laboratory for Manufacturing System Engineering, School of Mechanical Engineering, Xi'an Jiaotong University, Xi'an, China

National Medical Products Administration (NMPA) Key Laboratory for Research and Evaluation of Additive Manufacturing Medical Devices, Xi'an Jiaotong University, Xi'an, China

National Innovation Platform (Center) for Industry-Education Integration of Medical Technology, Xi'an Jiaotong University, Xi'an, China

Wenwen Liu Department of Orthopedics, Tangdu Hospital, Xi'an, China

Yingjie Liu State Key Laboratory for Manufacturing System Engineering, School of Mechanical Engineering, Xi'an Jiaotong University, Xi'an, China

National Medical Products Administration (NMPA) Key Laboratory for Research and Evaluation of Additive Manufacturing Medical Devices, Xi'an Jiaotong University, Xi'an, China

National Innovation Platform (Center) for Industry-Education Integration of Medical Technology, Xi'an Jiaotong University, Xi'an, China

Yanchi Li GBA Center for Medical Device Evaluation and Inspection, NMPA, Shenzhen, China

Minqi Lu GBA Center for Medical Device Evaluation and Inspection, NMPA, Shenzhen, China

Yanjun Pei Department of Orthopedics, People's Hospital of Shenzhen, Shenzhen, China

Hainan Shen GBA Center for Medical Device Evaluation and Inspection, NMPA, Shenzhen, China

Changning Sun State Key Laboratory for Manufacturing System Engineering, School of Mechanical Engineering, Xi'an Jiaotong University, Xi'an, China

National Medical Products Administration (NMPA) Key Laboratory for Research and Evaluation of Additive Manufacturing Medical Devices, Xi'an Jiaotong University, Xi'an, China

National Innovation Platform (Center) for Industry-Education Integration of Medical Technology, Xi'an Jiaotong University, Xi'an, China

Zhen Tang Department of Orthopedics, Tangdu Hospital, Xi'an, China

Jingjing Wang Wedo (Xian) Bio-Medical Technology Co., Ltd, Xi'an, China

Hao Wu Department of Orthopedics, Tangdu Hospital, Xi'an, China

Qi Wu Department of Orthopedics, Tangdu Hospital, Xi'an, China

Chang Yang GBA Center for Medical Device Evaluation and Inspection, NMPA, Shenzhen, China

Dongmei Yu Department of Orthopedics, Tangdu Hospital, Xi'an, China

Xuegui Yu GBA Center for Medical Device Evaluation and Inspection, NMPA, Shenzhen, China

Kun Zhang GBA Center for Medical Device Evaluation and Inspection, NMPA, Shenzhen, China

Xiangmei Zhang GBA Center for Medical Device Evaluation and Inspection, NMPA, Shenzhen, China

Xuefei Zhu State Key Laboratory for Manufacturing System Engineering, School of Mechanical Engineering, Xi'an Jiaotong University, Xi'an, China

Part I

3D-Printed Custom-Made Prostheses: From Design to Production

Design of 3D-Printed Custom-Made Prostheses

1

Changning Sun, Enchun Dong, and Ling Wang

1.1 Clinical Needs and Design Criteria for 3D-Printed Custom-Made Prostheses

1.1.1 Introduction

In clinical practice, custom-made prostheses are conventionally used to treat large bone defects caused by bone tumors or trauma. These custom-made prostheses partially or completely restore the original bone function by repairing the structural defects of the bone. The development of additive manufacturing, a technology commonly known as 3D printing, has facilitated the development of custom-made prostheses with complex structural morphologies and internal microstructural characteristics. Prostheses design must account for the entire life of the prostheses, which affects the safety and feasibility of the entire process, including clinical need assessment as well as prostheses manufacturing, implantation, and service. Therefore, the design of custom-made prostheses should elucidate the clinical needs and establish design criteria that meet these clinical needs and manufacturing requirements.

C. Sun · E. Dong · L. Wang (✉)
State Key Laboratory for Manufacturing System Engineering, School of Mechanical Engineering, Xi'an Jiaotong University, Xi'an, China

National Medical Products Administration (NMPA) Key Laboratory for Research and Evaluation of Additive Manufacturing Medical Devices, Xi'an Jiaotong University, Xi'an, China

National Innovation Platform (Center) for Industry-Education Integration of Medical Technology, Xi'an Jiaotong University, Xi'an, China
e-mail: sun.cn@xjtu.edu.cn; dongenchun@stu.xjtu.edu.cn; menlwang@mail.xjtu.edu.cn

Z. Guo et al. (eds.), *3D-Printed Prosthesis in Orthopedic Oncology*,
https://doi.org/10.1007/978-981-95-1454-0_1

1.1.2 Clinical Needs of 3D-Printed Custom-Made Prostheses

To restore the function of defective bone tissue, based on the bone's characteristics, 3D-printed custom-made prostheses should meet the following clinical needs (Sun et al. 2022a):

Anatomical matching: The most obvious advantage of 3D-printed custom-made prostheses compared with traditional prostheses is the ability to match anatomical shapes well; this was one of the initial reasons for the application of 3D printing technology in the field of orthopedic implants. At present, the process of designing custom-made prostheses primarily relies on medical image reconstructions from the original data. This provides a database that facilitates morphological matching from the beginning of the design process. Anatomical shape matching is a fundamental requirement for custom-made prostheses, and this technology has been successfully implemented.

Mechanical loading: After a custom-made prosthesis is implanted into a human body, it should be able to withstand physiological loads. Prostheses failure due to insufficient strength is typically indicated by a prosthetic fracture. Fractures of peripheral prostheses should be evaluated to determine if the failure was a matter of strength. According to data from joint registries in various countries, among the various types of artificial joints, periprosthetic fractures account for 5~10% of all revisions, and prosthetic fractures account for 1~3%. It is important to note that these fractures are often accompanied by serious incidental injuries, but they do not present obvious signs in the human body. Therefore, strict measures must be taken to prevent such safety issues.

Immediate stability: During prosthesis implantation surgery, immediate fixation with the surrounding bones, muscles, ligaments, and other tissues is essential. Bone cement, screws, wire binding, and other technologies are commonly used for immediate fixation in orthopedic surgery. Firm immediate fixation is necessary to ensure a stable mechanical connection and interfacial healing between the prosthesis and autologous bone and other tissues in the human body. This approach is the basis for stable long-term fixation.

Long-term stability: The long-term stability of orthopedic implants after implantation in the human body is crucial for their long-term effective service. Loosening and displacement of a prosthesis due to poor long-term stability are the main causes of long-term failure. After implantation, the prosthesis forms a new biomechanical system with the surrounding bones, and together, the components of this system bear the load and movement of the human body. Gradual loss of stable bony support is associated with severe bone loss around the prosthesis, which can cause loosening or lowering of the prosthesis. In contrast, the vigorous growth of surrounding bone can promote tight integration of the bone and the prosthesis.

Functional reconstruction: Restoring the function of defective bone is one of the core purposes of orthopedic implants. The mechanical functions of bone include support, protection, and movement. Therefore, during the design of orthopedic implants, the core function of the original bones must be considered. For example, the main function of the cranium is to protect the brain, so the safety of the implants should be considered when they are impacted. Moreover, the maxillofacial bone plays a role in supporting the shape of the face and forming the temporomandibular joint, and the match between the morphology of the implant and the original bone, as well as the role of chewing muscles, needs to be considered. When designing prostheses for long bones in the limbs, the physiological condition and whether the prosthesis can withstand human movement should be considered.

Surgical timeliness: When custom-made prostheses are used to repair bone defects due to trauma or bone tumors, timely surgery is crucial. Therefore, there are strict requirements for the timeline of 3D-printed custom-made prostheses design and manufacturing. That is, the design and manufacture of a prosthesis must be completed before the patient is scheduled for surgery.

1.1.3 Design Criteria for 3D-Printed Custom-Made Prostheses

The design of custom-made prostheses acts as a bridge between clinical needs and prosthetic manufacturing. Thus, the clinical requirements and constraints of addtive manufacturing (AM) must be considered when designing a custom-made prosthesis. Based on clinical and manufacturing needs, Sun et al. (2022a) proposed the design criteria, as shown in Fig. 1.1.

Geometric matching criterion: Geometric matching is an important criterion for the design of prostheses related to patient appearance, such as maxillofacial bone repair prostheses and cranial repair prostheses. Aesthetic restoration is the key factor in assessing the clinical efficacy of this type of prosthesis. However, when designing a custom-made prosthesis, it is not necessary to replicate all the geometrical characteristics of the tissue near the bone defect; this would make the

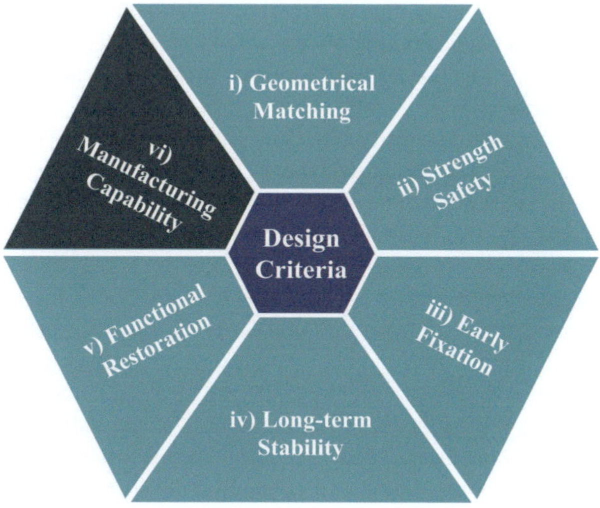

Fig. 1.1 Design criteria for 3D-printed custom-made prostheses (Sun et al. 2022a)

geometrical structure of the prosthesis too complicated or lead to the generation of unnecessary geometric features, which would reduce the quality of the prosthesis, cause stress concentration or even shorten its service life. For example, in the design of a custom rib prosthesis by Kang et al. (2018), the method of extracting the centerline and cross-sectional features of the natural rib was used to create a simplified rib prosthesis instead of reconstructing an accurate 3D model from computed tomography (CT) images, and this proved to be an effective and practical approach.

Mechanical safety criterion: The mechanical safety criterion must be considered throughout the entire design process, but the starting point for mechanical safety considerations is different for different types of prostheses. Custom-made prostheses, such as long bone prostheses, artificial vertebral bodies, and pelvic bone prostheses, play important roles in the human body by bearing physiological loads. Therefore, long-term durability must be assessed for these prostheses. For example, in the field of artificial joints, there are existing standards related to wear and fatigue, such as ISO 14242, ISO 14243, and ISO 7206. For other types of prostheses that are only loaded for a short period of time after implantation in the human body, such as bone plates, mechanical safety considerations can focus solely on static loading. The main function of some bones, such as the cranium and sternum, is to protect human organs. Therefore, safety considerations should focus on the toughness and safety of these materials during accidental impact.

Early stability criterion: In the design of a prosthesis, fixation structures, such as screw holes or shallow grooves for wire binding, should be designed based on the immediate fixation method that will be used during surgery. The extent of interface micromotion between the bone and the prostheses is a quantitative indicator of early fixation. Cameron et al. (1973) revealed for the first time the effect of micromovements on promoting fracture healing, and Maniatopoulos et al. (1986) proposed a micromotion threshold. That is, micromotions within an appropriate range promoted healing between the implant and bone, while greater micromotion led to poor early fixation and thus destruction of the healing interface. Li et al. (2018) reviewed previous studies on the micromotion threshold and concluded that micromotions in the range of 50–100 μm facilitate interfacial healing and bone ingrowth in porous implants.

Long-term stability criterion: Early fixation is typically achieved by mechanical fixation, which has a high risk of loosening with long-term movement in the human body. Stability can be achieved by osseointegration between the bone and the prosthesis and by the bone support that is provided by the surrounding tissues. Long-term stability is a more difficult challenge. The advantage of 3D printing technology in the design of custom-made prostheses lies in the manufacture of porous structures that can improve the long-term stability of prostheses in two ways. On the one hand, the porous structure provides space for the ingrowth of bone tissue, achieving integration between the bone and prosthesis. On the other hand, the porous structure reduces the equivalent elastic modulus of the prosthesis, which transfers more load to the bone tissue, thus providing the necessary mechanical stimulation for surrounding bone growth and enhancing the surrounding bony support.

Functional restoration criterion: The primary aim of custom-made prostheses is to restore the mechanical function of a defective bone. Due to the differences in the function of different bones, different considerations need to be given to the design of different prostheses. For example, the kinematics of reconstructed joints must be considered in the design of custom-made prostheses within articular surfaces. Prostheses of the lower extremities need to focus on bearing the static and dynamic loads of the human body. In addition, for sternocostal prostheses, the expansion of the thorax during breathing should be considered. The functional restoration criteria are related to the clinical application scenarios in design practice, and the close cooperation of design engineers and physicians is required.

Manufacturing capability criterion: Although 3D printing technology has high flexibility, limitations of manufacturing capabilities should be considered as a first step in the design of custom-made prostheses. Manufacturing constraints are mainly reflected in two aspects: whether the manufacturing capability of the corresponding 3D printing process can achieve the necessary porous structure and feature dimensions, and whether the design and manufacturing timeline of 3D-printed custom-made prostheses can match the surgical timeline. The expected delivery time must be confirmed when finalizing the treatment plan using custom-made prostheses.

Starting from clinical needs and summarizing the clinical needs of customized 3D-printed prostheses, six criteria for prosthesis design are proposed in this section. These criteria are not limited to the materials used for the prosthesis or its intended locations but are general criteria that need to be considered in the design of all custom-made prostheses, and these criteria should be considered at different stages of the design process. However, different design criteria require consideration from the perspectives of different disciplines during the design process. For example, the mechanical safety criterion and the manufacturing capability criterion should be considered from an engineering perspective, and the functional restoration criterion should be considered from a medical perspective. Therefore, both medical and engineering teams are required to work together in the design process. To ensure the safety and effectiveness of custom-made prostheses, strict processes need to be followed in the design, and the rights and responsibilities of the medical and engineering staff must be clarified.

1.2 Design Process and Medicine–Engineering Interaction of 3D-Printed Custom-Made Prostheses

The general process of customized prostheses design is shown in Fig. 1.2, and it generally includes six main steps: proposal, 3D reconstruction, implant design, mechanical analysis, design confirmation, and manufacturing. If the design of the prosthesis does not meet the performance requirements during mechanical analysis, the shape and structure of the prosthesis must be optimized until the design requirements are met. If the requirements are not met during the design evaluation, the design process needs to be restarted. To ensure the traceability of the design process, all the steps that are involved in the design process need to be documented, and

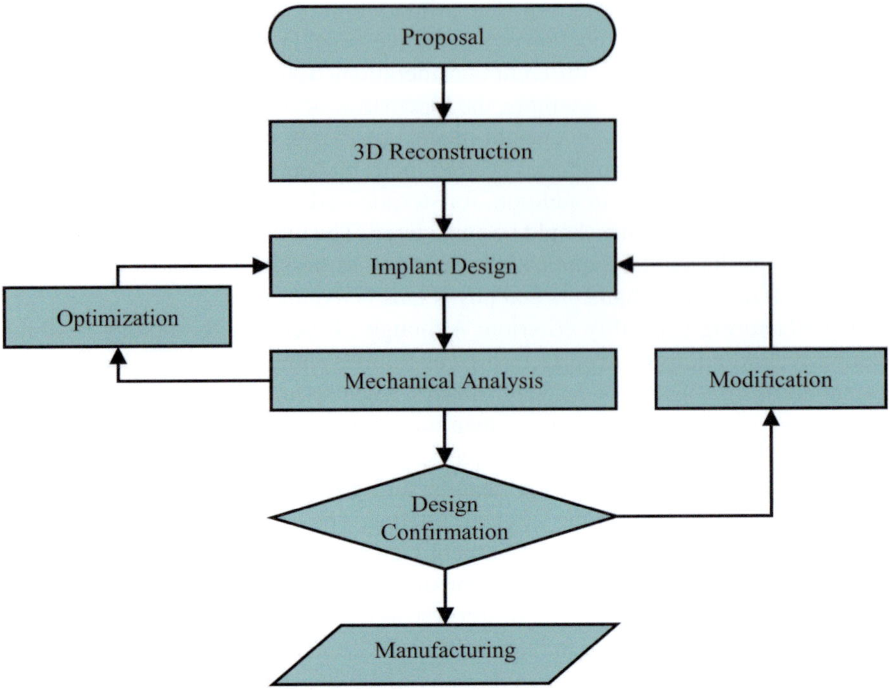

Fig. 1.2 General design process of custom-made prostheses (adapted from "guidance document of the National Medical Products Administration")

samples should be retained when appropriate. To improve the effectiveness of medicine–engineering interactions during the design process and to ensure that the rights and responsibilities of the medical and engineering staff are clear, the Center for Medical Device Evaluation (CMDE) of the National Medical Products Administration (NMPA) of China released the "Guiding Principles of Quality Control of Medical–Industrial Interaction of Personalized Matched Bone Implants and Instruments (No. 62, 2020)" in 2020, providing overall guidelines for the design and development of custom-made prostheses.

1.2.1 Planning and Approval of the Project

Each set of custom-made prosthesis for each patient is a custom-made prosthesis project, and planning and approval documents are formulated for each project. The planning and project approval documents serve two purposes. One is to clarify information that is closely related to the design process, such as the clinical condition and prosthesis design requirements, and the other is to demonstrate the necessity of the use of custom-made prostheses to avoid the risk of the overuse of custom-made prostheses.

Based on these two objectives, planning and project approval documents should include an overview of the clinical situation, expected performance, and evidence of necessity and feasibility. An overview of the clinical situation and the expected performance should be completed by the medical staff. The clinical situation includes the basic condition of the patient, the application range of the prosthesis, the medical function of the prosthesis, and the assumption of prosthesis implantation. The expected performance needs to clarify the requirements of the custom-made prosthesis, including the expected functional characteristics, use conditions, and service duration.

Then, based on the clinical situation and the description of the expected performance of the prosthesis, the medical team should demonstrate the necessity of a custom-made prosthesis from the following perspectives: first, whether there are registered commercial prostheses available for the proposed treatment plan; second, if commercial prostheses are already available, whether the clinical effects can be improved by using custom-made prostheses; and third, whether the risks of custom-made prostheses are controllable.

Ultimately, before the design process begins, the engineering team must demonstrate the feasibility of using 3D printing to customize the prosthesis based on the clinical situation and expected performance. At the material level, the biocompatibility, processability, and mechanical properties of the material must meet prosthesis requirements. At the process level, whether the capability of the additive manufacturing process can produce a prosthesis that meets the expected requirements is assessed in terms of minimum feature manufacturing capability, accuracy, and roughness. The design and manufacturing capabilities of the engineering team must be used to confirm the suitability of the custom-made prosthesis. The design and manufacturing timeline must be considered in light of the design and manufacturing capabilities of the engineering team to ensure that the clinical surgery timeline can be met.

1.2.2 Three-Dimensional Reconstruction

Custom-made prostheses require a personalized 3D model as input data. In clinical practice, the original data that is used to design most custom-made prostheses are computed tomography (CT) data. The design of custom-made prostheses heavily depends on the acquisition and processing of radiological data and the 3D reconstruction of the anatomical and structural component models; however, excessively fine 3D reconstruction is time-consuming and increases the number of geometric features unnecessarily. This approach may significantly increase the subsequent workload of prosthesis design and mechanical analysis. Therefore, during 3D data acquisition and reconstruction, medical and engineering personnel need to determine the source of the original radiological data, the extent of the tissues to be reconstructed, the allowable error range between the reconstructed model and the original data, and the anatomical features that can be omitted from the 3D model. The purpose of this approach is to efficiently and accurately acquire CT data and reconstruct a 3D model of the affected area.

During 3D reconstruction, the medical team usually acquires CT data and delivers the data to the engineering team for 3D reconstruction. To ensure the traceability of the process, the medical team needs to confirm the medical imaging data before delivering it to the engineering team.

1.2.3 Implant Design

The ultimate goal of prosthesis design is to design a prosthesis that matches the expected goal described in the planning and project approval documents. This section does not introduce the specific technologies that are used in prosthesis design but rather focuses on how to consider each element of prosthesis design based on the expected goals and design criteria of the prosthesis, as shown in Table 1.1.

In addition to the recovery of function, immediate fixation of the prosthesis to bone and soft tissues and long-term fixation structures are needed. For immediate fixation, a screw connection, binding, or interference fit is typically used; the anastomosis structure should be designed with the assistance of customized surgical tools or osteotomy guides, if necessary, to ensure the accuracy of screw installation and osteotomy during the surgical procedure. For long-term fixation, a partially porous structure is typically used in 3D-printed custom-made prostheses. When the prosthesis is in the human body, bone tissue gradually grows into the porous structure to form a stable bone–prosthesis biofixation system.

Table 1.1 Key points of functional recovery in prosthesis design

Function	Description
Morphological recovery	The prosthesis restores the appearance of the patient
Stability	The prosthesis performs part of the bone's load-bearing function for a long or short time period; the static strength, stiffness, and fatigue performance meet the requirements
Restriction or control of movement	The structure of the prosthesis limits or controls local relative movement; the local deformation and strain meet the requirements
Prevention of fracture, deformation, and dislocation	The strength and stiffness of the prosthesis limit deformation under physiological load
Fragment connections	The structural design of the prosthesis allows the fragments to be correctly anastomosed according to the anatomical relationship. The strength and stiffness of the prosthesis support the load of the human body and provide certain mechanical stimulation to promote fragment healing
Controlled extrusion or transfer	The strength and stiffness of the prosthesis limit deformation under human load
Protection of adjacent tissue structures	The strength and impact resistance of the prosthesis allow it to protect the adjacent tissue structures
Joint movement	The wear resistance of the prosthesis meets the expected friction life

1.2.4 Mechanical Analysis

Custom-made prostheses play roles in mechanical support, protection, and connection in the human body. Therefore, mechanical analysis of the prosthesis through physical testing or computer simulation is an important way to evaluate the service performance of the prosthesis before it is delivered for manufacturing. However, the anatomical morphological characteristics and loading environment of custom-made prostheses are complex, making it difficult to systematically evaluate product performance and function. To address this problem, the NMPA of China proposed a customized prosthesis equivalence model method, which was published in the "Guiding Principles for Technical Review of the Registration of Equivalence Models for Customized Personalized Bone Implants" that was released in 2020. Equivalence models should be used to assess the anatomical fit and biomechanical properties of custom-made prostheses. Equivalence models with clinical expectations and bioequivalence are evaluated in terms of function and clinical expectations. Equivalence can be used to identify risk factors, such as material properties, structural design, geometric size, intended use, usage methods, implant product application sites, human mechanical environments, and biological effects, combined with implantation risk assessment and clinical studies.

In the clinical application of custom-made prostheses, there are two difficulties in conducting equivalence model studies based on bench tests. On the one hand, due to the personal characteristics of prostheses, usually only 1–2 duplicates of each prosthesis are manufactured, which makes it difficult to perform bench tests with statistical significance. On the other hand, due to the complexity of the mechanical environment of custom-made prostheses, it is extremely difficult to design a bench test to simulate the *in vivo* mechanical environment, and this approach is not feasible given the limited timeline for product delivery. Therefore, in practice, computer simulation is typically used for the mechanical analysis of custom-made prostheses. The computer simulation of custom-made prostheses is mainly based on the finite element (FE) analysis method. The FE biomechanical analysis technique is described in detail in Sect. 1.3.1 of this chapter.

1.2.5 Design Confirmation

Design confirmation is a key step in the process of designing custom-made prostheses and needs to be completed by both the medical and engineering staff based on their own responsibilities. Design confirmation has two main aspects: the first aspect is the confirmation of the design results, including whether the shape and structure of the implant meet the expectations, and the mechanical analysis and calculation results of the prosthesis are used to determine whether the expected function can be performed. The medical team should be responsible for the design confirmation of the implantability of the prosthesis and whether the patient experienced significant changes in their condition during the period of prosthesis design that prevent the design results from meeting clinical needs. The second aspect of design confirmation is manufacturing feasibility; it is the responsibility of the engineering team to evaluate whether the designed prosthesis meets the requirements in terms of structure, mechanics, and manufacturing time.

Design confirmation is the key to ensuring the service performance and quality of custom-made prostheses. During this step, the medical and engineering teams must implement confirmation elements for different types of custom-made prostheses and create internal management documents for the enterprise or hospital, which must be included for each custom prosthesis that is developed. During the design process, the specific people who are responsible for each confirmation element are identified, and clear and traceable documentation is provided.

1.2.6 Manufacturing

The manufacturing step involves the transformation of custom-made prostheses from design to production, and this is also the last step in the design process. In this step, the medical and engineering teams responsible for prosthesis design must work together to formulate acceptance criteria for the final product, namely, the custom prosthesis. The acceptance criteria can be derived from the following aspects. The first aspect is the macro- and micro-accuracy of the prosthesis, which includes the macroscopic dimensional accuracy, the integrity and critical dimensions, such as pore size and microrod diameter, the microscopic porous structure, and the surface roughness. The second aspect is the internal defects of the prosthesis, such as internal microcracks, which can be detected by nondestructive testing techniques, such as micro-CT or ultrasonic flaw detection. The third aspect is the mechanical properties, for which standard samples are generally preserved during the manufacture of custom-made prostheses or accompanying products, and the mechanical properties of these specimens should be inspected when necessary.

This section summarizes the general process of custom prosthesis design and identifies the key elements of medicine–engineering interactions. On the one hand, the medical and engineering teams who are involved in the design of prostheses need to clarify the rights and responsibilities of all parties, that is, the team that is responsible for the implementation of each element; on the other hand, the effectiveness of the interaction process also needs to be ensured. The medical team should consider the overall details of prosthesis design. These details include the anatomical characteristics of the target region, the anatomical and biomechanical parameters of the adjacent region, and the factors of the uninjured side/contralateral side; considering these details can avoid any overarching issues about which the clinician is concerned during the prosthetic design process. Any deviation from the local design requires the involvement of the engineers. Therefore, it is necessary to clarify rights and responsibilities and to fully communicate in medicine–engineering interactions.

1.3 Key Technologies for 3D-Printed Customized Prostheses Design

1.3.1 Application of Biomechanical Analysis in the Design and Evaluation of Custom-Made Prostheses

Biomechanics is a branch of biophysics that applies mechanical theories and methods to the quantitative study of mechanical problems in living organisms, with an emphasis on studies of mechanical problems related to physiology and medicine. With the development of manufacturing technology, the demand for custom-made prostheses is increasing. However, due to the specificity of the morphology and performance of custom-made prostheses, it is usually difficult to evaluate and optimize the performance of custom-made prostheses through *in vitro* experiments. Biomechanical analysis methods based on finite element technology can perfectly simulate the *in vivo* mechanical environment of custom-made prostheses; therefore, this approach has gradually become an important means for optimizing the design and evaluating the performance of custom-made prostheses.

Currently, biomechanical analysis is mainly used for the design optimization and performance analysis of custom-made prostheses, as shown in Table 1.2. The optimization design can be applied to structural and design parameter optimization, material distribution optimization, internal fixation methods optimization, etc., so that the prostheses have optimal mechanical properties and *in vivo* service performance. The service performance analysis can be oriented toward strength, stiffness, and stability to ensure the safety and reliability of the prostheses. The worst-case analysis can be used to predict the fatigue performance, wear performance, and fracture failure performance of prostheses to verify whether the prosthesis design will meet the mechanical requirements *in vivo*.

1.3.1.1 Optimization Design

First, in terms of structure optimization, biomechanical analysis and topology optimization methods can be used to design custom-made prostheses or to quantitatively study the design parameters of custom-made prostheses to achieve the optimal

Table 1.2 Applications of biomechanical analysis

Application fields	Category
Optimization design	Optimization of structural parameters
	Optimization of materials
	Optimization of fixation method
Service performance analysis	Strength analysis
	Stiffness analysis
	Stability analysis
Worst-case analysis	Fatigue performance
	Wear performance
	Fracture failure

structural design. Kang et al. (2021) and Iqbal et al. (2019) constructed a finite element model of the lumbar spine and pelvis, and custom-made prostheses for vertebral body and pelvic defects were designed using the topology optimization method, respectively. Wang et al. (2018) constructed a mechanical model of lumbar spine reconstruction with a personalized artificial vertebral body, and the effects of parameters including the end surface topography, tilting angle, wall thickness, and implantation position of the custom-made artificial vertebral body on the anti-subsidence performance of the artificial vertebral body and the performance of bone graft fusion were analyzed (Fig. 1.3), and these results provided guidance, and these results provided guidance for the optimized design of artificial vertebral body structures.

In terms of material optimization design, biomechanical analysis methods can be used to optimize the material distribution of custom-made prostheses to control the mechanical properties of these custom-made prostheses and thus improve their *in vivo* performance. Pasini et al. (2017) and Sun et al. (2018, 2022b) optimized the internal material properties of a femoral stem based on the stress distribution of the femoral stem *in vivo*, and the designed prosthesis significantly reduced the stress shielding effect and improved the osteointegration of the prosthesis with the surrounding bone tissue.

In terms of fixation method optimization, Kang et al. (2021) systematically studied the effect of different connection structures of custom-made rib prostheses on

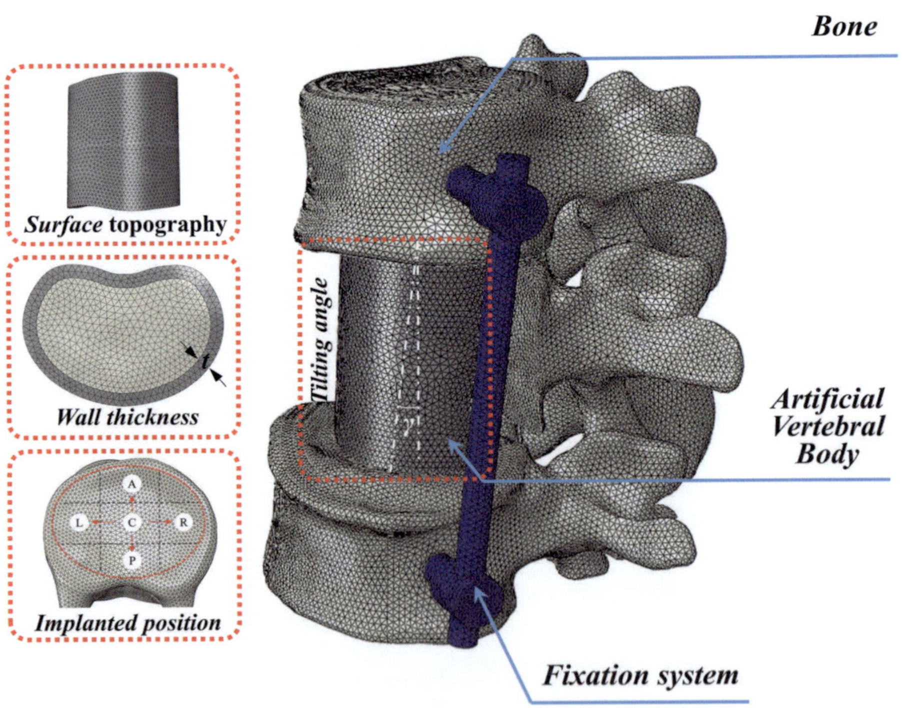

Fig. 1.3 Design parameters optimization of the artificial vertebral body (Wang et al. 2018)

the stress and deformation distribution between the prosthesis and the surrounding bone based on the rib finite element model, and the results provided guidance for designing the connection structure of custom-made rib prostheses. Dong et al. (2018) conducted a parametric analysis on the effect of the number and preloading force of custom-made pelvic prosthesis fixation screws on the stress distribution of custom-made prostheses, and they provided a method for optimizing screw preloading force and quantity. Güvenç et al. (2017) studied the effect of the pedicle screw installation angle on the screw stress distribution based on a cervical fusion finite element model; this work provided guidance for the optimization of spinal fixation methods. Therefore, biomechanical analysis is a low-cost and effective method to achieve the optimal design of custom-made prostheses.

1.3.1.2 Service Performance Analysis

The *in vivo* safety and stability of custom-made prostheses can be evaluated using biomechanical analysis methods. For safety, the structural strength and structural stiffness of the prosthesis are the two main aspects. Dong et al. (2020) calculated the stress distribution of a custom-made artificial vertebral body under human daily activity loads (Fig. 1.4a) based on the constructed spine finite element model, and the maximum stress of the artificial vertebral body was compared with the yield strength of the corresponding material. To evaluate the *in vivo* safety of the designed rib prosthesis, Kang et al. (2021) calculated the deformation distribution of poly-ether-ether-ketone (PEEK) rib prostheses (Fig. 1.4b) under chest compression loading conditions based on the constructed rib finite element model to evaluate the *in vivo* safety of the rib prosthesis.

The *in vivo* stability of the custom-made prosthesis was evaluated mainly in terms of short-term and long-term stability. Short-term stability was evaluated by calculating parameters such as the relative displacement of the interface between the bone

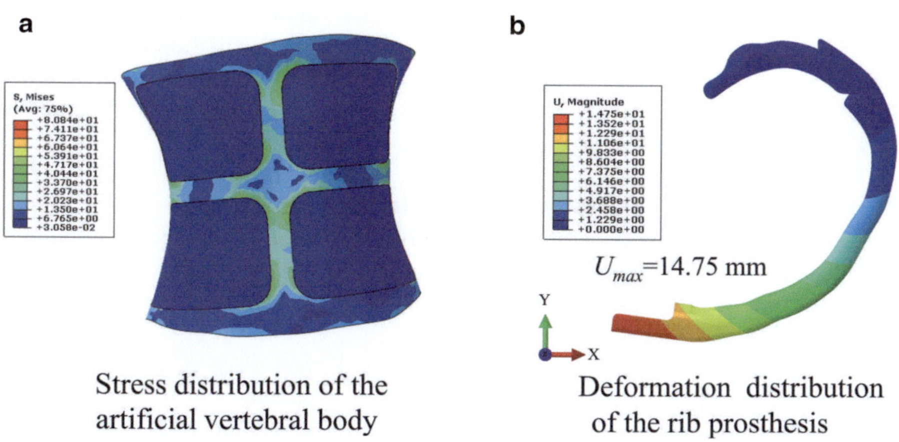

Fig. 1.4 Safety analysis of the custom-made prostheses (**a**) Stress distribution of the artifical vertebral body (Dong et al. 2020); (**b**) Deformation distribution of the rid prosthesis (Kang et al. 2021)

and the prosthesis or the range of motion (ROM) of the spinal fixation segment. Dong et al. (2020) calculated the ROM of a lumbar spine that was reconstructed with a custom-made artificial vertebral body and compared this ROM with the ROMs of the corresponding segments of the healthy lumbar spine. The results indicated that the ROM of the reconstructed lumbar spine was significantly lower than that of the healthy lumbar spine (68.1–92.6%), which indicated good lumbar reconstruction stability. For long-term stability, the strain distribution of the interface between the bone and prosthesis can be calculated because Wolff's law (Wolff et al. 1986) can be subsequently used to predict bone growth and reconstruction at the interface between the prosthesis and the host bone after implantation (Dong et al. 2020).

1.3.2 Application of Topology Optimization in the Design of Custom-Made Prostheses

Topology optimization is a mathematical method that optimizes the material distribution in a given area based on particular load conditions, constraint conditions, and performance indicators. The designed structure has the advantages of high strength, high stiffness, and low weight. In recent years, with the development of medical imaging, materials science, and additive manufacturing technology, topology optimization technology based on finite element analysis has been gradually applied to the innovative design of medical models, especially in the field of custom-made prosthesis design.

The construction of an optimization model is the most important basis for addressing topology optimization problems. Currently, commonly used mathematical modeling methods include the homogenization method, variable density method, variable thickness method, independent-continuous-mapping method, and progressive structural optimization method. The most frequently used methods in the medical field are the homogenization method and the variable density method. The variable density method has the advantages of a simple calculation process, high calculation efficiency, and a very high practical value; therefore, it is used by most topology optimization solvers, such as Abaqus, Ansys, and Optistruct, for the topology optimization design of prostheses.

1.3.2.1 Prostheses Topology Optimization Design Cases

Benefiting from the lightweight and high-stiffness design advantages of topology optimization methods, topology optimization has been applied to the optimization design of human prostheses, such as craniomaxillofacial, spinal, limb joint, pelvic, and bone plate prostheses, in recent years.

In the field of cranimaxillofacial prosthesis design, Park et al. (2021) and Sutradhar et al. (2016) designed custom-made maxillofacial prostheses for different maxillofacial defect morphologies using the topology optimization method. (Fig. 1.5a) *In vitro* mechanical property tests showed that a topology-optimized maxillofacial prosthesis could meet the strength requirements of human daily activities. These studies could lead to new insights into the innovative design of

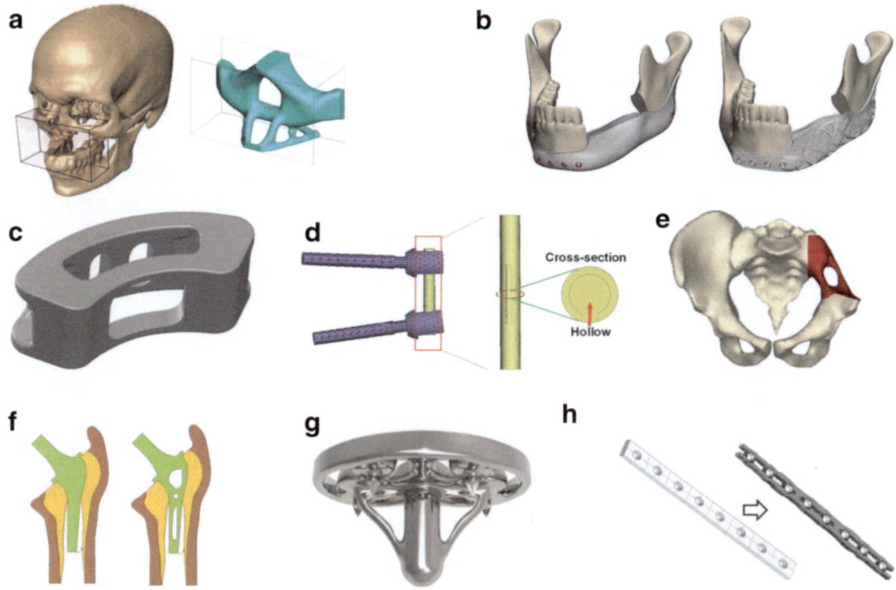

Fig. 1.5 Application of topology optimization in prosthetic design (**a**) Maxillofacial prosthesis; (**b**) Mandibular prosthesis; (**c**) Spinal cage; (**d**) Fixation rod; (**e**) Pelvic prosthesis; (**f**) Femoral stem; (**g**) Tibia tray; (**h**) Bone plate

craniofacial surgical prostheses. In addition, topology optimization design has been applied to the treatment of mandibular defects and fractures (Li et al. 2020; van Kootwijk et al. 2022) (Fig. 1.5b).

Regarding spinal prosthesis design, Sun et al. (2021) designed a topological cage with the advantages of being lightweight and having a better osseointegration effect at the bone and prosthesis interface (Fig. 1.5c). To design a spinal fixation device, Guo and Wang (2020) designed a hollow, slotted, low-stiffness posterior fixation rod through topology optimization (Fig. 1.5d). The finite element analysis results showed that the topological rod could reduce the stress on the fixation system as well as on the adjacent segment disc, thereby reducing the risk of adjacent segment degeneration.

In pelvic defect reconstruction, the topology optimization method was used in the design of pelvic prostheses and was successfully applied in clinical practice (Fig. 1.5e) by Iqbal et al. (2019). Compared with traditional pelvic prostheses, topology-optimized pelvic prostheses have the advantages of being lightweight and having high strength, and they can significantly improve the *in vivo* biomechanical properties of prostheses. The effectiveness and safety of the proposed topology optimization design method in the design of hemi-pelvis prostheses were also verified via finite element analysis.

The main use of the topology optimization method in designing limb joint prosthesis is in the design of prostheses for the femoral stem (Abdullah et al. 2023;

Kharmanda 2016; Xiao et al. 2023) (Fig. 1.5f) and tibia tray (Guoqing et al. 2021; Kladovasilakis et al. 2023; Rahimizadeh et al. 2018) (Fig. 1.5g). Through topology optimization, the weight and stiffness of the femoral stem and of the tibial tray prostheses can be reduced; therefore, the stress shielding effect can be improved, and the risk of prosthetic loosening or failure can be reduced.

In bone plate design, many studies have shown that using a topology-optimized bone plate (Fig. 1.5h) can greatly reduce stiffness while ensuring the structural strength of the bone plate, thereby improving the stress transfer at the bone/prosthesis interface and promoting the fracture's healing speed (Al-Tamimi et al. 2019, 2020; Kaymaz et al. 2022; Liu et al. 2020).

1.3.2.2 Topology Optimization Design and Clinical Application of Artificial Vertebral Body

This section introduces the topology optimization method and the clinical application process using a custom-made artificial vertebral body as an example. During the topology optimization design process of the artificial vertebral bodies, the loads of human daily spine activities, including flexion, extension, left/right bending, and left/right rotation, were considered to achieve the organic combination of artificial vertebral body structure design and human spine motion loads. The adaptability and stability of the artificial vertebral body were significantly improved to align with the complex mechanical environment of the human spine throughout its life cycle.

The overall process of artificial vertebral body topology optimization overall process of artificial vertebral body topology optimization is shown in Fig. 1.6.

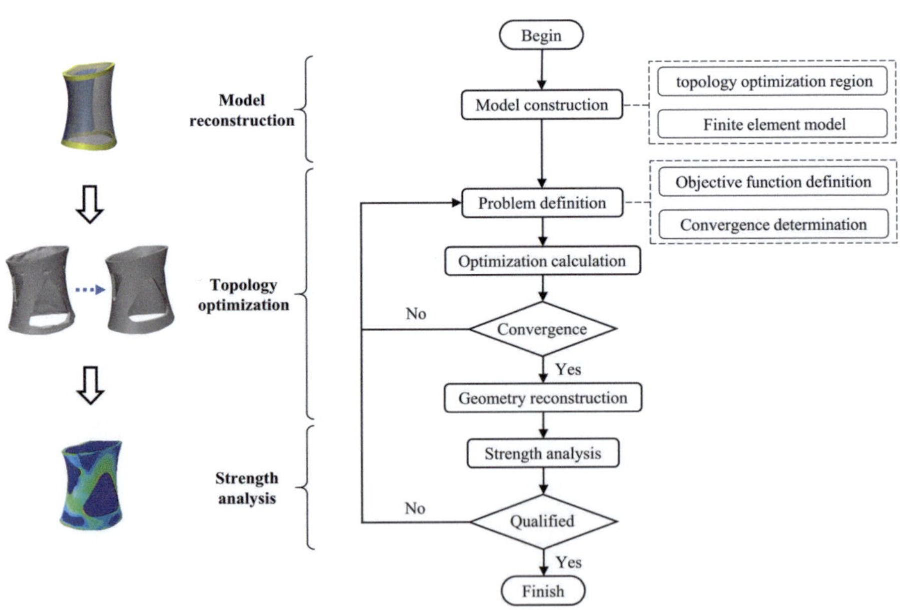

Fig. 1.6 Design process of the topology optimization

The process includes three steps: topology optimization model construction, topology includes three steps: topology optimization model construction, topology optimization calculation, and prosthesis strength analysis. Model construction is the basic premise of the topology optimization design process, and it includes the design of the topology optimization region of the artificial vertebral body and the construction of the finite element model of the spine. The topology optimization calculation is the main part of the topology optimization design process of the artificial vertebral body, and it includes the optimization problem definition, optimization calculation, convergence determination, and geometry reconstruction. Strength analysis is the final step in the optimization design process of artificial vertebral body topology. Only when the artificial vertebral structure obtained by topology optimization design meets the strength requirements of the human mechanical environment can the topology optimization design model of the artificial prosthesis be used for prosthesis manufacturing and clinical application.

Based on the abovementioned topology optimization design method for the artificial vertebral body, the research teams at the Air Force Medical University and Xi'an Jiaotong University collaborated on the design of a topology-optimized artificial vertebral body for use in clinical spinal tumor resection, and it was successfully implanted into the patient.

Patient Li SL, a 53-year-old female, was admitted to Xijing Hospital of the Air Force Medical University for spinal pain. The attending physician showed that a tumor had eroded the L5 segment of the patient's lumbar spine, and the patient experienced vertebral collapse accompanied by scoliosis. Vertebral body segment and adjacent discectomy at the L5 segment were performed, and a topology-optimized artificial vertebral body was used to reconstruct the spine resection area. Internal fixation with the screw and rod fixation system was performed to achieve stable reconstruction. The design and clinical application of the topology optimized artificial vertebral body are shown in Fig. 1.7.

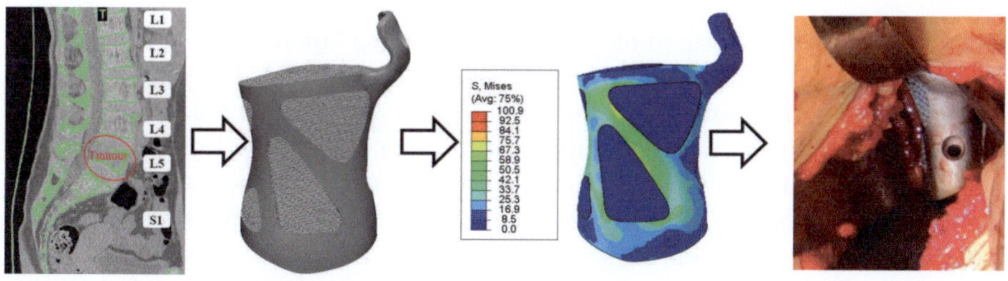

Fig. 1.7 Topology optimization design and clinical application of artificial vertebral body

1.3.3 Porous Structure Design in Customized Prostheses

1.3.3.1 The Significance of Designing Porous Structures in Custom-Made Prostheses

The advent of 3D printing technology not only provides the ability to produce custom-made prostheses of any shape but also provides the only viable manufacturing technology for producing prostheses with controllable porous structures. An increase in the porosity reduces the macroscopic elastic modulus of a material, and the porosity also generates a prosthesis with mechanical properties that are similar to those of native bone tissue by constructing a biomimetic gradient porous structure. Additionally, porous structures can provide space for the growth of bone tissue and are more conducive to the close combination of the prosthesis and the surrounding bone, making porous structures ideal internal interfaces for orthopedic prostheses.

1.3.3.2 Evaluation of the Mechanical Properties of Porous Prostheses

There are two main mechanical problems in the design of porous prostheses: mechanical safety and stress shielding. In the design of porous prostheses, these two issues place conflicting demands on the design of the pore structure. Typically, increasing the porosity of a porous prosthesis helps to reduce the structural elastic modulus, thereby weakening the stress shielding effect but simultaneously reducing the structural strength of the prosthesis. Therefore, when designing porous prostheses, it is necessary to quantitatively evaluate the mechanical safety and stress conduction of the prosthesis.

(a) Mechanical Safety Assessment

In material mechanics, the safety factor of a component is used to evaluate its safety. The safety factor is defined as the ratio of the allowable stress of the component to the yield strength of the material, as shown in Eq. (1.1):

$$N = \frac{\sigma_s}{[\sigma]} \tag{1.1}$$

where N is the safety factor of the component; σ_s is the failure stress of the material, usually the yield strength; and $[\sigma]$ is the allowable stress of the component. The allowable stress of a component is artificially specified based on the environment in which it is used, such as the maximum load-bearing mass of the load-bearing component. However, the environment and load conditions of orthopedic implants in the human body cannot be completely limited. Therefore, the maximum stress σ_{max} experienced by the prosthesis during service replaces the allowable stress $[\sigma]$ as a safety factor to ensure implant safety. The prosthesis safety factor is defined as follows:

$$N = \frac{\sigma_s}{[\sigma_{max}]} \tag{1.2}$$

However, calculating the safety factor for custom-made prostheses with porous structures is difficult. On the one hand, the maximum stress that a prosthesis can withstand in the human biomechanical environment is unknown; on the other hand, the mechanical properties of the materials with porous structures are also unclear. Therefore, to predict the safety of this type of prosthesis and ensure its safety after implantation, two aspects must be considered. First, a stress analysis method for customized prostheses based on the human biomechanical environment should be established. Second, the porous structure should be studied. Only by studying the relationship between the microstructural characteristics and the macroscopic mechanical properties of the material can we accurately assess the safety of implants during use. More importantly, for implants subjected to alternating loads in the human body over a long period of time, the failure stress σ is the fatigue limit stress of the material when considering the safety factor. In addition, in the mechanical analysis model of customized prostheses, the stress on the bone around the prosthesis should also be considered to ensure that the maximum stress on the surrounding bone is less than the strength limit of the bone.

(b) Evaluation of Stress Conduction

Long-term loosening of the prosthesis caused by peripheral bone loss and a lack of stable bony support are the most important factors that limit the service life of prostheses. Therefore, periprosthetic bone reconstruction has a significant impact on the long-term stability of prostheses. Bone reconstruction is a process of continuous bone tissue self-renewal to maintain the optimal tissue structure and load-bearing capacity in different mechanical and biological environments. The reconstruction of bone tissue that is subjected to mechanical stimulation was first described in Wolff's law (Wolff et al. 1986). In recent years, various more detailed theories of bone reconstruction based on Wolff's law have been proposed, among which the mechanical stability theory has been widely accepted and has led to subsequent experiments. The methods used for authentication are shown in Fig. 1.8.

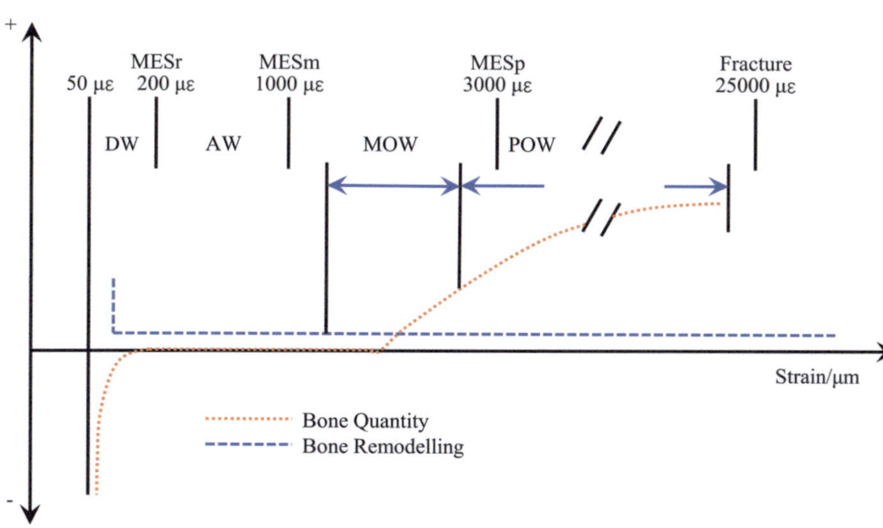

Fig. 1.8 Theoretical schematic diagram of a mechanically stability system

The mechanical stability theory of bone (Frost 2003) states that strain is the mechanical stimulus for bone remodeling. There are three important strain thresholds in the mechanical stability system: the threshold range for disuse-mode BMU-based bone remodeling (MSEr) is approximately 200 με, the bone modeling threshold (MESm) is approximately 1000 με, and the bone operational microdamage threshold (MSEp) is approximately 3000 με. As shown in Fig. 1.8, these three thresholds divide the strain range into four zones: the disuse window (DW), the adapted window (AW), the mild overload window (MOW), and the pathological overload window (POW).

According to the theory of the relationship between bone reconstruction and mechanical stimuli, bone reconstruction criteria for periprosthetic implants have been proposed. In the design of orthopedic prostheses, these prostheses can effectively conduct stress to the bone when they bears the physiological loads of the human body. Therefore, mechanical stimulation of the surrounding bone within this range can promote bone growth and reconstruction as much as possible to guide the reconstruction and remodeling of the bone tissue at the interface to ensure stable osseointegration and stable bony support of the prostheses.

1.3.3.3 Design of Gradient Porous Prosthesis

Porous prostheses need to meet the following requirements: the material must have good biocompatibility and osteoinductive ability to promote the differentiation and propagation of bone cells, the structure must have a suitable pore size and porosity to ensure the attachment of bone cells, the prosthesis must have sufficient strength and fatigue life, and the elastic modulus must be similar to that of the original bone tissue to avoid the stress shielding effect. Among these indicators, compatibility and osteoinduction ability are characteristics of the material itself, while the porosity, strength, and elastic modulus can be adjusted by modulating the porosity of the implant.

However, in the design of porous prostheses, different indicators place different demands on porosity. To avoid stress shielding of the prostheses in the human body, the macroscopic elastic modulus needs to be reduced, and the porosity should be increased. To ensure sufficient strength and safety of the implant, the porosity should be reduced. To promote the ingrowth of bone tissue, the pore size should be approximately 400–800 μm. These requirements cannot be met by a single porous structure. According to the principles of biomimetic design and the structure of the human bone tissue, gradient porosity design was developed to balance the different needs of implants.

Prostheses with gradient porosity can be considered functionally graded materials; that is, composite materials in which the components and/or the microstructure vary with space. Functional gradient design was first proposed in the field of orthopedic prostheses in 1997 by Kuiper and Huiskes (1997). Prostheses designed using functionally graded materials were found to have the potential to meet the mechanical requirements of prostheses at different locations. A numerical optimization method was proposed to determine the elastic modulus distribution, and a simplified 2D model of the femoral stem was optimized. To date, there has been substantial research on functionally graded designs in the field of orthopedic implants, and these designs have been applied to joint, spine, and trauma implants. The optimization of various gradient porous prostheses commonly involves optimizing the distribution of the mechanical properties of a component to optimize its microscopic porous structure (Sola et al. 2016). The typical literature on the optimization design of gradient porous prostheses is reviewed in Table 1.3. The results show that the elastic modulus, which is one of the most important properties in material mechanics, is the most common variable in the design of functionally gradient prostheses.

A high-strength, fully porous femoral stem with adjustable mechanical properties was designed by Pasini et al. (2017). A systematic method for 3D printing a fully porous femoral prosthesis was established. From the initial concept, multiscale mechanics of porous materials, material microstructure modification, additive manufacturing, and *in vitro* performance evaluation were proposed. The results showed that, compared to solid prostheses, optimized fully porous prostheses could reduce stress shielding by 75%, playing a critical role in reducing bone resorption.

Sun et al. (2018, 2022b) established a gradient porous structure design method based on the stress environment of the prostheses. The relationship between the equivalent elastic modulus of the prosthesis and the prosthesis stress was optimized, and an iterative calculation was used to ensure that the prosthesis had the characteristics of a prosthesis while improving the stress transfer capacity and achieving an adequate safety factor. As shown in Fig. 1.9, the elastic modulus distribution of the designed prosthesis is higher elastic modulus/low porosity inside, a lower elastic modulus/high porosity on the outside, and a high elastic modulus in the inner region. The material gradually transitions to a lower elastic modulus from the inside to the outside to evenly conduct stress to the surrounding bone, while the porous structure on the surface integrates with the bone tissue.

Although the previously reported design of the gradient porous prostheses was intended for non-custom-made prostheses, the design concept and the methods are applicable to custom-made prostheses. On the one hand, the design of gradient porous prostheses is based on the evaluation of safety and stability. These two indicators are also required for custom-made prostheses. Therefore, according to the design criteria, a gradient porous design can be used for custom-made prostheses. On the other hand, the stress distribution of a prosthesis served as the data on which the gradient design was based, and this approach is also suitable for custom-made prostheses. Therefore, the gradient porous design method is universally applicable to both standard and customized prostheses.

Table 1.3 Design methods for typical gradient porous prostheses

Design objects and distribution mode	Author, citation, and year	Design objective	Design methods
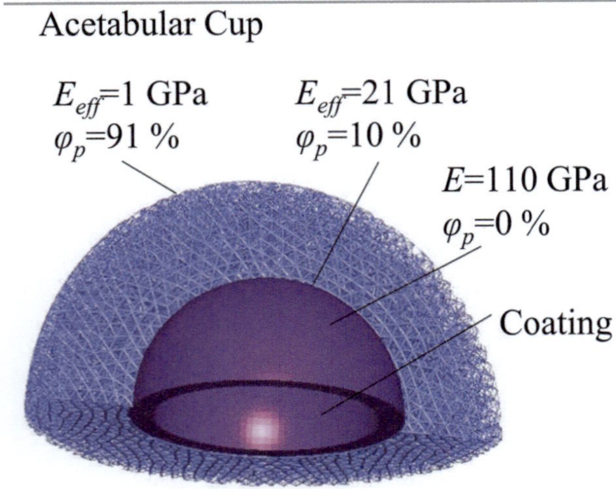	Johnston et al., (Johnston et al. 2006), 2006	① Improve the stability of the acetabular cup	① The porosity of the acetabular cup increased from the inside to the outside, while the elastic modulus decreased

Design objects and distribution mode	Author, citation, and year	Design objective	Design methods
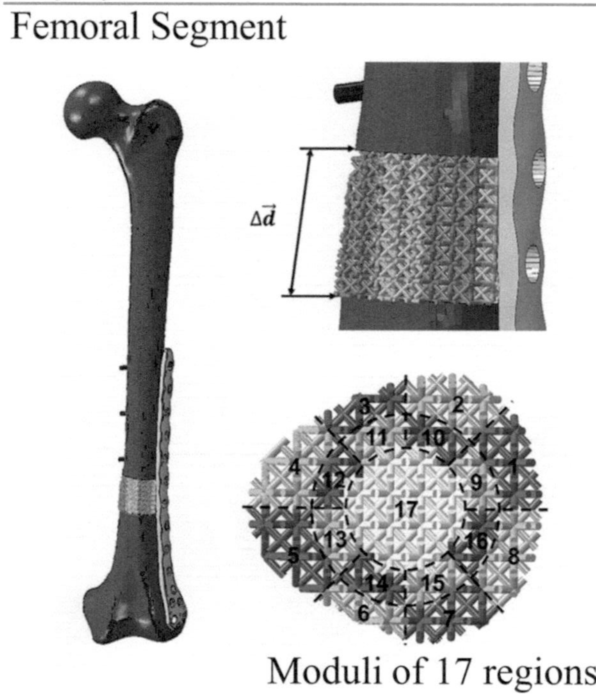	Wieding et al., (Wieding et al. 2014), 2014	① The gap between the fractured femoral prosthesis and the cross section of the femur during bending and torsion	① The femoral segmental prosthesis was divided into 17 regions along the cross section, and the elastic modulus of each region simulated the distribution of the elastic modulus of the femur on the cross section

Table 1.3 (continued)

Design objects and distribution mode	Author, citation, and year	Design objective	Design methods
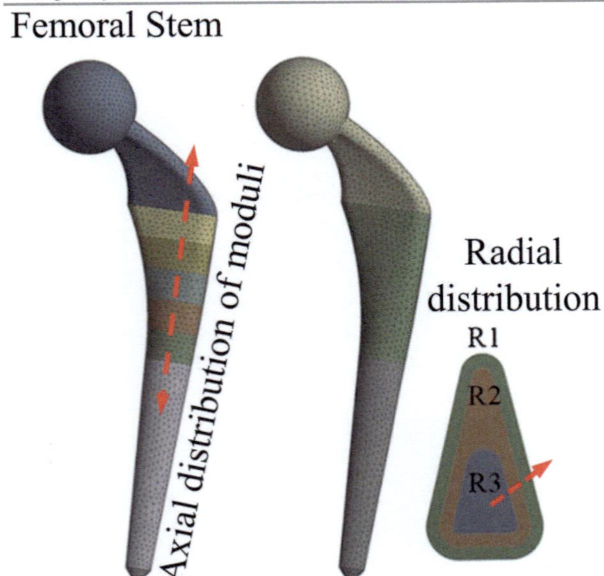 	Limmahakhun et al., (Limmahakhun et al. 2017), 2017	① Control micromotion; ② Increase the stress on the bone around the prosthesis	① The proximal end of the femoral stem was divided into five parts along the axial direction, each with different elastic moduli ② The proximal end of the femoral stem was divided into three parts from the inside to the outside, and the elastic modulus of each was different

From Literature: Johnston et al. (2006), Gabbrielli et al. (2008), Wieding et al. (2014), and Limmahakhun et al. (2017)

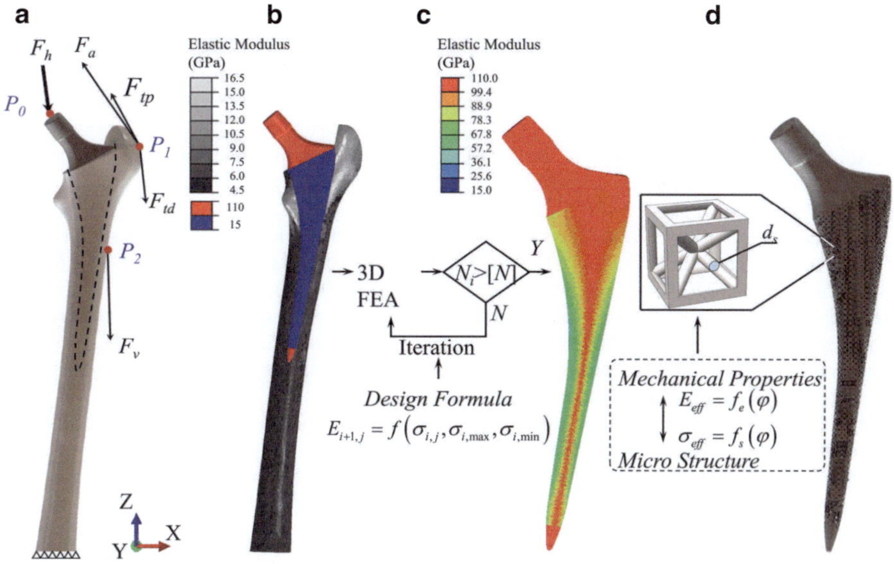

Fig. 1.9 Design method for gradient porous structures based on the stress environment of the prosthesis (Sun et al. 2018; Sun et al. 2022b)

1.4 Conclusions

3D printing technology provides accurate manufacturing methods for controlling the macro- and microstructure of custom-made prostheses. As a bridge between clinical needs and prosthetic manufacturing, the design of 3D-printed, custom-made prostheses is particularly important. In this chapter, the clinical requirements of custom-made prostheses were analyzed, design criteria with common characteristics were proposed, a standardized medicine–engineering interaction design process was summarized, and the key technologies in the design of custom prostheses were reviewed. The design criteria, medical–industrial interaction process, and key technologies proposed in this chapter form a general, theoretical, and methodological basis for the design of custom-made prostheses. The design of specific prostheses requires specific analyses according to specific issues. For example, geometric matching is particularly important in maxillofacial prostheses; rib defects lack protection for the chest cavity, and mechanical safety analysis should focus on impact resistance, and additional consideration of the resistance of the interface surfaces is needed for prostheses involving articular surfaces. The relevant content is reflected in the subsequent chapters of this book.

References

Abdullah M, Mubashar A, Uddin E. Structural optimization of orthopedic hip implant using parametric and non-parametric optimization techniques. Biomed Phys Eng Express. 2023;9(5):055026.

Al-Tamimi AA, Huang B, Vyas C, et al. Topology optimised metallic bone plates produced by electron beam melting: a mechanical and biological study. Int J Adv Manuf Technol. 2019;104(1–4):195–210.

Al-Tamimi AA, Hernandez MA, Omar A, et al. Mechanical, biological and tribological behaviour of fixation plates 3D printed by electron beam and selective laser melting. Int J Adv Manuf Technol. 2020;109(3–4):673–88. https://doi.org/10.1007/s00170-020-05676-1.

Arabnejad S, Johnston B, Tanzer M, et al. Fully porous 3D printed titanium femoral stem to reduce stress-shielding following total hip arthroplasty. J Orthop Res. 2017;35(8):1774–83.

Cameron HU, Pilliar RM, Macnab I. The effect of movement on the bonding of porous metal to bone. J Biomed Mater Res Part A. 1973;7(4):301–11.

Dong EC, Wang L, Iqbal T, et al. Finite element analysis of the pelvis after customized prosthesis reconstruction. J Bionic Eng. 2018;15:443–51.

Dong EC, Shi L, Kang JF, et al. Biomechanical characterization of vertebral body replacement in situ: effects of different fixation strategies. Comput Methods Prog Biomed. 2020;197:105741. https://doi.org/10.1016/j.cmpb.2020.105741.

Frost HM. Bone's mechanostat: a 2003 update. Anat Rec A Discov Mol Cell Evol Biol. 2003;275(2):1081–101.

Gabbrielli R, Turner IG, Bowen CR. Development of modelling methods for materials to be used as bone substitutes. Key Eng Mater. 2008;361–363:903–6. https://doi.org/10.4028/www.scientific.net/KEM.361-363.903.

Guo L-X, Wang Q-D. Biomechanical analysis of a new bilateral pedicle screw fixator system based on topological optimization. Int J Precis Eng Manuf. 2020;21(7):1363–74. https://doi.org/10.1007/s12541-020-00336-6.

Guoqing Z, Junxin L, Chengguang Z, et al. Design optimization and manufacturing of bio-fixed tibial implants using 3D printing technology. J Mech Behav Biomed Mater. 2021;117:104415.

Güvenç Y, Akyoldaş G, Şentürk S, et al. How to reduce stress on the pedicle screws in thoracic spine? Importance of screw trajectory: a finite element analysis. Turkish Neurosurgery; 2017.

Iqbal T, Wang L, Li D, et al. A general multi-objective topology optimization methodology developed for customized design of pelvic prostheses. Med Eng Phys. 2019;69:8–16. https://doi.org/10.1016/j.medengphy.2019.06.008.

Johnston SR, Rosen DW, Wang HV. Design of a graded cellular structure for an acetabular hip replacement component. Georgia Institute of Technology; 2006. https://doi.org/10.26153/tsw/7122.

Kang JF, Wang L, Yang CC, et al. Custom design and biomechanical analysis of 3D-printed PEEK rib prostheses. Biomech Model Mechanobiol. 2018;17(4):1083–92. https://doi.org/10.1007/s10237-018-1015-x.

Kang JF, Dong E, Li X, et al. Topological design and biomechanical evaluation for 3D printed multi-segment artificial vertebral implants. Mater Sci Eng C Mater Biol Appl. 2021;127:112250. https://doi.org/10.1007/s10237-018-1015-x.

Kaymaz I, Murat F, Korkmaz IH, et al. A new design for the humerus fixation plate using a novel reliability-based topology optimization approach to mitigate the stress shielding effect. Clin Biomech. 2022;99:105768.

Kharmanda G. Integration of multi-objective structural optimization into cementless hip prosthesis design: improved Austin-Moore model. Comput Methods Biomech Biomed Engin. 2016;19(14):1557–66. https://doi.org/10.1080/10255842.2016.1170121.

Kladovasilakis N, Bountourelis T, Tsongas K, et al. Computational investigation of a tibial implant using topology optimization and finite element analysis. Technologies. 2023;11(2):58. https://doi.org/10.3390/technologies11020058.

Kuiper JH, Huiskes R. Mathematical optimization of elastic properties: application to cementless hip stem design. J Biomech Eng. 1997;119(2):166.

Li ZH, Muller R, Ruffoni D. Bone remodeling and mechanobiology around implants: insights from small animal imaging. J Orthop Res. 2018;36(2):584–93.

Li C, Wu C, Lin C. Design of a patient-specific mandible reconstruction implant with dental prosthesis for metal 3D printing using integrated weighted topology optimization and finite element analysis. J Mech Behav Biomed Mater. 2020;105:103700.

Limmahakhun S, Oloyede A, Chantarapanich N, et al. Alternative designs of load−sharing cobalt chromium graded femoral stems. Mater Today Commun. 2017;12(1):1–10. https://doi.org/10.1016/j.mtcomm.2017.05.002.

Liu HC, Jiang J-S, Lin C-L. Biomechanical investigation of a novel hybrid dorsal double plating for distal radius fractures by integrating topology optimization and finite element analysis. Inj Int J Care Inj. 2020;51(6):1271–80.

Maniatopoulos C, Pilliar RM, Smith DC. Threaded versus porous-surfaced designs for implant stabilization in bone-endodontic implant model. J Biomed Mater Res Part A. 1986;20(9):1309–33.

Park J, Zobaer T, Sutradhar A. A two-scale multi-resolution topologically optimized multi-material design of 3D printed craniofacial bone implants. Micromachines. 2021;12(2):101. https://doi.org/10.3390/mi12020101.

Rahimizadeh A, Nourmohammadi Z, Arabnejad S, et al. Porous architected biomaterial for a tibial-knee implant with minimum bone resorption and bone-implant interface micromotion. J Mech Behav Biomed Mater. 2018;78:465–79.

Sola A, Bellucci D, Cannillo V. Functionally graded materials for orthopedic applications – an update on design and manufacturing. Biotechnol Adv. 2016;34(5):504–31.

Sun CN, Wang L, Kang JF, et al. Biomechanical optimization of elastic modulus distribution in porous femoral stem for artificial hip joints. J Bionic Eng. 2018;15(4):693–702.

Sun J, Wang Q, Cai D, et al. A lattice topology optimization of cervical interbody fusion cage and finite element comparison with ZK60 and Ti-6Al-4V cages. BMC Musculoskeletal Disorders. 2021;22(1):1–14.

Sun C, Kang J, Yang C, et al. Additive manufactured polyether-ether-ketone implants for orthopaedic applications: a narrative review. Biomater Transl. 2022a;3(2):116. https://doi.org/10.12336/biomatertransl.2022.02.001.

Sun C, Kang J, Wang L, et al. Stress-dependent design and optimization methodology of gradient porous implant and application in femoral stem. Comput Methods Biomech Biomed Eng. 2022b;26(11):1308–19. https://doi.org/10.1080/10255842.2022.2115291.

Sutradhar A, Park J, Carrau D, et al. Designing patient-specific 3D printed craniofacial implants using a novel topology optimization method. Med Biol Eng Comput. 2016;54(7):1123–35.

van Kootwijk A, Moosabeiki V, Saldivar MC, et al. Semi-automated digital workflow to design and evaluate patient-specific mandibular reconstruction implants. J Mech Behav Biomed Mater. 2022;132:105291. https://doi.org/10.1016/j.jmbbm.2022.105291.

Wang L, Kang JF, Shi L, et al. Investigation into factors affecting the mechanical behaviours of a patient-specific vertebral body replacement. J Eng Med. 2018;232:378–87. https://doi.org/10.1177/0954411918754926.

Wieding J, Wolf A, Bader R. Numerical optimization of open-porous bone scaffold structures to match the elastic properties of human cortical bone. J Mech Behav Biomed Mater. 2014;37:56–68. https://doi.org/10.1016/j.jmbbm.2014.05.002.

Wolff J, Maquet P, Furlong R. The law of bone remodelling. Berlin: Springer; 1986.

Xiao Z, Wu L, Wu W, et al. Multi-scale topology optimization of femoral stem structure subject to stress shielding reduce. Materials. 2023;16(8):3151.

Porous Structure of 3D-Printed Custom-Made Prostheses

2

Jianfeng Kang, Yingjie Liu, Jiayin Liu, Xuefei Zhu, and Ling Wang

2.1 Introduction

2.1.1 Effect of Porous Structures

The human skeletal system performs essential functions, such as support, protection, and movement, in daily life. The performance of these functions is closely related to the external anatomical morphology and internal porous structure of bone tissue. When patients require bone defect repair, custom-made prostheses with multiple advantages, such as morphological adaptation, performance matching, and functional restoration, can achieve accurate and personalized treatment through biomimetic design and 3D printing technology. These approaches have gradually been applied and recognized. As shown in Fig. 2.1, the clinical applications of 3D-printed porous prostheses have been demonstrated. The rational design of the porous structures for these custom-made prostheses can effectively overcome existing problems

J. Kang
School of Mechatronic Engineering and Automation, Foshan University, Foshan, China

Y. Liu · J. Liu · L. Wang (✉)
State Key Laboratory for Manufacturing System Engineering, School of Mechanical Engineering, Xi'an Jiaotong University, Xi'an, China

National Medical Products Administration (NMPA) Key Laboratory for Research and Evaluation of Additive Manufacturing Medical Devices, Xi'an Jiaotong University, Xi'an, China

National Innovation Platform (Center) for Industry-Education Integration of Medical Technology, Xi'an Jiaotong University, Xi'an, China
e-mail: lyj263333@stu.xjtu.edu.cn; menlwang@mail.xjtu.edu.cn

X. Zhu
State Key Laboratory for Manufacturing System Engineering, School of Mechanical Engineering, Xi'an Jiaotong University, Xi'an, China

Z. Guo et al. (eds.), *3D-Printed Prosthesis in Orthopedic Oncology*,
https://doi.org/10.1007/978-981-95-1454-0_2

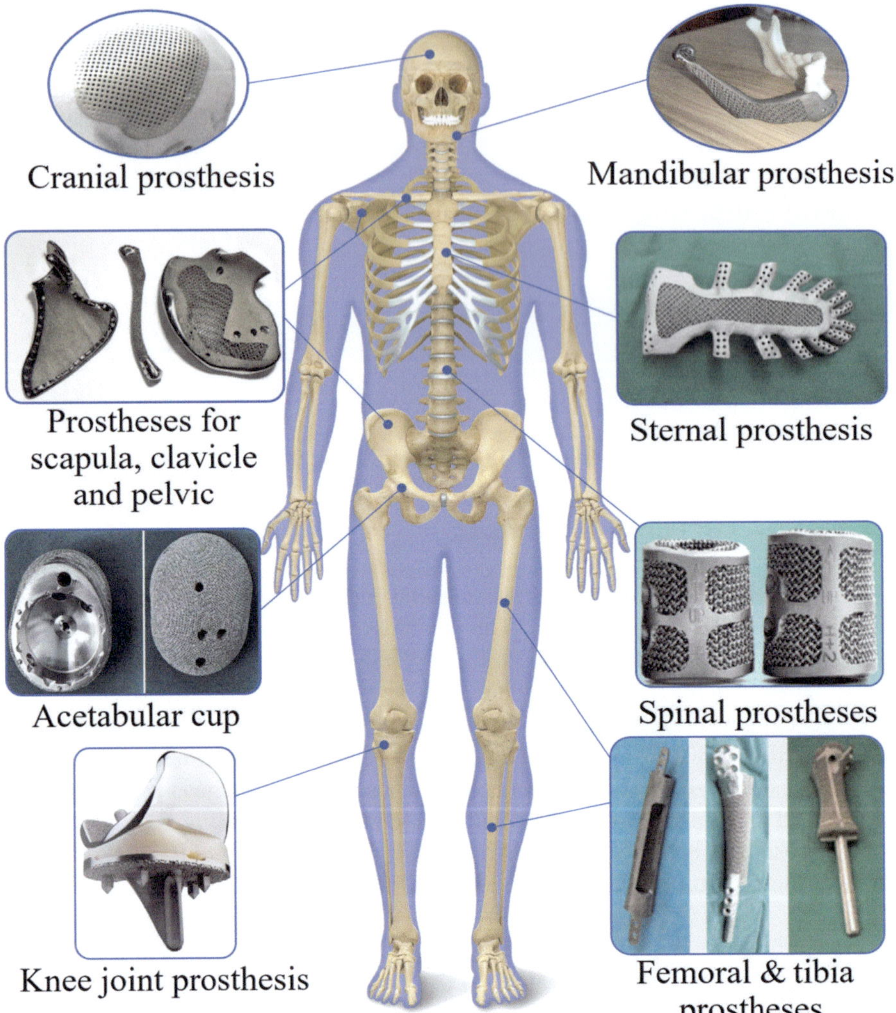

Fig. 2.1 3D-printed porous metal prostheses for different parts of the human body (Peng et al. 2022; Wei et al. 2022; Yu et al. 2022)

associated with conventional metal prostheses after implantation, such as stress shielding and the weak bonding strength of bone/prosthesis interfaces. Hence, the potential risk of prosthesis loosening and fracture is reduced, which is an important benefit for bone defect repair and functional restoration.

In general, the effects of the porous structures of 3D-printed, custom-made prostheses can be explained mainly in the following ways.

(a) *A porous structure improves the modulus compatibility between the metal specimen and the host bone, and the rational design of pore distribution promotes the stress transfer of the bone/prosthesis system and restores the dynamic balance of mechanical stimulation for bone growth.*

The elastic modulus of biomedical metallic materials is much higher than that of human cortical bone (approximately 12–20 GPa). For example, the elastic modulus of the Ti-6Al-4V material is 110 GPa, and that of the CoCrMo alloy is 210 GPa. When a dense metal prosthesis is implanted, the large difference in modulus easily causes a lack of effective mechanical stimulation around the bone/prosthesis interface, which further results in bone resorption and prosthesis loosening. Therefore, the effective elastic modulus of the metal specimen can be successfully reduced and regulated by designing a porous structure that more closely matches the modulus of the host bone. Moreover, Pasini et al. proposed a design and optimization method for the gradient porous distribution of metal femoral stems (Arabnejad et al. 2017). The results showed that, compared with solid prostheses, prostheses with optimized porous distributions reduce the proportion of bone loss around the implant by 75%, playing a crucial role in reducing bone absorption and stress shielding. Therefore, rational design of the distribution of the porous structure inside a prosthesis effectively improves the stress transfer of the bone/prosthesis system during load-carrying and movement and improves the safety of the prosthesis in service.

(b) *A porous structure enhances the osseointegration capability of the bone/prosthesis interface, promoting biological fixation and improving the medium- to long-term stability of the prosthesis.*

A porous structure provides favorable space for the host bone ingrowth around the prosthesis, playing a prominent role in enhancing osseointegration at the bone/prosthesis interface and biological fixation. The responses of bone ingrowth and osseointegration to a porous structure are manifested as follows. Osteogenic cells migrate to the surface of the pores where they proliferate and differentiate, promoting the regeneration of new bone; a porous structure allows for the transfer of nutrients and oxygen and the removal of metabolic waste; and a porous structure supports the ingrowth of vascular networks and neovascularization within the scaffold. The excellent bone integration effect of 3D-printed porous implants has been confirmed in clinical applications. Guo Zheng and colleagues completed the world's first 3D-printed porous titanium alloy clavicles and scapulae for repairing bone defects after tumor resection surgery. These researchers also conducted various clinical studies on titanium alloy 3D-printed artificial vertebral bodies, limb segment bone implants, intervertebral fusion devices, and femoral head support rods. These implants have been used in more than 100 cases, with the longest follow-up time of 7 years, and the results have shown tight connections between the implants and bones without any related complications such as implant loosening. Eric So and colleagues used 3D-printed porous titanium alloy implants to reconstruct extensive bone defects in the feet of three patients (So et al. 2018). One year later, the follow-up results showed that the implants had bonded with the surrounding cortical and cancellous bone, with no complications observed in the patients who were able to resume normal daily activities.

(c) *Porous structures have expanded the breadth and depth of the functional requirements for bone defect repair and treatment, enhancing multiple functional synergistic effects, such as antibacterial, antitumor, and bone formation effects.*

To meet the functional requirements for the clinical treatment of bone defect repair, 3D-printed, custom-made porous prostheses face new challenges related to synergizing multiple effects, such as improving antibacterial, antitumor, and osteogenic effects. The high specific surface area of porous structures provides favorable prerequisites for the attachment of bioactive factors, and the release of bioactive factors through the degradation of porous structures can achieve good synergistic therapeutic effects. Van Hengel et al. (2020) explored surface biofunctionalized 3D-printed porous Ti-6Al-4V scaffolds using plasma electrolytic oxidation technology, and these scaffolds locally release bone-forming agents containing strontium and antibacterial agents containing silver ions. Evaluation of the antibacterial activity in in vitro and ex vivo mouse models revealed very strong bactericidal effects against highly toxic and multidrug-resistant strains of *Staphylococcus aureus* and the complete eradication of planktonic bacteria and adherent bacteria. Furthermore, porous structures constructed with advanced functional materials to achieve physical stimulation, such as electrothermal stimulation, can also enhance the therapeutic effects of implants. Fan et al. (2020) coated piezoelectric barium titanate ceramics onto the surface of porous titanium alloy scaffolds, resulting in an approximately 30% increase in new bone formation within the titanium alloy scaffolds and good bone defect repair effects.

Therefore, the porous structures of 3D-printed, custom prostheses play a very important role in the treatment of bone defect repair, greatly increasing the safety, stability, and functionality in service and laying a solid foundation for functional restoration in the clinical treatment of bone defect repair.

2.1.2 Principles of Porous Structure Design

2.1.2.1 Differences in Bone Structure and Mechanical Properties

The porous structural characteristics and mechanical properties of different parts of host bones vary significantly. When designing porous prostheses to repair bone defects based on biomimetic theory, it is essential to understand the differences in the structural morphology and mechanical properties of human bones. Figure 2.2 and Table 2.1 summarize and compare different bones from the perspectives of anatomical structure and mechanical properties, respectively. The structural differences of bones determine their distinct mechanical properties, which are closely

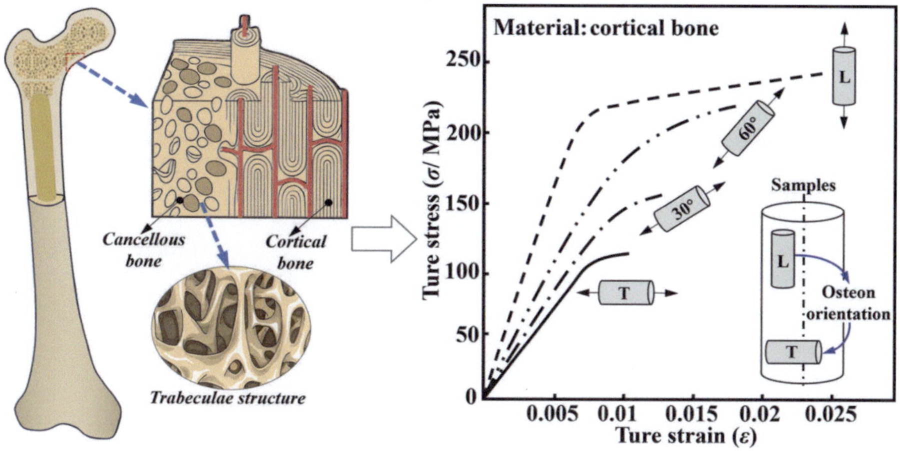

Fig. 2.2 Macro- and micro-structure of the human femur and its mechanical properties (Wang et al. 2016)

related to their physiological functions. The skull has a high bending modulus and bending strength to withstand external impact loads. The femur and tibia have high stiffness and compressive strength to support the body's weight and maintain upright walking and movement. In addition to compressive properties, the spine and pelvis also have good shear resistance and torsion resistance to maintain the balance and stability of the human trunk and enable the human body to perform various movements, such as bending and rotation.

In addition to these differences, the discrepancy in the mechanical properties in different directions caused by differences in porous structures also needs sufficient attention to achieve better bone replacement and repair. For example, the significant mechanical anisotropy caused by the nonuniform trabecular structure of long bones results in noticeable changes in Young's modulus and yield strength. Additionally, it is important to consider the differences in porosity and bone strength that occur due to different bone qualities in the human body; additionally, age, sex, and function can all contribute to bone quality variances. Hence, when designing customized 3D-printed porous prostheses, it is essential to completely consider the differences and specificities of different bones, combined with the actual physiological characteristics of the patient's bone tissue.

2.1.2.2 Basic Principles of 3D-Printed Porous Structure Design

According to the functional needs of bone defect repair and the differences in structure and performance of different human host bones, the manufacture of porous bone implants through biomimetic design principles and 3D printing technology effectively improves the safety and stability of prostheses and ensures the precision and personalized treatment of bone defect repair. However, various types of porous structures are currently used to generate 3D-printed custom prostheses, and

Table 2.1 Physiological structure and mechanical properties of different host bones

Human bones	Physiological structure		Mechanical properties	
	Bone density (g/cm^3)	Porosity (%)	Elastic modulus (GPa)	Strength (MPa)
Skull	1.56–1.91 (Auperrin et al. 2014)	6.52–17.96 (Motherway et al. 2009)	B: 3.81–9.7 (Auperrin et al. 2014)	B: 213–243 (Maloul et al. 2013)
Spine	0.09–0.38* (Gilsanz et al. 1994; Kopperdahl et al. 2002)	82–93* (Thomsen et al. 2002)	T: 0.13–0.508* (Kopperdahl et al. 2002) C: 0.244–0.668* (Ogurkowska and Blaszczyk 2020) B: 0.053–0.124* (Ogurkowska and Blaszczyk 2020)	C: 0.5–5.2* (Mosekilde and Mosekilde 1986)
Pelvis	0.32–0.38 (Zhang et al. 2009) 0.04–0.22* (Dalstra et al. 1993)	58.11–76.35 (Zhang et al. 2009) 62–91* (Thomsen et al. 2002)	C: 0.225–0.616* (Dalstra et al. 1993) S: 0.0129–0.026* (Dalstra et al. 1993)	TS: 4.4–7.5 (Zhang et al. 2009) C: 9.2–10.7 (Zhang et al. 2009) B: 13.4–18.1 (Zhang et al. 2009)
Femur	0.63–0.87$^+$ (Duchemin et al. 2008)	11.0~11.8$^+$ (Yeni et al. 1997) 69~77* (Nauman et al. 1999)	T: 14.78–18.44$^+$ (Dong and Guo 2004) S: 4.09–5.39$^+$ (Dong and Guo 2004) C: 8.2–15.4$^+$ (Duchemin et al. 2008)	TS: 33.5–74.1$^+$ (Duchemin et al. 2008) C: 77.0–135.8$^+$ (Duchemin et al. 2008)
Tibia	0.98–1.07$^+$ (Ward et al. 2005)	10.0~10.8$^+$ (Yeni et al. 1997) 37~57* (Nauman et al. 1999)	T: 18.4$^+$ (Chen 1989) B: 12.2$^+$ (Chen 1989)	TS: 173–175$^+$ (Chen 1989) C: 162$^+$ (Chen 1989) B: 204$^+$ (Chen 1989)

From literature: Auperrin et al. (2014), Motherway et al. (2009), Maloul et al. (2013), Gilsanz et al. (1994), Kopperdahl et al. (2002), Thomsen et al. (2002), Ogurkowska and Blaszczyk (2020), Mosekilde and Mosekilde (1986), Dalstra et al. (1993), Duchemin et al. (2008), Yeni et al. (1997), Nauman et al. (1999), Dong and Guo (2004), Ward et al. (2005)

Abbreviations: *B* bending testing, *T* tensile testing, *C* compressive testing, *S* shear testing, *TS* torsion testing

Note: Superscript (*) indicates that the data are from cancellous bone, and superscript (+) indicates that the data are from cortical bone

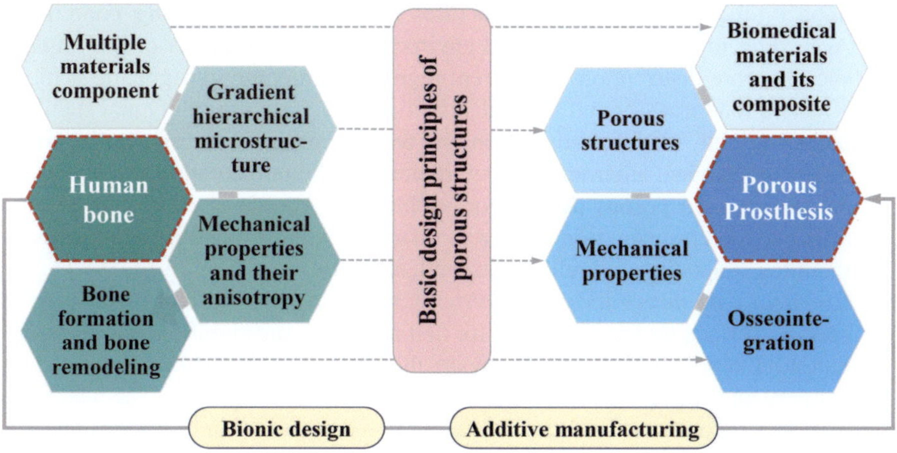

Fig. 2.3 Basic principles of porous structure design based on the functionalization needs of human bone

different pore structure designs have unique differences in performance, which affect their function in vivo after implantation. Therefore, as shown in Fig. 2.3, the basic principles that should be followed when designing the porous structures of 3D-printed custom prostheses are as follows:

(a) *Good biocompatibility*: Biocompatibility evaluations usually include assessments of biological safety and biological functionality. Good biocompatibility requires that the raw materials of porous structural samples and their physical or chemical byproducts have very low or no toxicity during preparation and that these materials contribute to appropriately stimulating the body's corresponding functions in specific applications. Biomaterials that are currently commonly used for porous prostheses mainly include metal, ceramic, and polymer materials. The biocompatibility of these materials, which is influenced by their inherent physicochemical characteristics, still needs to be enhanced. Consequently, many studies (Bandyopadhyay et al. 2023) have aimed to improve the biocompatibility of porous prostheses through surface modification, bulk modification, and bioagent incorporation.
(b) *Mechanical property matching*: The mechanical property matching and good load transfer capability between the porous structure of a prosthesis and the bone in the defect area are crucial. Due to the significant differences in the elastic modulus and yield strength between human cortical bone and cancellous bone, the elastic modulus of porous metal samples can be effectively regulated by modulating the porosity, which is designed to be close to that of the host bone, further alleviating or even preventing the stress shielding effect but also reducing the mechanical strength to a certain extent. Therefore, it is essential to comprehensively evaluate the anisotropy and mechanical properties, such as the elastic modulus, tensile/compressive/bending/torsional/fatigue strength, and

impact toughness of porous structures under different loading conditions. According to the mechanical and environmental requirements of the implant site, the pore distribution in different regions is rationally designed to achieve effective load transfer and stress distribution and to ensure safety and stability, including both modulus adaptation and reliable strength. Subsequently, based on the mechanical environment requirements of the implantation site, the rational design of a porous distribution within a prosthesis is crucial to achieve effective load transmission and stress distribution, ensuring a balance between modulus adaptation and reliable strength stability.

(c) *Excellent osseointegration capability*: A highly porous structure with a large specific surface area is necessary for cell adhesion, proliferation, and differentiation. Interconnected pores provide the necessary foundation for nutrient delivery and waste removal, which are essential for cell growth. The host bone around a porous structure grows into the pores, resulting in biological fixation that significantly enhances the medium to long-term stability of the prosthesis. According to existing research (Germaini et al. 2022), the pore size and porosity of porous structures have significant impacts on osseointegration capability. Pore sizes of 300–500 μm are favorable for new bone ingrowth, while pores of 0.7–1.2 mm exhibit excellent bone conductivity. Pores larger than 1.5 mm hinder bone conduction and connection, while pores smaller than 300 μm promote vascular ingrowth, with approximately 100 μm being favorable for cell migration. In addition, since the delivery of cells, nutrients, and growth factors required for bone ingrowth depends on blood flow through the porous structure, the permeability of the porous structure is particularly important for promoting osseointegration. Studies have shown (Wang et al. 2016) that high permeability helps to enhance osseointegration.

(d) *Printability*: A variety of materials are used for customizing porous prostheses according to clinical needs, which determine the selection of 3D printing technology. The conventional printing methods mainly include selective laser melting (SLM), electron beam melting (EBM), stereolithography (SLA), selective laser sintering (SLS), and fused filament fabrication (FFF). According to the raw materials of the prosthesis and the characteristics of the designed porous structure, as well as the basic principles and manufacturing process of 3D printing, a porous structure should have good printability.

2.2 Design and Characterization of Porous Structures for 3D Printed Customized Prostheses

2.2.1 Design Methodology for the Porous Structures of 3D-Printed, Custom-Made Prostheses

The design of porous structures is an important step in custom prosthesis design. As shown in Table 2.2, commonly used methods for designing porous structures include the medical imaging-based design method, CAD-based design method, implicit surface-based design method, and print path-based design method.

Table 2.2 Comparison of porous structure design methods

Method/content	Medical imaging-based design method	CAD-based design method	Implicit surface-based design method	Print path-based design method
Design principle	Construction of Voronoi units based on medical images	Construction of crystal unit cells based on CAD technology	Construction of porous surface shapes based on mathematical functions	Construction of spatial porous structures based on printing paths
Structures	Bone-like trabecular structure	Various crystal lattice structures	Complex curved surface structures	Intersecting line structure
Design efficiency	Low	High	High	Exceptionally high
Material	Metal, ceramic	Metal, ceramic	Metal, ceramic	Polymer materials
Manufacturing method	SLM, EBM	SLM, EBM	SLM, EBM	FFF
Advantage	The structure designed by this method has a larger surface area and allows the continuous gradient porous structures	This method has a wide range of applicability, and the designed structure exhibits high controllability	This method can construct continuous gradient porous structures, and the designed structure has a larger surface area	This method is efficient and cost-effective
Disadvantage	This method requires the collaboration of computed tomography and magnetic resonance imaging (CT/MRI) has a complex design process, and high printing difficulty	It is difficult to construct continuous gradient porous structures using this method, and the permeability performance of the designed structure is poor	The structures designed by this method are prone to the formation of internal voids and other defects during the manufacturing process	The structures designed by this method have a single geometric configuration

The medical imaging-based design method is a commonly used approach for designing biomimetic, irregular porous structures. The raw bone tissue data of patients are acquired through medical imaging techniques such as computed tomography (CT) and magnetic resonance imaging (MRI). Based on the obtained medical images, it is possible to directly reconstruct three-dimensional porous models of trabeculae (Yao et al. 2015) or to determine the microscopic structural parameters of bone porous structures through image processing and establish corresponding mathematical models for the design of three-dimensional porous structures (Chen et al. 2007). The most commonly used mathematical model is Voronoi-Tessellation, which transforms medical scan data to generate 2D Voronoi point coordinates (x, y)

and then constructs 3D Voronoi point coordinates (*x*, *y*, *z*) by evenly processing the average spacing between trabeculae in the *z* direction to ultimately generate 3D Voronoi porous structures, as shown in Fig. 2.4. The Voronoi-Tessellation method enables precise control of the pore distribution, pore gradient, porosity, and specific surface area of the porous structures, making the main morphological parameters of the porous structures highly consistent with those of natural trabecular bone structures. This is considered an ideal method for pore structure design.

The CAD-based design method involves obtaining individual crystal unit structures through geometric modeling and then expanding them through an array of crystal units to form periodic porous structures. Various methods are used to construct crystal unit structures. Common crystal unit structures include the following: standard crystal unit structures constructed through Boolean operations (intersection, union, and difference) using standard polyhedra, such as cubes, spheres, cylinders, and hexagons; wireframe crystal unit structures constructed based on Archimedean/Platonic polyhedral structures (Wettergreen et al. 2005), wireframe crystal unit structures constructed based on body-centered cubic (BCC) and face-centered cubic (FCC) structures; and crystal unit structures constructed based on topological optimization. Professor and colleagues Chua (Cheah et al. 2003; Chua et al. 2003) from Nanyang Technological University in Singapore constructed a

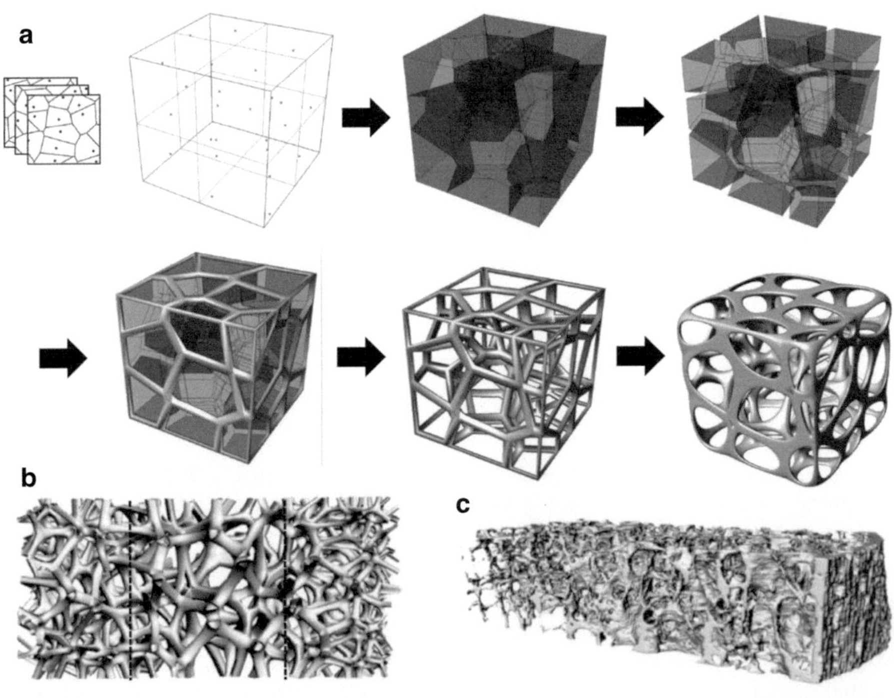

Fig. 2.4 (**a**) Design process of 3D Voronoi units. (**b**) Biomimetic continuous gradient porous structures generated based on the gradient Voronoi-Tessellation method. (**c**) Natural trabecular bone structure (Gómez et al. 2016)

parameter library for CAD crystal units called CASTS (computer-aided system for tissue scaffolds), *as shown in* Fig. 2.5, to automatically create the required porous structures, reducing design time. The CAD crystal unit was an effective attempt at early porous structure design, and it continues to be frequently used in the design of porous structures for implants or scaffolds. However, it also has disadvantages such as excessively high porosity in the unit cell, leading to poor mechanical and permeation properties. Topological optimization of CAD crystal units often targets mechanical performance or permeability. Through topological optimization calculations, it is possible to achieve an elastic modulus closer to that of natural bone as well as improved permeability (Hollister 2005).

The implicit surface-based design method uses mathematical functions to freely introduce pore shapes, thereby controlling the generation of porous structures. Triply periodic minimal surfaces (TPMS) are the most commonly used types of control functions and possess highly interconnected and periodic structures in all three independent spatial directions. According to their different functional patterns, common TPMS units can be divided into Schwartz Primitive (P-type), Schwartz Diamond (D-type), and Schoen Gyroid (G-type) units. By changing the functional parameters, it is possible to flexibly and accurately control the pore size, porosity, and other parameters of TPMS porous structures. Furthermore, continuous gradient design or anisotropic design targeting the overall pores is possible. In addition, another significant advantage of TPMS porous structures is their larger specific surface area, which positively influences cell adhesion, growth, migration, and tissue ingrowth into the scaffold interior.

The print path-based design method is a porous structure design method that is unique to fused filament fabrication (FFF). This method controls the nozzle's path, direction, and spacing between paths during printing to construct porous structures with different pore shapes, sizes, and porosities. Common porous structures include straight-line intersecting structures and helical 24-hedron structures, where the helical 24-hedron structure is essentially an implicit surface structure based on the Schoen Gyroid surface function to control the printing path. The printing path design method is characterized by its simplicity and efficiency. It allows for direct top-down design and manufacturing of porous structures on solid implant models. The other three methods mentioned above typically require Boolean operations between the solid implant model and the constructed porous structure model to

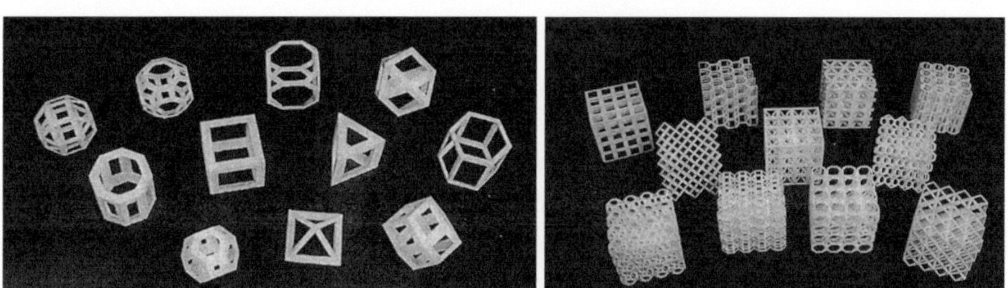

Fig. 2.5 Unit cells and their arrays based on CASTS (Cheah et al. 2003)

obtain the final porous implant model that is used for manufacturing. However, because the porous structures generated by the printing path design method must be expressible as two-dimensional lines that can be stacked to form three-dimensional structures, the shapes of the pores that can be constructed are relatively limited.

In addition to the aforementioned porous structures, another common type of porous structure is the sponge/foam structure. This structure typically consists of irregular voids formed on the surface of 3D-printed prostheses during postprocessing. Its pore morphology resembles that of trabecular bone and has been shown to facilitate bone tissue growth. Although the porosity and the pore size of sponge/foam structures can be adjusted to some extent through process parameters, it is difficult to design or precisely control detailed features, such as geometric shape, pore connectivity, and pore distribution.

2.2.2 Characterization of the Geometric Parameters of Porous Structures in 3D-Printed Customized Prostheses

The characterization of porous structures is an important focus of research on 3D-printed prostheses because structural parameters, especially porosity, pore size, and specific surface area, directly or indirectly affect the mechanical performance of scaffolds and their interactions with cells.

In the initial stages of prosthesis research and development, it is necessary to have effective technologies that can provide information on scaffold morphology characteristics. This allows for the design of implants that are tailored to specific applications and that meet the corresponding performance requirements. Common methods for testing porous structures are shown in Table 2.3. The most common method for high-resolution nondestructive testing of porous structures is X-ray Computed Tomography (X–CT). Through projection imaging, X–CT reconstructs three-dimensional in situ images of porous structures, allowing the analysis and characterization of their spatial distribution and morphological features.

Porosity is the space within a porous structure that is constrained by solid surfaces (Pennella et al. 2013). The porosity directly affects the mechanical performance of a prosthesis. An appropriate porosity can provide suitable space for cell proliferation while regulating the mechanical strength of the prosthesis, making it similar to a natural bone and preventing stress shielding. The porosity η can be obtained from CT scan images, and it is calculated by the following formula:

$$\eta = \frac{V_{\mathrm{P}}}{V} \times 100\% = \frac{1 - V_{\mathrm{S}}}{V} \times 100\%$$

where V_{P} is the volume of the void space in the porous structure, V_{s} is the volume of the solid in the porous structure, and V is the total volume of the porous structure.

Table 2.3 Commonly used techniques for characterizing three-dimensional porous structures: comparison table

Technology	Measurable structural parameters	Advantage	Disadvantage
X-ray computed tomography (X-CT)	Pore morphology, porosity, pore size, pore size distribution, pore connectivity, specific surface area, etc.	This technique allows for high-resolution nondestructive testing of porous structures and three-dimensional reconstruction	This technique is expensive, not suitable for materials with insufficient imaging capabilities, and the analysis process is relatively complex
Microscopic observation methods (optical microscopy, scanning electron microscopy, transmission electron microscopy)	Pore morphology, pore size, porosity, pore connectivity	These techniques are simple, time-efficient, and have high resolution	These techniques yield two-dimensional plane images, which do not fully characterize the three-dimensional morphology of the pores
Gas adsorption technique (Brunauer-Emmett-Teller method)	Specific surface area, pore size distribution	The technique has a fast analysis speed and high accuracy, and is suitable for most materials	This technique is not suitable for large pore size analysis and can only analyze open pores
High-pressure mercury intrusion porosimetry	Pore connectivity, porosity, pore size, pore size distribution	This technique is simple, has low sample requirements, and can measure a wide range of pore sizes	This technique involves high toxicity of mercury, poses high experimental risks, and can only analyze open pores

For low-density materials with limited imaging capabilities, the porosity can also be determined by the weighing method. The formula for the weighing method is as follows:

$$P\% = \left(1 - \frac{\rho}{\rho_{\mathrm{m}}}\right) \times 100\% = \left(1 - \frac{m}{\rho_{\mathrm{m}} \cdot V}\right) \times 100\%$$

where ρ is the apparent density of the porous structure, which is equal to the actual mass m of the porous structure divided by the total volume V of the porous structure, and ρ_{m} is the density of the material of the porous structure.

When discussing porosity, pore characteristics such as open and closed pores, as well as pore connectivity, are also important topics of discussion. Based on CT images, pores that are connected to the external contour are considered open pores, whereas pores that are not connected are considered closed pores. Closed pores have no significant effects on the growth of biological tissues or the transport of nutrients. In cases where the closed pore ratio is high and the pore connectivity is low, even if the porous implant has a high porosity, it cannot have a beneficial effect on tissue ingrowth. Therefore, researchers (Chor and Li 2007) have defined the effective porosity (η_e) to highlight the actual effective pores in porous structures that are conducive to nutrient transport. This value is the ratio of the volume of pores in the porous structure that can achieve fluid circulation to the total volume of the porous structure. It is calculated by the following formula:

$$\varepsilon_{\mathrm{e}} = \frac{V_{\mathrm{mw}}}{V} = \frac{V_{\mathrm{mw}}}{V_{\mathrm{mw}} + V_{\mathrm{s}} + V_{\mathrm{iw}}}$$

where $V = V_w + V_s$ is the total volume of the porous structure, $V_w = V_{iw} + V_{mw}$ is the volume of the liquid phase inside the pores, V_{iw} is the volume of the liquid phase that cannot move freely, including the liquid that is adsorbed on the porous surface and the liquid that is found in dead-end pores, and V_{mw} is the volume of the liquid phase that can move freely.

Pore size represents the amount of three-dimensional space within the pore structure. Due to the variety of pore structure morphologies, there are certain differences in the definition of pore size for porous structures. For irregular porous structures, such as sponge structures and biomimetic trabecular structures, the pore size is typically defined based on two-dimensional images (microscopic/scan images) using the hydraulic diameter D (Innocentini et al. 2010). For crystalline cell porous structures and TPMS porous structures, the pore size is typically defined using the diameter of the largest inscribed circle in the three-dimensional space of the pore structure (Ambu and Morabito 2019). For porous structures constructed based on FFF pathways, the pore size is typically defined using the spacing between two parallel rods in the two-dimensional plane (Shanjani et al. 2017). Based on extensive research on porous bone tissue engineering materials, Peng et al. (2023) defined pore size as the maximum three-dimensional spatial dimension that the smallest pore in the porous structure can accommodate. Furthermore, they defined pore throat size as the maximum two-dimensional planar dimension between adjacent pores within the porous structure; this value is used to evaluate the maximum size of cells that can grow inwardly into the porous structure, directly determining whether cells can enter the pore structure, as shown in Fig. 2.6.

Most studies on implant pore size are conducted through CT scans or microscopic observations combined with corresponding analysis software to directly calculate the pore size of porous implants.

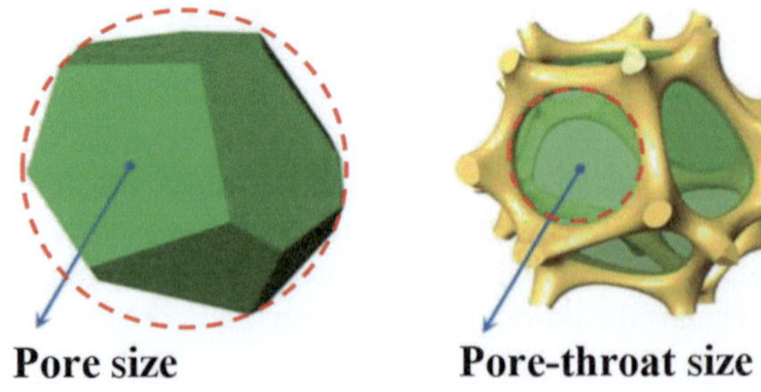

Fig. 2.6 The definition of pore size and pore throat size in porous structures (Wang et al. 2018a)

Although indirect measurement techniques, such as gas adsorption or high-pressure mercury intrusion, can provide more efficient and rapid measurements of pore size, the obtained data may not necessarily correspond to the numerical value of the defined pore size. Based on the results of calculating the pore size of porous structures, corresponding statistical intervals can be set according to the statistical requirements to analyze the pore size distribution and the average pore size of the porous structure. The pore size directly affects the activity of cells within tissue scaffolds. Excessively large pores are not conducive to cell adhesion and growth within the scaffold, while excessively small pores may restrict cell movement within the scaffold. Direct measurements are conducted through optical instruments such as scanning electron microscopy (SEM), and indirect measurements rely on techniques such as X-ray computed tomography (CT).

The specific surface area is an index that is used to evaluate the surface area of the pore space within a porous structure. A larger specific surface area can provide more sites for protein and cell adsorption, which is advantageous for cell adhesion, migration, and proliferation. Additionally, a larger specific surface area provides ample space for extracellular matrix secretion and deposition, enhancing the bioactivity of the implant (Murphy et al. 2010). The specific surface area (ε) can be obtained from CT scan images, and the formula is as follows:

$$\varepsilon = \frac{S_{\mathrm{P}}}{V_{\mathrm{P}}} \times 100\% = \frac{V_{\mathrm{P}}}{V - V_{\mathrm{S}}} \times 100\%$$

where S_{P} is the surface area of the pores and V_{P} is the volume of the pores in the porous structure. V_{S} is the volume of the solid phase in the porous structure. V is the total volume of the porous structure. Additionally, the specific surface area can be obtained by the Brunauer-Emmett-Teller (BET) method, which is based on gas adsorption principles. A certain amount of gas (often nitrogen) is adsorbed onto the material surface, and by measuring the amount of adsorbed gas and the pressure, the specific surface area of the material can be calculated. A certain amount of gas (often nitrogen) is adsorbed onto the material surface, and by measuring the amount of adsorbed gas and the pressure, the specific surface area of the material can be calculated.

2.3 Evaluation of the Mechanical Properties of Porous Structures for 3D-Printed Custom-Made Prostheses

A comprehensive and accurate evaluation of the mechanical properties of biomimetic porous structures facilitates the construction of microstructural models that are compatible with the mechanical properties of human host bones. This approach also provides essential data to support the design of 3D-printed, custom-made porous prostheses for use in bone defect repair. This section introduces methods for evaluating the static and dynamic mechanical properties of porous structures, summarizes the mechanical properties of some typical porous structures and their interrelation rules, and finally provides guidance for the controllable design of the mechanical properties of porous structures through comprehensive comparisons with the mechanical properties of the human host bones.

2.3.1 Methods for Analyzing Mechanical Properties

A porous structure is subjected to different types of static and dynamic loads in vivo, such as tension, compression, bending, torsion, and combinations of these loads. The closely related mechanical properties mainly include the effective elastic modulus, yield strength, fatigue strength, and anisotropy. Currently, common methods for analyzing the mechanical properties of porous structures include theoretical calculations, numerical simulations, and experimental testing. Each method has its own advantages and disadvantages. The methods for analyzing the static and dynamic mechanical properties of porous structures are summarized below.

2.3.1.1 Static Mechanical Properties

According to the study (Gibson and Ashby 1988), the deformation of porous structures under uniaxial compressive loading includes three stages, namely, elastic deformation, yield plateau, and densification, as shown in Fig. 2.7a. By analyzing the stress–strain curve, the effective elastic modulus and yield strength can be

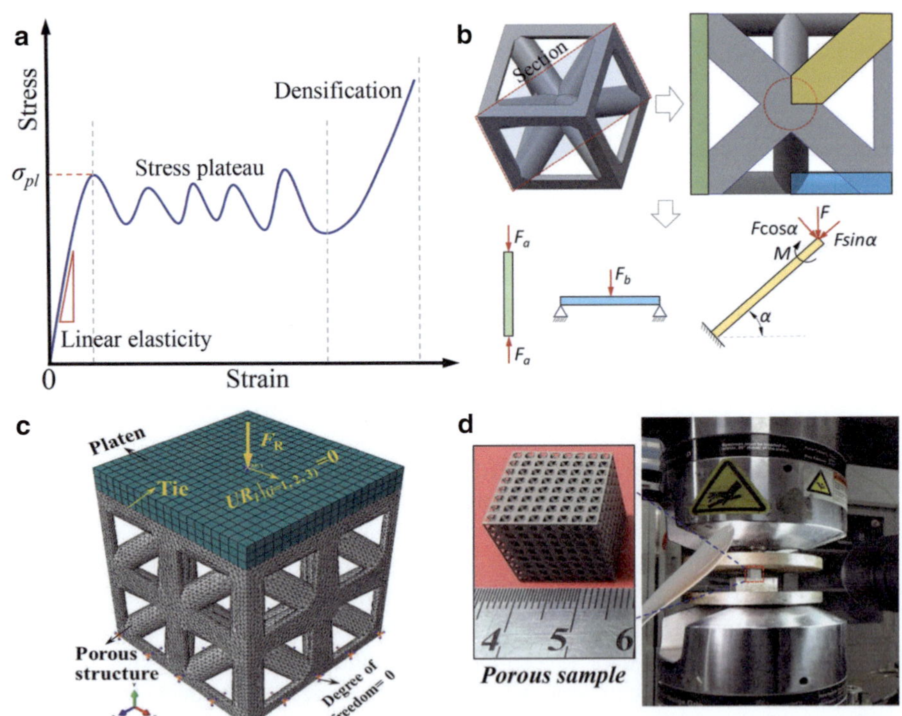

Fig. 2.7 Methods for analyzing the static mechanical properties of porous structures: (**a**) stress–strain curve of a porous sample under compression test; (**b**) theoretical calculation method; (**c**) finite element analysis method; (**d**) experimental testing method (Wang et al. 2017)

determined, providing an important foundation for subsequent evaluations of the dynamic mechanical properties.

In the elastic deformation stage, three different methods for calculating the effective elastic modulus are used, as shown in Fig. 2.7b–d. Theoretical calculation methods mainly rely on Euler–Bernoulli or Timoshenko beam theory, and the specific processes are performed by stepwise decomposition of each component of the porous structure to obtain the effective elastic modulus and establish a mathematical relationship between the elastic modulus and geometrical parameters. However, the derivation of the theoretical method is complicated and limited to rod-shaped structures, and it is difficult to determine the influence of deviation on the actual size and surface morphology of printed porous samples, which in turn affects their applicability and prediction accuracy.

Moreover, the combination of finite element analysis and experimental testing has been widely used to calculate the effective elastic modulus. The fundamental principles of these two methods are primarily based on Hooke's law, which calculates the equivalent elastic modulus from the linear relationship between stress and strain in materials under uniaxial compressive or tensile loading. For the finite element method, the response deformation of porous structures under various types of loads can be analyzed. This method has advantages such as low cost, ease of operation, high efficiency, and visual display of the results of structural mechanics analysis (Gibson and Ashby 1988). However, the prediction accuracy of finite element analysis is also affected by various factors, such as the deviation of geometrical size and surface topography between the design model and the printed sample, the internal defects of the printed sample, and the preprocessing settings for finite element analysis. Therefore, experimental testing is still needed to validate the numerical results. Currently, the standards for the experimental testing of the quasistatic mechanical properties of porous structures include ISO 13314-2011 and ASTM F3122-2014. According to these standards, different mechanical property tests have been performed on porous structure samples manufactured using 3D printing technology. The test conditions are set according to the experimental requirements, and then the data from experimental tests on porous samples are obtained to further calculate the equivalent static mechanical properties.

During the plastic deformation stage, porous structures usually undergo irreversible deformation until fracture failure occurs, with the yield strength being an important indicator for evaluating the safety of porous prostheses. Most previous studies used a combination of finite element analysis and experimental testing to analyze the yield strength of porous structures (Gibson and Ashby 1988). In the process of finite element analysis, by setting the plastic stress–strain data or relevant parameters of control equations for porous structure material, different types of loading conditions are applied to the designed CAD models or the reverse geometric model of the 3D printing sample to simulate the yield strength of porous structures and analyze their deformation response mechanisms. The yield strength of a porous structure can be calculated, and its deformation response mechanism can be analyzed. Additionally, the mechanical properties of porous structure samples can be further tested experimentally and evaluated in accordance with relevant standards.

The mechanical properties of porous structures are anisotropic due to the influence of various factors, such as the complex geometric shape, the combination type and spatial arrangement of the porous structure, the layer-by-layer manufacturing principle of 3D printing, and the geometrical size deviation or irregular morphology of the fabricated sample. Therefore, rational design and optimization of porous structures are expected to further adapt to the anisotropy of the mechanical properties of the human host bones. At present, through numerical analysis or experimental testing, the mechanical anisotropy of porous structures is usually evaluated according to the ratio of the effective elastic modulus or yield strength in different directions or the Zener anisotropic coefficient obtained by calculating the stiffness matrix coefficients (Gibson and Ashby 1988). This method reflects the anisotropy of the elastic modulus well. However, the evaluation of mechanical anisotropy focuses more on the elastic modulus.

2.3.1.2 Dynamic Mechanical Properties

When 3D-printed porous prostheses are subjected to long-term cyclic loading, with prolonged service time, these conditions may lead to fatigue failure issues, such as crack initiation, propagation, and eventual fracture, even if the maximum repeated alternating stress is lower than the material's yield strength. In general, the fatigue life of a porous structure usually changes with applied stress; the fatigue life can be divided into low-cycle fatigue and high-cycle fatigue, which represent fatigue with and without plastic deformation, respectively. In low-cycle fatigue analysis, the Coffin–Manson strain–life fatigue model is often utilized to assess fatigue life. Fatigue tests are conducted under various degrees of strain to determine the relevant parameters of the fatigue model based on the test data. In contrast, high-cycle fatigue is evaluated mainly using the stress model. According to the Basquin equation, the relationship between different cyclic stresses and fatigue life can be tested, and the stress–life curve (also known as the stress-number curve) can be drawn. It is worth noting that porous prostheses actually bear alternating loads with non-zero mean stress, so the equation proposed by Goodman and Gerber is often used to determine fatigue test results.

The fatigue strength of porous structures is mostly determined by uniaxial compression–compression testing according to the ISO 13314:2011 standard. According to this standard, the sample size should be at least 10 times the average pore diameter to reduce edge effects, and it is advisable to build a solid plate at both ends of the porous sample to ensure better flatness of contact between the sample and the pressure plate. Based on the static mechanical properties of the porous samples obtained from the experimental tests, the yield and ultimate strength are selected as reference stress values for fatigue experiments. Generally, the cyclic frequency ranges from 10 to 50 Hz, with a load ratio (the ratio of the absolute values of both the maximum and minimum loads) of 0.1. The global maximum absolute stress used is generally between 10% and 80% of the yield stress. The fatigue life of porous specimens is tested under cyclic loading from the initial stage to 1–2 million cycles. In addition, compression–tension and tension–tension fatigue performance tests have been conducted on porous structures.

Overall, previous studies on the fatigue properties of porous structures were limited to uniaxial loading and quasistatic torsion analysis (Benedetti et al. 2021), while porous prostheses exhibit multiaxial stress states under complex mechanical environmental conditions in vivo, as well as the influence of varying amplitude loads under different gait conditions. Therefore, in response to the real application needs of porous prostheses, the analysis and evaluation of their fatigue properties still face numerous challenges.

2.3.2 Strategy for Controlling Mechanical Properties

With respect to the biomimetic design of the porous structures for custom-made prostheses, the mechanical properties of different types of porous units are summarized in Table 2.4. In comparison with the human host bones, some suitable porous structures can be selected. This approach provides important data for the controllable design of custom-made porous prostheses.

2.3.2.1 Factors That Affect the Mechanical Properties of Porous Structures

The mechanical properties of porous structures, including the elastic modulus, yield strength, and fatigue strength, are weakened with increasing porosity due to changes in the geometric size or modulation of parameters. Generally, the Gibson–Ashby power function is used to determine the mapping relationship between mechanical properties and porosity. Due to the complex geometric morphology of porous structures, the uniqueness of manufacturing technologies and processes, and the diversity of materials that are used, different types of porous structures exhibit significant discrepancies in their equivalent mechanical properties. This necessitates thorough consideration of the tensile/compressive stress states that act on prostheses when designing 3D-printed custom-made porous prostheses. Therefore, it is essential to systematically explore the fundamental mechanical properties of porous structures to ensure the mechanical restoration of bone defects and the safety of prostheses.

Moreover, previous studies on the mechanical anisotropic properties of porous units have focused mainly on the effective elastic modulus, and the yield strength has mostly been evaluated by the strength ratio in different directions. There is still a need to explore advanced evaluation methods that can comprehensively and accurately reflect the spatial variation in the mechanical properties of porous units, further enhancing the safety and stability of prostheses in service. Additionally, dynamic fatigue performance is affected by the high number of test cycles, high cost, difficulty in reconstructing complex mechanical environments in vivo, and time-varying characteristics of bone ingrowth into pores; for these reasons, there are significantly fewer studies on fatigue performance than on static mechanical properties.

Table 2.4 Mechanical properties of 3D-printed porous structures

Methods of porous structure design	Porous units	Porosity (%)	Materials	Analytical methods	Mechanical properties: Effective elastic modulus (GPa)	Mechanical properties: Yield strength (MPa)	Ref.
Image-based reverse design	Voronoi	50–85	Ti_6Al_4V	EXP	2.13–3.97	78.99–130.5	Du et al. (2020)
	Biomimetic trabecula structure	16.2 ± 2.9	Ti_6Al_4V	EXP	3.693 ± 0.027	–	Cheng et al. (2014)
		38.5 ± 3.9			3.522 ± 0.052		
		70.0 ± 3.5			2.579 ± 0.106		
Constructive solid geometry	Body-centered cubic	33.78	Ti_6Al_4V	EXP	9.0 ± 0.6	392 ± 14	Onal et al. (2018)
		53.06	Ti_6Al_4V		4.6 ± 0.4	192 ± 14	
		71.87	Ti_6Al_4V		1.6 ± 0.2	53 ± 4	
	Diamond	60–90	Ti_6Al_4V	FEA	0.98–6.74	51.95–186.05	Ataee et al. (2018a)
	Rhombic dodecahedron	70.6	Tantalum	EXP	1.43 ± 0.1	25.04 ± 1.38	Guo et al. (2022)
	Rhombic dodecahedron	63.29	Ti_6Al_4V	EXP	6.7	209.96	Gurkan et al. (2023)
	Octahedral	83.06	Ti_6Al_4V	EXP	1.7	35.46	
	Cube	65	Ti_6Al_4V	EXP	2.6	96	Deng et al. (2021)

Minimal surface based on an implicit function	Gyroid	82–85	Ti_6Al_4V	EXP	0.637–1.084	13.18–19.2	Ataee et al. (2018b)
	Gyroid	68.7–72.4	CP-Ti	EXP	1.465–2.676	44.9–56.5	Yan et al. (2015)
	Gyroid	5–10	Ti_6Al_4V	FEA	17.45–19.14	1342–1581	Ataee et al. (2018a)
	Gyroid	80–95	Ti_6Al_4V	EXP	0.13–1.25	6.501–81.30	
	Diamond	5–10	Ti_6Al_4V	FEA	15.73–17.19	1403–1559	
	Diamond	80–95	Ti_6Al_4V	EXP	0.12–1.25	4.662–69.12	
Printed path planning	Square structure	37.8 ± 0.37	PEEK	EXP	0.675 ± 0.03	43.5 ± 0.95	Zheng et al. (2021)
		51.9 ± 0.67			0.493 ± 0.02	28.7 ± 0.61	
		61.1 ± 0.25			0.329 ± 0.03	21.9 ± 1.40	
		75.7 ± 0.42			0.103 ± 0.01	6.1 ± 0.42	
	Wheel structure	38.1 ± 0.86	PEEK	EXP	0.562 ± 0.02	39.2 ± 0.5	
		51.4 ± 0.65			0.344 ± 0.02	25.3 ± 0.6	
		62.2 ± 1.1			0.212 ± 0.01	15.6 ± 0.4	
		74.4 ± 0.39			0.167 ± 0.0	8.1 ± 0.3	

From literature: Deng et al. (2021), Du et al. (2020), Cheng et al. (2014), Liu et al. (2020), Ataee et al. (2018a, b), Guo et al. (2022), Onal et al. (2018), Gurkan et al. (2023), Yan et al. (2015), Zheng et al. (2021)

Abbreviations: *EXP* experimental testing, *FEA* finite element analysis

2.3.2.2 Strategy to Control the Mechanical Properties of Porous Structures

Two approaches are employed to address variations in the mechanical properties and dynamic responses of human bones in different body parts, and to match the mechanical properties of porous structures with those of host bone. First, by altering the geometric dimensions or control parameters of a porous structure, a similar equivalent elastic modulus can be achieved. Second, through the rational design of the porous structure gradients or nonuniform configurations, effective mechanical transfer and stress distributions are established. This ensures the safety and stability requirements of custom porous prostheses during their service.

Most studies have established mathematical relationships between the mechanical properties of porous structures and their geometric parameters, allowing for the selection of prosthetics for bone defect repair based on the mechanical performance requirements of different areas. However, these relationships are primarily based on uniform structures constructed from single lattice periodic arrays. For gradient or nonuniform porous structures, some strategies can be adopted to change the gradient porosity in the axial or radial direction, to alter pore shapes, and to adjust the spatial arrangement and distribution of different pore shapes or porous lattices. The macroscopic equivalent mechanical properties and the response mechanism between the porous structure and the properties vary. Therefore, in research on the controllable design of the mechanical properties of porous structures, it is essential to delineate the adjustable range of mechanical properties for various types of porous structures. Subsequently, consideration should be given to the gradient or nonuniform design involving different pore shapes or porous unit combinations. This approach aims to achieve the overarching objective of matching the mechanical properties of porous structures with those of the host bone.

2.4 Evaluation of the Osseointegration Properties of 3D-Printed Customized Prostheses with Porous Structures

The concept of osseointegration was first proposed by Professor Brånemark et al. (2001) and refers to the persistent osseous contact of an implant with an active bone tissue without fiber intervention at the interface. Numerous animal experiments and clinical studies have shown that good implant osseointegration contributes to clinical success and long-term stability after implantation (Engh et al. 1987). There are many methods for evaluating the osseointegration performance of implants, including histological evaluation, cellular and molecular biology evaluation, medical imaging evaluation, and biomechanical analysis. However, most of these methods can only be applied to in vitro cell experiments and animal experiments, and effective clinical evaluation methods remain limited. Moreover, most studies on the osseointegration of implants and their conclusions are based on in vitro cellular and animal experiments.

2.4.1 Influence of the Geometric Characteristics of Porous Structures on Osteointegration

2.4.1.1 Porosity

A large volume of pores provides space for cell and blood vessel growth. A highly interconnected pore structure facilitates cell migration and proliferation. In studies on porous titanium alloy scaffolds, porosities typically range from 30% to 90%. Liu et al. designed and manufactured Ti-6Al-4V biomimetic bone scaffolds with porosities of 85%, 75%, 65%, and 55% and average pore sizes of 550–1150 μm to study their osseointegration properties (Liu et al. 2023). This study revealed that decreasing the average pore size enhanced the adhesion and proliferation of osteoblasts when the porosity remained constant. The Ti-6Al-4V biomimetic bone scaffold, with a porosity of 65% and an average pore size of 550 μm, had the most favorable effects on osteoblast adhesion and proliferation. Chen et al. designed and manufactured Ti-6Al-4V ELI porous scaffolds with octahedral lattices with porosities of 60% and 70% and pore sizes of 500 μm, 600 μm, and 700 μm to study their effects on cell proliferation, osteogenesis, and inward bone growth (Chen et al. 2020). In vitro and in vivo experiments revealed that the scaffold with a porosity of 60% and a pore size of 500 μm resulted in the best cell proliferation, osteogenesis, and inward bone growth. Li et al. designed and manufactured porous spinal implants with porosities ranging from 55% to 90% and pore sizes ranging from 300 to 1500 μm for implantation in adult female sheep (Li et al. 2018). The study revealed that a pore size of 600 μm and a porosity of 76% resulted in better osseointegration. Nune et al. designed and manufactured three types of porous titanium alloy scaffolds with porosities ranging from 76% to 90% and pore sizes ranging from 700 to 1500 μm (Nune et al. 2015). They found that as the porosity increased, the osteoblast seeding efficiency significantly decreased. However, there is no unified conclusion on the effect of porosity on osteointegration.

2.4.1.2 Pore Size

The pore size of a porous structure is a key parameter that affects the mechanical strength and the nutrient transport of scaffolds, which in turn affects the bone tissue growth. Karageorgiou et al. proposed that the pore size of a porous scaffold should be more than 100 μm, and a pore size greater than 300 μm can significantly promote the generation of the bone tissue and the capillaries (Karageorgiou and Kaplan 2005). Cheng et al. manufactured titanium alloy porous scaffolds with pore sizes of 177, 383, and 653 μm and studied the osteogenesis of osteoblasts on the scaffolds in vitro (Cheng et al. 2014). They found that increasing the pore size significantly enhanced the expression of osteogenic proteins and that a pore size of approximately 600 μm is conducive to promoting osteoblast differentiation. However, in vitro studies usually cannot represent the complex process of bone tissue growth in the in vivo environment. Table 2.5 summarizes the osseointegration performance of scaffolds with different pore sizes after implantation *in vivo*. The optimal pore sizes of titanium alloy and bioceramic scaffolds have been studied the most.

Table 2.5 Effect of pore size on osseointegration

Material	Pore geometry	Pore size (μm)	Optimal pore size (μm)	Bone volume/ bone area (%)	Reference
Aluminum alloy	Diamond unit cell	300 600 900	600	–	Taniguchi et al. (2016)
Aluminum alloy	Diamond unit cell	800	1000	9.2	Wang et al. (2021)
Aluminum alloy	Spherical unit cell	400 600 800	600	13.5	Ran et al. (2018)
Tantalum alloy	Hexahedron unit cell	100 200 400 600	400	18.8	Luo et al. (2021)
Calcium phosphate	Square structure	100 200 300	300	41.7	Hayashi et al. (2020)
Calcium phosphate	Trabecular-like structure	200–300 300–450 450–600	200–300	35.4	Zhao et al. (2017)
HA	Trabecular-like structure	500–600 750–900 1100–1250	750–900	37.08	Li et al. (2016)
HA	–	50–150 100–250 300–500	100–250	–	Zhu et al. (2009)

From literature: Taniguchi et al. (2016), Wang et al. (2021), Ran et al. (2018), Luo et al. (2021), Hayashi et al. (2020), Zhao et al. (2017), Li et al. (2016), Zhu et al. (2009)

In studies of the optimal pore size for titanium alloys, the pore sizes typically vary within the range of 200–1200 μm, with unit types including diamond, circular, and square unit cells. The influence of pore size on bone growth was investigated by implanting the relevant scaffolds into the femurs and tibias of animals. According to a previous study, titanium scaffolds with pore sizes of approximately 600 μm were found to promote bone tissue growth into scaffolds and achieve better interface bonding and bone ingrowth depth (Taniguchi et al. 2016).

In studies of the optimal pore size for bioceramic scaffolds, Zhao et al. manufactured porous calcium phosphate scaffolds with pore sizes ranging from 200 to 300 μm, 300 to 450 μm, and 450 to 600 μm (Zhao et al. 2017). After implanting the scaffolds with different pore sizes into rabbits, it was found that porous scaffolds with pore sizes in the range of 200–300 μm resulted in greater bone ingrowth, demonstrating good effects on bone ingrowth. Numerous studies have shown that for porous calcium phosphate and hydroxyapatite scaffolds, a pore size of approximately 300 μm significantly promotes bone ingrowth. When the pore size exceeds 300 μm, the effect of promoting bone ingrowth decreases. It is generally believed that for bioceramic porous scaffolds, a pore size between 300 and 400 μm has a better effect on osseointegration (Li et al. 2016; Tarafder et al. 2013).

These results indicate that variation in the scaffold pore size has an important effect on scaffold osseointegration performance. It is widely accepted that the optimal pore size for porous titanium alloys is 400–600 μm, while that for bioceramics is 300–400 μm. Therefore, there is a certain difference in the optimal pore size for porous implants that are made of different materials. Currently, research on the effect of pore size on osseointegration has mostly focused on titanium alloys and ceramic materials, while studies on the optimal pore size of new materials such as PEEK are rare, and a general conclusion has not yet been reached.

2.4.1.3 Pore Geometry

The geometric shape of pores in porous scaffolds can alter the mechanical stiffness and strength of the scaffold and can alter vascular growth and nutrient diffusion in the scaffold, thereby affecting the osseointegration of the porous scaffold (Wang et al. 2016). Table 2.6 summarizes relevant studies on the effect of pore geometry on osseointegration. Deng et al. designed scaffolds with DIA, TC, CIR, and CU structures (Deng et al. 2021). After implantation into rabbit femoral condyles, the DIA structure was shown to have a better effect on improved bone tissue growth, and the difference in structure permeability between the different structures may be a key factor that influences bone ingrowth. Li et al. designed and fabricated uniform and gradient minimal surface structures and found that the gradient minimal surface

Table 2.6 Effect of pore geometry on osseointegration

Material	Pore geometry	Pore size (μm)	Bone volume/bone area (%)	Reference
Aluminum alloy	Diamond unit cell Square unit cell Spherical unit cell Tetrahedral unit cell	600	23.1	Deng et al. (2021)
Aluminum alloy	Minimal surface structure	450–650	–	Li et al. (2023)
Aluminum alloy	Uniform diamond unit Uneven diamond unit Gradient diamond unit Uniform tetrahedral unit	427–458	37	Wang et al. (2018b)
HA	Mosaic-like structure	22	–	Teraoka et al. (2013)
Bioactive borate glass	Cubic unit cell Spherical unit cell X unit cell Gyroid unit cell Diamond unit cell	500–1300	6.2	Kolan et al. (2020a)

From literature: Deng et al. (2021), Li et al. (2023), Wang et al. (2018b), Teraoka et al. (2013), Kolan et al. (2020a)

structure had better load transfer efficiency, preventing stress shielding and promoting new bone generation (Li et al. 2023). Kolan et al. fabricated implants with cubic and diamond unit cells with bioactive borate glass and implanted these scaffolds into rat cranial bone defects for 6 weeks (Kolan et al. 2020b). The results showed that there was no significant difference in bone formation between the two structures. However, more fibrous tissue was formed within scaffolds with the diamond unit cell, which may further promote bone formation.

Changes in curvature caused by pore shape variation also have a significant effect on tissue integration. Rumpler et al. showed that the magnitude relations between the geometric curvature of pores and the curvature of cells affect cell behavior (Rumpler et al. 2008). When the curvature of pores is much greater than the cell radius, cell proliferation can be promoted. Scarano et al. manufactured tibial scaffolds with grooves using apatitic calcium phosphate (a TCP/HA blend) and implanted these scaffolds into rabbits (Scarano et al. 2014). They found that the degree of neovascularization was significantly higher in grooves with greater curvature. Zhang et al. manufactured porous scaffolds with different curvatures to study the influence of curvature on cell growth (Zhang et al. 2022). They found that the curvature of the porous structure affects the distribution of growth factors, subsequently inducing the migration of cells of the osteoblast lineage and bone deposition to locations with greater curvature.

2.4.2 Influence of the Mechanical Properties of Porous Structures on Osseointegration

The mechanical properties of the porous structure can be regulated by changing the geometric characteristics of the porous structure, subsequently influencing osseointegration. For example, changes in the elastic modulus of porous structures can alter the mechanical environment of bone tissue, thereby affecting the generation and loss of bone tissue. The elastic modulus of metal materials is much greater than that of natural bone tissue. A mismatch in the modulus results in a lack of effective mechanical stimulation of the surrounding bone tissue, leading to bone loss. The mechanical stress of bone tissues can be changed by controlling the elastic modulus of the porous structures. Table 2.7 summarizes the relevant studies on improving the mechanical stimulation of the bone by regulating the geometrical parameters of porous structures. Li et al. designed P-type, D-type, and G-type porous structures and adjusted their elastic modulus to between 3.5~7.3 GPa by controlling their porosity (Li et al. 2019). Finite element analysis showed that increasing the porosity significantly changed the stress in the tissues surrounding the scaffold, reduced the stress shielding effects, and promoted early integration between the porous structures and surrounding tissues. Peng et al. designed mandibular porous bone implants using topology optimization methods and found that compared to solid implants, implants designed with porous structures had better load transfer efficiency and lower stress shielding effects (Peng et al. 2021). In conclusion, regulating the mechanical properties of porous

Table 2.7 Effect of the mechanical properties of porous structures on mechanical stimulation of tissue

Material	Object	Modulation method	Elastic modulus	Effect	Reference
Aluminum alloy	Scaffold	Minimal surface structure	3.5~7.3 GPa	Reduce stress shielding	Li et al. (2019)
Aluminum alloy	Mandibular	Topology optimization	269.5~541.3 MPa		Peng et al. (2021)
Carbon fiber-polysulfone composite	Intervertebral disk	Gradient porous structure	0.35~2.91 GPa		Migacz et al. (2014)
Aluminum alloy	Splint	Gradient porous structure	20~110 GPa		Fouad (2010)
Aluminum alloy	Femoral stem	Gradient porous structure	20~110 GPa		Hedia et al. (2006)
Aluminum alloy	Scaffold	Porosity modulation	–		San Cheong et al. (2018)

From literature: Li et al. (2019), Peng et al. (2021), Migacz et al. (2014), Fouad (2010), Hedia et al. (2006), San Cheong et al. (2018)

structures over a wide range can be achieved by the design of geometric characteristics. By making the mechanical properties of porous implants more similar to those of natural bone tissue, the mechanical stimulation of the surrounding bone tissue can be improved to promote bone growth.

In addition, researchers have conducted studies on the mechanism underlying cell activity and bone tissue growth under external load conditions (Zhang and Habibovic 2022). As shown in Table 2.8, Steinmetz fabricated hydrogels with hierarchical mechanical properties using photopolymerization and loaded human mesenchymal stem cells (hMSCs) into the hydrogels to study the effect of mechanical stimulation on hMSC differentiation (Steinmetz et al. 2015). By comparing cell differentiation in naturally swollen gels and gels to which 15% compressive strain was applied, it was found that mechanical stimulation significantly increased the protein expression of collagen and calcium deposition in hMSCs, thus promoting the differentiation of hMSCs to chondrocytes. This study confirmed the positive role of mechanical stimulation in cell differentiation. Subramony et al. fabricated porous nanofiber scaffolds using electrospinning technology (Subramony et al. 2013). Human mesenchymal stem cells (MSCs) were implanted on the surface of the scaffolds, and 10% strain was applied twice daily. The results showed that the loads on the oriented aligned nanofibrous structures promoted the differentiation of MSCs into ligament fibroblasts, while applying loads on the nonoriented nanofiber structure only changed the cell adhesion morphology without promoting directional

Table 2.8 Effect of mechanical stimulation on the osteogenesis of cells

Cell	Mechanical stimulation	Effect	Reference
hMSCs	Compressive stress	Promoted early osteogenic differentiation	Jung et al. (2008)
Mouse smooth muscle cell	Shear stress	Promoted calcium deposition and osteogenesis	Ahn et al. (2015)
MC3T3-E1 osteoblast-like cells	Shear stress	Induced oriented cell alignment and enhanced expression of phosphatase	Prodanov et al. (2013)
Myoblasts	Tensile stress	Promoted cell proliferation	Li et al. (2009)
NIH 3T3 fibroblasts	Tensile stress	Promoted cell proliferation and osteogenic protein expression	Steward et al. (2010)

From literature: Jung et al. (2008), Ahn et al. (2015), Prodanov et al. (2013), Li et al. (2009), Steward et al. (2010)

differentiation, indicating that cell differentiation is influenced by both the structure of the scaffold and external loads.

These studies indicate that a consensus similar to Wolff's Law has been reached regarding the influence of external loading on the growth of bone tissue. Mechanical stimulation plays an important role in cell proliferation, differentiation, and osteogenic function. The proper application of external mechanical stimulation has great potential for improving the integration of implants and tissues. However, the current lack of methods to accurately assess prestress in vivo limits relevant in vivo/in vitro studies and further clinical applications.

2.4.3 Influence of Porous Structure Permeability on Osseointegration

An increase in the permeability of a porous structure can effectively improve the fluid microenvironment within scaffolds, providing the blood circulation and nutrient supply that are necessary for cell growth and enhancing cell adhesion and proliferation on porous scaffolds. In addition, the shear stress of fluid flow on cells also has an important impact on the migration and differentiation of cells inside the scaffold (Takebe et al. 2012).

The factors that affect the permeability of scaffolds include pore geometry, porosity, connectivity, and pore size. A summary of relevant studies on the effect of geometric characteristics on permeability is shown in Table 2.9. It can be seen that porous structures with higher porosities and larger pore sizes exhibit superior permeability.

When the porosity is the same, the pore geometry has a significant impact on the permeability. For example, the permeability of porous structures with diamond-shaped units and body-centered cubic units is greater than that of structures with minimally porous surface structures. In addition, for structures with minimally

Table 2.9 Effect of the geometrical characteristics of porous structures on the permeability

Pore geometry		Analysis method	Porosity (%)	Permeability/10^{-9} m^2	Reference
Rec-L unit cell	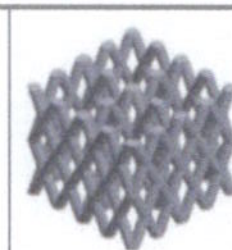	FEM	65–90	5.1–36.3	Ali and Sen (2017)
Primitive structure	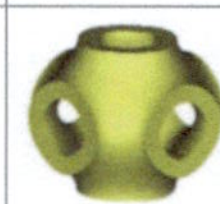	EXP	65	0.55	Yu et al. (2020)
Gyroid structure	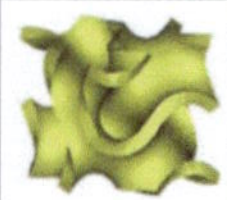	EXP	65	0.30	Yu et al. (2020)
BCC structure	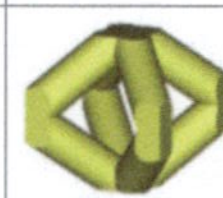	EXP	65	1.48	Yu et al. (2020)
Gradient porous structure with minimal surface	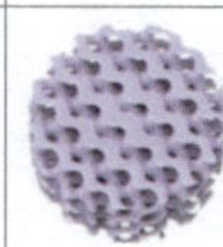	FEM	28–76	0.16–4.1	Montazerian et al. (2019)
Voronoi unit cell	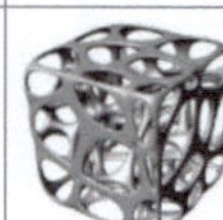	FEM	39.8–87.8 38.9–87.1 38.5–87.8	9.9–44.4 5.7–32.3 4.3–25.2	Gómez et al. (2016)

From literature: Ali and Sen (2017), Yu et al. (2020), Montazerian et al. (2019), Gómez et al. (2016)

porous surfaces, the permeability of the P-type structure is greater than that of the G-type structure. The design of gradient porous structures has different effects on different pore geometries. A gradient porous structure can enhance the permeability of a G-type structure, while the effect on the permeability of a P-type structure is relatively small (Ali and Sen 2017; Yu et al. 2020).

Therefore, the design of geometrical characteristics enables the modulation of the permeability of scaffolds with metal and bioceramic materials. However, no studies have systematically investigated the specific role of scaffold permeability in osteointegration, and there is no consensus on the effective range of permeability for bone ingrowth to the scaffold.

The mechanical properties and permeability of porous structures are key factors that influence osseointegration. By adjusting the geometric characteristics of porous structures, the mechanical properties and permeability can be controlled within a wide range. However, porous structures with higher permeabilities often correspond to structures with lower moduli and strengths. These two factors influence and restrict each other. However, the mechanisms by which the mechanical properties and permeability of porous structures affect tissue growth are not clear, hindering the precise design of porous structures with optimized permeability and mechanical properties to better promote osteointegration.

2.5 Summary

To address the personalized, precise, and functional demands of treatments to repair human bone defects, custom-made porous prostheses designed with biomimetic microstructures and manufactured by 3D printing technology can effectively solve clinical issues, such as loosening and fractures, that are observed after the use of traditional prostheses. This significantly enhances the safety and stability throughout the service life of the prostheses, offering a viable and superior solution for clinical repair treatments. Consequently, this chapter concentrates on the porous structures of 3D-printed, custom prostheses and their characteristics and elaborates on the main effects of porous structures and the basic principles of design from the perspective of the structure-performance-function interaction with the human host bone. Four approaches for designing commonly used porous structures in custom-made prostheses and methods for characterizing geometrical parameters are summarized. The evaluation methods for the static and dynamic mechanical properties of porous structures are generalized, and the results of the mechanical properties for different types of porous structures are presented. Some strategies to control mechanical properties by changing the geometrical size, gradient, or nonuniform distribution of the pores are proposed. Finally, the methods for evaluating the osseointegration capability of porous structures and methods for analyzing the effects are outlined.

Overall, custom-made porous prostheses that are rationally designed and fabricated by 3D printing can meet various requirements, including shape adaptation, performance matching, and functional restoration. Clinical follow-ups have also demonstrated excellent therapeutic effects. However, it is crucial to recognize that the mechanical and osseointegration capabilities of porous structures exhibit varying responses based on their geometric design. For instance, a higher porosity can reduce the equivalent elastic modulus of porous metal specimens to mitigate stress shielding and enhance permeability, facilitating the transport of the nutrients necessary for bone ingrowth. Nonetheless, a compromise in strength could decrease safety. Therefore, in the process of designing porous structures of customized prostheses, on the premise of ensuring printability and safety, it is still necessary to further explore the synergistic regulation and optimization of the mechanical properties and bone integration properties by changing the geometric shape, characteristic parameters, and distribution design of the porous structure.

References

Ahn H, Ju YM, Takahashi H, et al. Engineered small diameter vascular grafts by combining cell sheet engineering and electrospinning technology. Acta Biomater. 2015;16:14–22. https://doi.org/10.1016/j.actbio.2015.01.030.

Ali D, Sen S. Finite element analysis of mechanical behavior, permeability and fluid induced wall shear stress of high porosity scaffolds with gyroid and lattice-based architectures. J Mech Behav Biomed Mater. 2017;75:262–70. https://doi.org/10.1016/j.jmbbm.2017.07.035.

Ambu R, Morabito AE. Modeling, assessment, and design of porous cells based on Schwartz primitive surface for bone scaffolds. Sci World J. 2019;2019:7060847.

Arabnejad S, Johnston B, Tanzer M, et al. Fully porous 3D printed titanium femoral stem to reduce stress-shielding following total hip arthroplasty. J Orthop Res. 2017;35(8):1774–83.

Ataee A, Li Y, Brandt M, et al. Ultrahigh-strength titanium gyroid scaffolds manufactured by selective laser melting (SLM) for bone implant applications. Acta Mater. 2018a;158:354–68. https://doi.org/10.1016/j.actamat.2018.08.005.

Ataee A, Li Y, Fraser D, et al. Anisotropic Ti-6Al-4V gyroid scaffolds manufactured by electron beam melting (EBM) for bone implant applications. Mater Des. 2018b;137:345–54. https://doi.org/10.1016/j.matdes.2017.10.040.

Auperrin A, Delille R, Lesueur D, et al. Geometrical and material parameters to assess the macroscopic mechanical behaviour of fresh cranial bone samples. J Biomech. 2014;47(5):1180–5. https://doi.org/10.1016/j.jbiomech.2013.10.060.

Bandyopadhyay A, Mitra I, Goodman SB, et al. Improving biocompatibility for next generation of metallic implants. Prog Mater Sci. 2023;133:101053.

Benedetti M, du Plessis A, Ritchie RO, et al. Architected cellular materials: a review on their mechanical properties towards fatigue-tolerant design and fabrication. Mater Sci Eng. 2021;144:R-Reports 144.

Brånemark R, Brånemark PI, Rydevik B, et al. Osseointegration in skeletal reconstruction and rehabilitation: a review. J Rehabil Res Dev. 2001;38(2):175–81.

Cheah CM, Chua CK, Leong KF, et al. Development of a tissue engineering scaffold structure library for rapid prototyping. Part 2: parametric library and assembly program. Int J Adv Manuf Technol. 2003;21(4):302–12.

Chen JH. 骨骼机械性能 (Bone mechanical properties). Changchun: Jilin Science and Technology Press. 1989. ISBN: 7-5384-0339-6..

Chen Z, Su Z, Ma S, et al. Biomimetic modeling and three-dimension reconstruction of the artificial bone. Comput Methods Prog Biomed. 2007;88(2):123–30.

Chen Z, Yan X, Yin S, et al. Influence of the pore size and porosity of selective laser melted Ti-6Al-4V ELI porous scaffold on cell proliferation, osteogenesis and bone ingrowth. Mater Sci Eng C-Mater Biol Appl. 2020;106:110289.

Cheng A, Humayun A, Cohen DJ, et al. Additively manufactured 3D porous Ti-6Al-4V constructs mimic trabecular bone structure and regulate osteoblast proliferation, differentiation and local factor production in a porosity and surface roughness dependent manner. Biofabrication. 2014;6(4):045007.

Chor MV, Li W. A permeability measurement system for tissue engineering scaffolds. Meas Sci Technol. 2007;18(1):208–16.

Chua CK, Leong KF, Cheah CM, et al. Development of a tissue engineering scaffold structure library for rapid prototyping. Part 1: investigation and classification. Int J Adv Manuf Technol. 2003;21(4):291–301.

Dalstra M, Huiskes R, Odgaard A, et al. Mechanical and textural properties of pelvic trabecular bone. J Biomech. 1993;26(4–5):523–35.

Deng F, Liu L, Li Z, et al. 3D printed Ti-6Al-4V bone scaffolds with different pore structure effects on bone ingrowth. J Biol Eng. 2021;15(1):4. https://doi.org/10.1186/s13036-021-00255-8.

Dong XN, Guo XE. The dependence of transversely isotropic elasticity of human femoral cortical bone on porosity. J Biomech. 2004;37(8):1281–7. https://doi.org/10.1016/j.jbiomech.2003.12.011.

Du Y, Liang H, Xie D, et al. Design and statistical analysis of irregular porous scaffolds for orthopedic reconstruction based on voronoi tessellation and fabricated via selective laser melting (SLM). Mater Chem Phys. 2020;239:121968. https://doi.org/10.1016/j.matchemphys.2019.121968.

Duchemin L, Bousson V, Raossanaly C, et al. Prediction of mechanical properties of cortical bone by quantitative computed tomography. Med Eng Phys. 2008;30(3):321–8. https://doi.org/10.1016/j.medengphy.2007.04.008.

Engh CA, Bobyn JD, Glassman AH. Porous-coated hip-replacement—the factors governing bone ingrowth, stress shielding, and clinical-results. J Bone Joint Surg. 1987;69(1):45–55.

Fan B, Guo Z, Li X, et al. Electroactive barium titanate coated titanium scaffold improves osteogenesis and osseointegration with low-intensity pulsed ultrasound for large segmental bone defects. Bioact Mater. 2020;5(4):1087–101.

Fouad H. Effects of the bone-plate material and the presence of a gap between the fractured bone and plate on the predicted stresses at the fractured bone. Med Eng Phys. 2010;32(7):783–9. https://doi.org/10.1016/j.medengphy.2010.05.003.

Germaini MM, Belhabib S, Guessasma S, et al. Additive manufacturing of biomaterials for bone tissue engineering—a critical review of the state of the art and new concepts. Prog Mater Sci. 2022;130:100963.

Gibson LJ, Ashby MF. Cellular solids—structure and properties. 2nd ed. Cambridge: Cambridge University Press; 1988.

Gilsanz V, Boechat MI, Gilsanz R, et al. Gender differences in vertebral sizes in adults—biomechanical implications. Radiology. 1994;190(3):678–82. https://doi.org/10.1148/radiology.190.3.8115610.

Gómez S, Vlad MD, López J, et al. Design and properties of 3D scaffolds for bone tissue engineering. Acta Biomater. 2016;42:341–50. https://doi.org/10.1016/j.actbio.2016.06.032.

Guo Y, Chen C, Tan L, et al. The role of pore structures on the fatigue properties of additively manufactured porous tantalum scaffolds produced by electron beam powder bed fusion. J Mater Res Technol. 2022;19:3461–73.

Gurkan D, Sagbas B, Dalbayrak B. Investigating mechanical and biological properties of additive manufactured Ti6Al4V lattice structures for orthopedic implants. J Mater Res. 2023;38(2):507–18. https://doi.org/10.1557/s43578-022-00837-2.

Hayashi K, Munar ML, Ishikawa K. Effects of macropore size in carbonate apatite honeycomb scaffolds on bone regeneration. Mater Sci Eng C-Mater Biol Appl. 2020;111:110848. https://doi.org/10.1016/j.msec.2020.110848.

Hedia HS, Shabara MAN, El-Midany TT, et al. Improved design of cementless hip stems using two-dimensional functionally graded materials. J Biomed Mater Res Part B. 2006;79B(1):42–9. https://doi.org/10.1002/jbm.b.30509.

Hollister SJ. Porous scaffold design for tissue engineering. Nat Mater. 2005;4(7):518–24.

Innocentini MDM, Faleiros RK, Pisani R Jr, et al. Permeability of porous gelcast scaffolds for bone tissue engineering. J Porous Mater. 2010;17(5):615–27.

Jung Y, Kim SH, Kim SH, et al. Cartilaginous tissue formation using a mechano-active scaffold and dynamic compressive stimulation. J Biomater Sci-Polym Ed. 2008;19(1):61–74. https://doi.org/10.1163/156856208783227712.

Karageorgiou V, Kaplan D. Porosity of 3D biomaterial scaffolds and osteogenesis. Biomaterials. 2005;26(27):5474–91.

Kolan KCR, Huang YW, Semon JA. 3D-printed biomimetic bioactive glass scaffolds for bone regeneration in rat calvarial defects (vol 6, pg 274, 2020). Int J Bioprint. 2020a;6(4):133. https://doi.org/10.18063/ijb.v6i2.274.

Kolan KCR, Huang YW, Semon JA, et al. 3D-printed biomimetic bioactive glass scaffolds for bone regeneration in rat calvarial defects. Int J Bioprint. 2020b;6(2):274.

Kopperdahl DL, Morgan EF, Keaveny TM. Quantitative computed tomography estimates of the mechanical properties of human vertebral trabecular bone. J Orthop Res. 2002;20(4):801–5. https://doi.org/10.1016/S0736-0266(01)00185-1.

Li Y, Zhao ZH, Song JL, et al. Cyclic force upregulates mechano-growth factor and elevates cell proliferation in 3D cultured skeletal myoblasts. Arch Biochem Biophys. 2009;490(2):171–6. https://doi.org/10.1016/j.abb.2009.08.016.

Li JY, Zhi W, Xu TT, et al. Ectopic osteogenesis and angiogenesis regulated by porous architecture of hydroxyapatite scaffolds with similar interconnecting structure in vivo. Regener Biomater. 2016;3(5):285–97. https://doi.org/10.1093/rb/rbw031.

Li S, Li X, Hou W, et al. Fabrication of open-cellular (porous) titanium alloy implants: osseointegration, vascularization and preliminary human trials. Sci China Mater. 2018;61(4):525–36.

Li L, Shi JP, Zhang KJ, et al. Early osteointegration evaluation of porous Ti6Al4V scaffolds designed based on triply periodic minimal surface models. J Orthop Translat. 2019;19:94–105. https://doi.org/10.1016/j.jot.2019.03.003.

Li L, Wang P, Liang H, et al. Design of a Haversian system-like gradient porous scaffold based on triply periodic minimal surfaces for promoting bone regeneration. J Adv Res. 2023;54:89–104. https://doi.org/10.1016/j.jare.2023.01.004.

Liu F, Ran Q, Zhao M, Zhang T, Zhang DZ, Su Z. Additively manufactured continuous cell-size gradient porous scaffolds: Pore characteristics, mechanical properties and biological responses in vitro. Materials. 2020;13(11):2589. https://doi.org/10.3390/ma13112589.

Liu J, Wang R, Gong X, et al. Ti6Al4V biomimetic scaffolds for bone tissue engineering: fabrication, biomechanics and osseointegration. Mater Des. 2023;234:112330.

Luo CQ, Wang CR, Wu XD, et al. Influence of porous tantalum scaffold pore size on osteogenesis and osteointegration: a comprehensive study based on 3D-printing technology. Mater Sci Eng C-Mater Biol Appl. 2021;129:112382. https://doi.org/10.1016/j.msec.2021.112382.

Maloul A, Fialkov J, Whyne CM. Characterization of the bending strength of craniofacial sutures. J Biomech. 2013;46(5):912–7. https://doi.org/10.1016/j.jbiomech.2012.12.016.

Migacz K, Chlopek J, Morawska-Chochol A, et al. Gradient composite materials for artificial intervertebral discs. Acta Bioeng Biomech. 2014;16(3):3–12. https://doi.org/10.5277/abb140301.

Montazerian H, Mohamed MGA, Montazeri MM, et al. Permeability and mechanical properties of gradient porous PDMS scaffolds fabricated by 3D-printed sacrificial templates designed with minimal surfaces. Acta Biomater. 2019;96:149–60. https://doi.org/10.1016/j.actbio.2019.06.040.

Mosekilde L, Mosekilde L. Normal vertebral body size and compressive strength—relations to age and to vertebral and iliac trabecular bone compressive strength. Bone. 1986;7(3):207–12. https://doi.org/10.1016/8756-3282(86)90019-0.

Motherway JA, Verschueren P, Van der Perre G, et al. The mechanical properties of cranial bone: the effect of loading rate and cranial sampling position. J Biomech. 2009;42(13):2129–35. https://doi.org/10.1016/j.jbiomech.2009.05.030.

Murphy CM, Haugh MG, O'Brien FJ. The effect of mean pore size on cell attachment, proliferation and migration in collagen-glycosaminoglycan scaffolds for bone tissue engineering. Biomaterials. 2010;31(3):461–6.

Nauman EA, Fong KE, Keaveny TM. Dependence of intertrabecular permeability on flow direction and anatomic site. Ann Biomed Eng. 1999;27(4):517–24. https://doi.org/10.1114/1.195.

Nune KC, Misra RDK, Gaytan SM, et al. Interplay between cellular activity and three-dimensional scaffold-cell constructs with different foam structure processed by electron beam melting. J Biomed Mater Res A. 2015;103(5):1677–92.

Ogurkowska MB, Blaszczyk A. Distribution of Young's modulus at various sampling points in a human lumbar spine vertebral body. Spine J. 2020;20(11):1861–75. https://doi.org/10.1016/j.spinee.2020.06.013.

Onal E, Frith JE, Jurg M, et al. Mechanical properties and in vitro behavior of additively manufactured and functionally graded Ti6Al4V porous scaffolds. Metals. 2018;8(4):200.

Peng WM, Cheng KJ, Liu YF, et al. Biomechanical and mechanostat analysis of a titanium layered porous implant for mandibular reconstruction: the effect of the topology optimization design. Mater Sci Eng C-Mater Biol Appl. 2021;124:112056. https://doi.org/10.1016/j.msec.2021.112056.

Peng W, Huang X, Xu H, et al. Clinical efficacy of 3D printed anatomical titanium alloy tibial prosthesis in reconstruction of bone defects in the lower tibia. J Army Med Univ. 2022;44(15):1531–7.

Peng W, Liu Y, Wang C. Definition, measurement, and function of pore structure dimensions of bioengineered porous bone tissue materials based on additive manufacturing: a review. Front Bioeng Biotechnol. 2023;10:1081548.

Pennella F, Cerino G, Massai D, et al. A survey of methods for the evaluation of tissue engineering scaffold permeability. Ann Biomed Eng. 2013;41(10):2027–41.

Prodanov L, Semeins CM, van Loon J, et al. Influence of nanostructural environment and fluid flow on osteoblast-like cell behavior: a model for cell-mechanics studies. Acta Biomater. 2013;9(5):6653–62. https://doi.org/10.1016/j.actbio.2013.02.011.

Ran QC, Yang WH, Hu Y, et al. Osteogenesis of 3D printed porous Ti6Al4V implants with different pore sizes. J Mech Behav Biomed Mater. 2018;84:1–11. https://doi.org/10.1016/j.jmbbm.2018.04.010.

Rumpler M, Woesz A, Dunlop JWC, et al. The effect of geometry on three-dimensional tissue growth. J R Soc Interface. 2008;5(27):1173–80.

San Cheong V, Fromme P, Mumith A, et al. Novel adaptive finite element algorithms to predict bone ingrowth in additive manufactured porous implants. J Mech Behav Biomed Mater. 2018;87:230–9. https://doi.org/10.1016/j.jmbbm.2018.07.019.

Scarano A, Perrotti V, Artese L, et al. Blood vessels are concentrated within the implant surface concavities: a histologic study in rabbit tibia. Odontology. 2014;102(2):259–66.

Shanjani Y, Kang Y, Zarnescu L, et al. Endothelial pattern formation in hybrid constructs of additive manufactured porous rigid scaffolds and cell-laden hydrogels for orthopedic applications. J Mech Behav Biomed Mater. 2017;65:356–72.

So E, Mandas VH, Hlad L. Large osseous defect reconstruction using a custom three-dimensional printed titanium truss implant. J Foot Ankle Surg. 2018;57(1):196–204.

Steinmetz NJ, Aisenbrey EA, Westbrook KK, et al. Mechanical loading regulates human MSC differentiation in a multi-layer hydrogel for osteochondral tissue engineering. Acta Biomater. 2015;21:142–53.

Steward RL, Cheng CM, Wang DL, et al. Probing cell structure responses through a shear and stretching mechanical stimulation technique. Cell Biochem Biophys. 2010;56(2–3):115–24.

Subramony SD, Dargis BR, Castillo M, et al. The guidance of stem cell differentiation by substrate alignment and mechanical stimulation. Biomaterials. 2013;34(8):1942–53.

Takebe T, Kobayashi S, Kan H, et al. Human elastic cartilage engineering from cartilage progenitor cells using rotating wall vessel bioreactor. Transplant Proc. 2012;44(4):1158–61.

Taniguchi N, Fujibayashi S, Takemoto M, et al. Effect of pore size on bone ingrowth into porous titanium implants fabricated by additive manufacturing: an in vivo experiment. Mater Sci Eng C-Mater Biol Appl. 2016;59:690–701. https://doi.org/10.1016/j.msec.2015.10.069.

Tarafder S, Balla VK, Davies NM, et al. Microwave-sintered 3D printed tricalcium phosphate scaffolds for bone tissue engineering. J Tissue Eng Regen Med. 2013;7(8):631–41.

Teraoka K, Kato T, Hattori K, et al. Evaluation of the capacity of mosaic-like porous ceramics with designed pores to support osteoconduction. J Biomed Mater Res Part A. 2013;101(12):3571–9. https://doi.org/10.1002/jbm.a.34663.

Thomsen JS, Ebbesen EN, Mosekilde L. Static histomorphometry of human iliac crest and vertebral trabecular bone: a comparative study. Bone. 2002;30(1):267–74.

van Hengel IAJ, Gelderman FSA, Athanasiadis S, et al. Functionality-packed additively manufactured porous titanium implants. Mater Today Bio. 2020;7:100060.

Wang X, Xu S, Zhou S, et al. Topological design and additive manufacturing of porous metals for bone scaffolds and orthopaedic implants: a review. Biomaterials. 2016;83:127–41.

Wang L, Kang J, Sun C, et al. Mapping porous microstructures to yield desired mechanical properties for application in 3D printed bone scaffolds and orthopaedic implants. Mater Des. 2017;133:62–8.

Wang G, Shen L, Zhao J, et al. Design and compressive behavior of controllable irregular porous scaffolds: based on voronoi-tessellation and for additive manufacturing. ACS Biomater Sci Eng. 2018a;4(2):719–27.

Wang H, Su KX, Su LZ, et al. The effect of 3D-printed Ti6Al4V scaffolds with various macropore structures on osteointegration and osteogenesis: a biomechanical evaluation. J Mech Behav Biomed Mater. 2018b;88:488–96. https://doi.org/10.1016/j.jmbbm.2018.08.049.

Wang C, Xu DL, Lin L, et al. Large-pore-size Ti6Al4V scaffolds with different pore structures for vascularized bone regeneration. Mater Sci Eng C-Mater Biol Appl. 2021;131:112499. https://doi.org/10.1016/j.msec.2021.112499.

Ward KA, Roberts SA, Adams JE, et al. Bone geometry and density in the skeleton of pre-pubertal gymnasts and school children. Bone. 2005;36(6):1012–8. https://doi.org/10.1016/j.bone.2005.03.001.

Wei X, Tang Z, Wu H, Guo Z, et al. Innovation to advance and courage to transcend. Meta World. 2022;(4):1–7.

Wettergreen MA, Bucklen BS, Starly B, et al. Creation of a unit block library of architectures for use in assembled scaffold engineering. Comput Aided Des. 2005;37(11):1141–9.

Yan C, Hao L, Hussein A, et al. Ti-6Al-4V triply periodic minimal surface structures for bone implants fabricated via selective laser melting. J Mech Behav Biomed Mater. 2015;51:61–73.

Yao Q, Wei B, Guo Y, et al. Design, construction and mechanical testing of digital 3D anatomical data-based PCL–HA bone tissue engineering scaffold. J Mater Sci Mater Med. 2015;26(1):51.

Yeni YN, Brown CU, Wang Z, et al. The influence of bone morphology on fracture toughness of the human femur and tibia. Bone. 1997;21(5):453–9. https://doi.org/10.1016/s8756-3282(97)00173-7.

Yu GS, Li ZB, Li SJ, et al. The select of internal architecture for porous Ti alloy scaffold: a compromise between mechanical properties and permeability. Mater Des. 2020;192:108754. https://doi.org/10.1016/j.matdes.2020.108754.

Yu D, Wu S, Zhao J, et al. Exploration and clinical application of 3D printed personalized titanium alloy for bone repair prosthesis. Meta World. 2022;(4):55–67.

Zhang YG, Habibovic P. Delivering mechanical stimulation to cells: state of the art in materials and devices design. Adv Mater. 2022;34(32):2110267.

Zhang Z-h, Luo F, Zhang J-s, et al. Study on properties of freeze-dried iliac crest bone allografts scaffold material. Acta Acad Med Mil Tertiae. 2009;31(11):1069–72.

Zhang Y, Wang P, Jin JY, et al. In silico and in vivo studies of the effect of surface curvature on the osteoconduction of porous scaffolds. Biotechnol Bioeng. 2022;119(2):591–604.

Zhao YN, Fan JJ, Li ZQ, et al. Effects of pore size on the osteoconductivity and mechanical properties of calcium phosphate cement in a rabbit model. Artif Organs. 2017;41(2):199–204. https://doi.org/10.1111/aor.12742.

Zheng J, Zhao H, Dong E, et al. Additively-manufactured PEEK/HA porous scaffolds with highly-controllable mechanical properties and excellent biocompatibility. Mater Sci Eng C-Mater Biol Appl. 2021;128:112333. https://doi.org/10.1016/j.msec.2021.112333.

Zhu WM, Xiao JD, Wang DP, et al. Experimental study of nano-HA artificial bone with different pore sizes for repairing the radial defect. Int Orthop. 2009;33(2):567–71. https://doi.org/10.1007/s00264-008-0572-5.

Production and Quality Control of 3D-Printed Custom-Made Prostheses

3

Jingjing Wang and Suhua Wu

3.1 Production of 3D-Printed Custom Prostheses

3.1.1 3D Printing Process Used in the Production of Custom Prostheses

3D printing, also known as additive manufacturing, is an emerging manufacturing technology that produces solid objects through layer-by-layer deposition. There are numerous types of 3D printing processes based on different layering and deposition methods. However, only a few 3D printing processes are currently directly applicable to the production of custom orthopedic implants. This is primarily due to the specific requirements of orthopedic implants in terms of manufacturing processes and materials.

First, custom orthopedic implants are primarily used to repair bone defects, requiring the implants to have mechanical properties that match the bone defect area. This must be considered when selecting the fabrication process and materials. Second, since most orthopedic implants are permanently implanted in the body, the selected implant materials must exhibit excellent biocompatibility. It is also important to avoid introducing additives, solvents, or auxiliary materials with high biological safety risks during the process of implant fabrication. Last, there is a high demand for a short timeline for fabricating custom implants. Prolonged fabrication periods may result in changes in the extent of tumor invasion, delaying the optimal treatment window and rendering the original surgical plan and implant design unsuitable.

The personnel who are involved in the design and production of 3D-printed custom implants should comprehensively consider factors such as the site of implant

J. Wang · S. Wu (✉)
Wedo (Xian) Bio-Medical Technology Co., Ltd, Xi'an, China
e-mail: wedo-clinical@wedo-bio.com

Z. Guo et al. (eds.), *3D-Printed Prosthesis in Orthopedic Oncology*,
https://doi.org/10.1007/978-981-95-1454-0_3

use, the expected function, and the specific development of the patient's condition to select the most suitable 3D printing process.

Currently, there are three main types of 3D printing processes that are used in the preparation of custom orthopedic implants. The first type is powder bed-based fabrication technologies, including selective laser melting (SLM), selective laser sintering (SLS), and electron beam melting (EBM). The second type is material extrusion technologies, including fused deposition modeling (FDM) and direct ink writing (DIW). The third type is photopolymerization-based technologies, including stereolithography apparatus (SLA) and digital light processing (DLP).

3.1.1.1 Powder Bed-Based Fabrication Technology

Metal materials such as titanium and tantalum have excellent mechanical properties, corrosion resistance, and biocompatibility and are currently the materials that are most commonly used for custom orthopedic prostheses. The mainstream 3D printing processes that are used for these metal materials include powder bed-based forming technologies, such as selective laser melting (SLM) and electron beam melting (EBM). The two forming principles are basically the same: first, a thin layer of metal powder is spread on the platform by a squeegee or a powder roller, and then, a high-energy laser beam or electron beam selectively melts the powder according to the cross-sectional model design. Once the solid layer has formed, the platform is lowered by one layer of thickness, the squeegee or powder roller spreads another layer of metal powder on top of the current layer, and the high-energy laser beam or electron beam selectively melts the powder with the data information of the next layer until the entire layer is manufactured (Fig. 3.1).

There are a few main differences between SLM and EBM. (1) The energy sources that are used are different. SLM uses a laser, while EBM uses an electron beam. Metal materials reflect laser light to different degrees, so the energy utilization of SLM is lower than that of EBM. The high energy utilization rate of EBM makes this approach more suitable for the manufacture of high thermal conductivity metals, superalloys, and refractory metal parts. (2) The printing accuracy is different. When preparing parts with the same specifications, the printing accuracy of SLM was better than that of EBM. Printing accuracy is determined by various factors, among which the size of the light spot or beam spot has a more significant impact. The

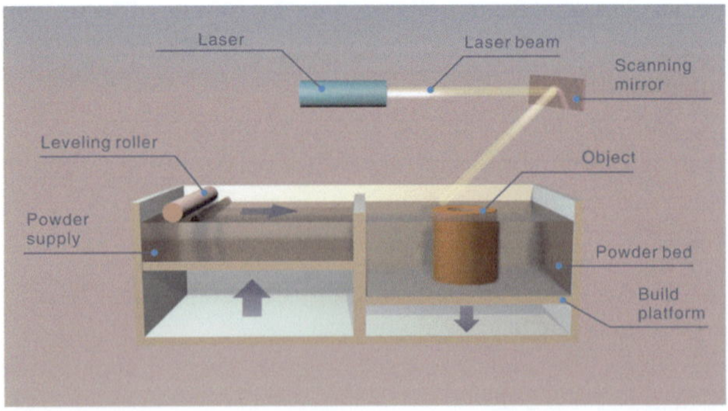

Fig. 3.1 Schematic diagram of the basic principle of laser powder bed fusion forming technology

diameter of the laser spot in typical SLM equipment can reach 60–80 μm, while the diameter of the electron beam spot in EBM equipment is 140–160 μm. A smaller spot diameter is conducive to the formation of fine features (such as microporous structures with pore sizes less than 400 μm) and a smoother surface. The average surface roughness of the parts prepared by the typical SLM process is Ra 9~12 μm, while the surface roughness of the parts prepared by the EBM process can reach Ra 25~35 μm. A greater surface roughness means that more machining allowances need to be left in the design, which will cause more difficulty in processing complex structures (Fig. 3.2). (3) The forming environment is different. The SLM forming chamber generally includes an inert gas environment (argon or nitrogen), while the EBM forming chamber consists of a high-vacuum environment. A high-vacuum chamber means higher equipment and maintenance costs. The use of inert gas can reduce the cost of 3D printing equipment, but the long-term cost of inert gas and the risk of gas leakage should not be ignored. (4) The postbuild treatment processes are different. During SLM, the powder is generally not preheated or is preheated only to 200–300 °C. After the laser melts the powder, the molten pool quickly transfers heat away and causes rapid cooling, and stress concentration likely occurs inside the parts. Therefore, SLM-processed parts generally require annealing treatment to relieve internal residual stresses. EBM technology uses an electron beam to scan and preheat each layer of metal powder so that the part can be processed and formed in the range of 600~1200 °C, which can greatly reduce the residual stress in the formed part. Therefore, parts formed by EBM generally no longer undergo heat treatment. (5) The demand for support is different. Due to the stronger support capability of the powder bed in the EBM process, the EBM process not only requires fewer support structures during printing but also allows for the stacking of parts in the printing direction, resulting in a greater quantity of parts being formed in one print compared to the SLM process.

Selective laser sintering (SLS) operates on the same basic principle as SLM, with the key difference being that SLS does not directly melt the powder to form a molten pool; instead, it sinters the powder particles together. One of the primary

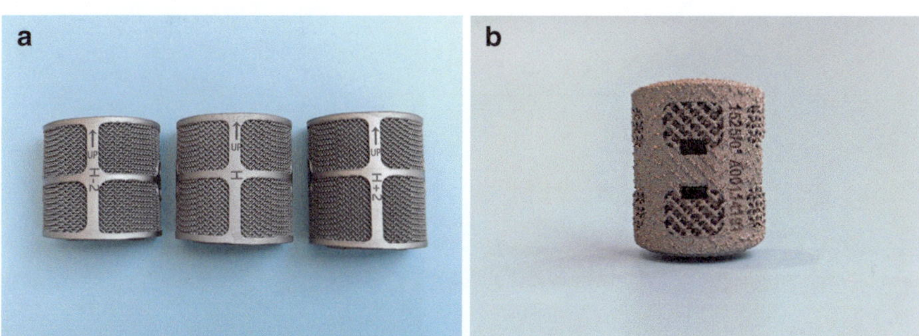

Fig. 3.2 (**a**) Titanium alloy artificial vertebral body printed by SLM; (**b**) titanium alloy artificial vertebral body printed by EBM

applications of SLS in the field of customized orthopedic implants is the production of bone defect repair implants using polyether ether ketone (PEEK) materials, such as cranial and maxillofacial repair implants (Fig. 3.3a). Compared to traditional injection molding and machining methods, SLS offers greater material utilization, and during the printing process, it can utilize powder for support, thus eliminating the need for most additional support structures, which is highly advantageous when printing complex structures (Fig. 3.3b).

Another application of SLS in the field of customized orthopedic implants is the 3D printing of bioceramic materials. However, due to the high-melting-point of ceramics, it is necessary to coat the ceramic powder particles with a layer of low-melting-point organic binder or to uniformly mix ceramic powder with a low-melting-point organic binder powder. During the printing process, the low-melting-point binder melts and binds the high-melting-point ceramic powder particles together to form a green body. Subsequently, the organic binder is removed through a debinding process, and the ceramic particles are sintered at high temperatures to form the final product. The two main issues with ceramic SLS are the high shrinkage and high porosity of the final workpiece, which can affect the appearance and mechanical properties of the final product. Currently, SLS is mostly used for printing tissue engineering scaffolds or for generating bioceramic bone defect fillers with less stringent mechanical requirements, such as hydroxyapatite tricalcium phosphate (HA-TCP) materials (Gao et al. 2013) and hydroxyapatite phosphate glass (Lorrison et al. 2005).

3.1.1.2 Material Extrusion Technology

The typical technology for material extrusion is fused deposition modeling (FDM), which uses filamentous thermoplastic materials as raw materials. The filament is first heated to a semimolten state within the extrusion head. Under computer control, the extrusion head moves along the contours and fills the trajectories of the

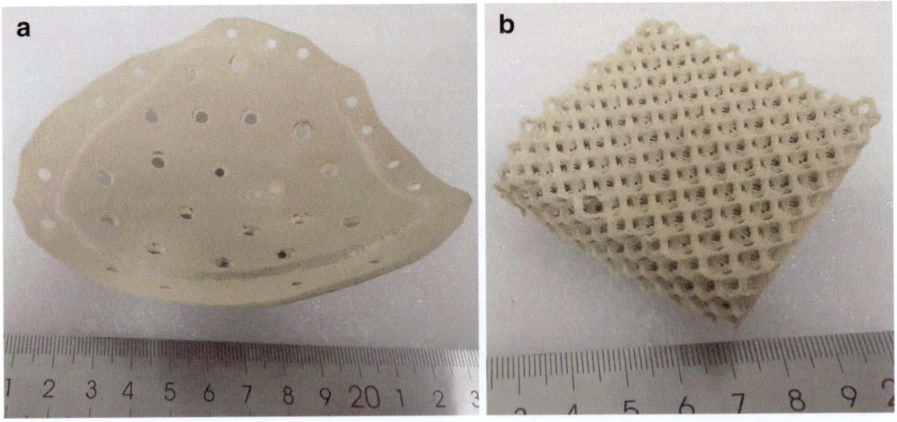

Fig. 3.3 (**a**) PEEK skull repair prosthesis printed by the SLS process; (**b**) PEEK porous structure printed by the SLS process

workpiece profile, continuously extruding the semimolten filament. As the material is extruded, it rapidly solidifies and bonds with the surrounding material due to a decrease in temperature. Once a layer is formed, the build platform descends by a layer thickness, and the process is repeated to form new layers until the entire workpiece is complete (Fig. 3.4). Due to its simple structure and low usage and maintenance costs, FDM has become one of the most widely used 3D printing technologies.

In bone tumor resection and reconstruction surgery, FDM is commonly used to print bone models or surgical guides made of polylactic acid (PLA) or nylon materials to assist in surgical planning or precise tumor resection. In custom implant manufacturing, FDM is mainly used to print bone repair and reconstruction implants made of PEEK material (Fig. 3.5). Compared to SLS technology, the use of FDM to manufacture PEEK implants results in greater material utilization and lower manufacturing costs. Additionally, FDM can control the crystallinity of PEEK components, providing better toughness and fatigue resistance. On the other hand, SLS is better for printing more complex microporous structures with better surface quality and without step-like layering. However, both methods have issues of warping and decreased mechanical performance when printing large-sized PEEK components, which is a major limitation for further clinical applications.

FDM is also used to print composite materials consisting of thermoplastic polymers and bioceramics, such as PEEK-HA and PCL-TCP (Wu et al. 2023). Implants that are printed from these composite materials have good biocompatibility and

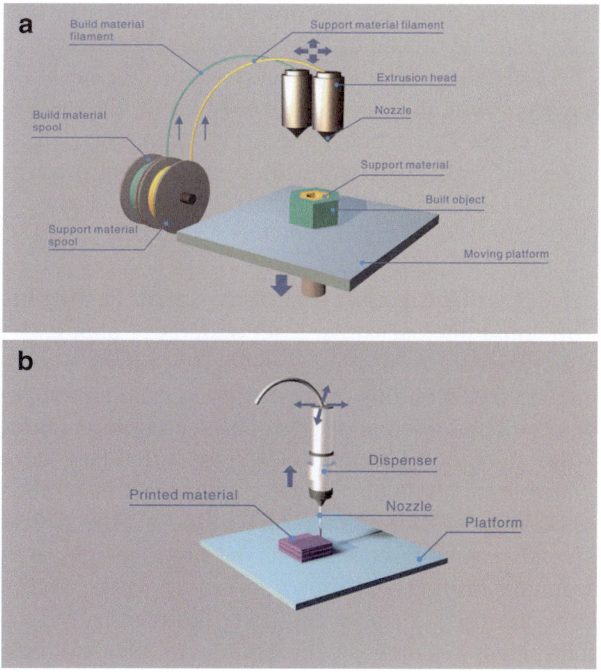

Fig. 3.4 Schematic diagrams of the FDM and direct ink writing technologies (**a**) Fused Deposition Modeling (FDM) (**b**) Direct Ink Writing (DIW)

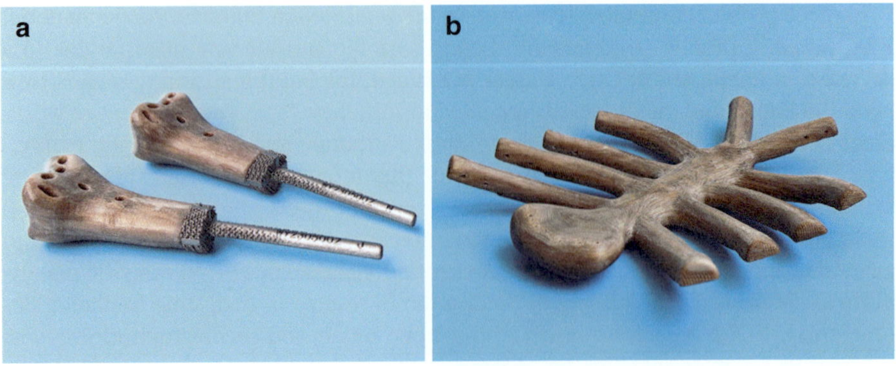

Fig. 3.5 (**a**) Prosthesis of the distal end of the radius printed by the FDM process; The connection between the prosthesis and the radial shaft was the porous titanium intramedullary fixation device printed by SLM; (**b**) sternal rib repair prosthesis with low-crystallinity printed by the FDM process

good mechanical properties, and some can gradually degrade and be completely replaced by bone tissue after implantation, showing promise for large bone defect repair and reconstruction. However, long-term follow-up results for clinical applications are currently lacking. For a more detailed discussion of 3D printing composite materials, please refer to Chap. 11 of this book.

Another representative material extrusion technology is direct ink writing (DIW), which is also known as robocasting. Its advantage lies in the wide range of printable materials, such as conductive gels, elastomers, and hydrogels. DIW is mainly used for printing tissue engineering scaffolds and can facilitate the printing of living cells, which is crucial for the repair and reconstruction of bone and cartilage tissues. This technology achieves direct movement in the *X*–*Y* and *Z* directions by connecting the nozzle directly to the robotic arm, thus not requiring a platform that can move in the *Z* direction, as in FDM technology. The technique involves extruding semisolid "ink" materials with shear-thinning properties from the printing nozzle and laying the "ink" to construct a predesigned three-dimensional structure (Fig. 3.4).

3.1.1.3 Photopolymerization-Based Technology

The liquid photosensitive resin undergoes photopolymerization to become solid after exposure to specific wavelengths of light. The layer-by-layer manufacturing method based on this phenomenon is called photopolymerization molding technology. The principle of photopolymerization molding technology was first proposed by Hideo Kodama in 1981. Charles Hull developed the first commercial system based on the principle of photopolymerization molding in 1984, and this technology is referred to as stereolithography apparatus (SLA). SLA technology uses ultraviolet laser beams as the forming light source, which are controlled by scanning mirrors and move according to the sectional data of the workpiece, either on the surface of the liquid photosensitive resin (Fig. 3.6a) or through a transparent window on the bottom of the photosensitive resin (Fig. 3.6b), to

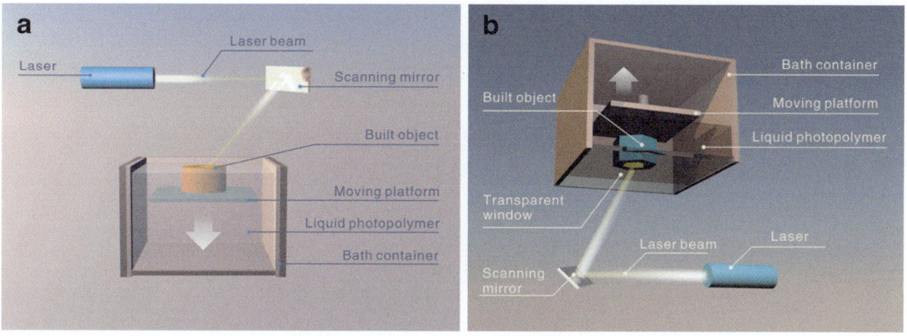

Fig. 3.6 Schematic diagram of the principle of photocuring technology (**a**) Laser beam scanning layer-by-layer on the upper surface of the photosensitive resin (b) Laser beam scanning layer-by-layer on the bottom surface of the photosensitive resin through a transparent window

achieve line-by-line scanning. The thin layer of resin in the scanning area undergoes a polymerization reaction to solidify and form a thin layer of the workpiece. The worktable then moves up or down by a layer thickness to cover the previously solidified resin surface with a new layer of liquid resin. This process is repeated until the entire workpiece is stacked, resulting in a complete three-dimensional workpiece. SLA uses a laser as the forming light source, providing high forming accuracy with a resolution of 25–100 μm.

Digital light processing (DLP) is another photopolymerization technology. The raw materials and forming accuracy of DLP are similar to those of SLA. The difference is that DLP can project the entire layer onto the photosensitive resin at a time using a special digital micromirror device (DMD). Therefore, DLP is faster than SLA. However, due to the resolution of the DMD, compared to SLA technology, DLP can only print products with smaller *X*–*Y* plane areas. Currently, commercial SLA equipment can form workpieces with a maximum *X*–*Y* plane area of more than 1000 mm, but DLP equipment of the same level (referring to similar forming accuracy and equipment price) can only form workpieces with a maximum *X*–*Y* plane area of approximately 1/5 to 1/3 the area that is achievable by SLA.

In 2015, a team led by Professor DeSimone developed an improved DLP technology called continuous liquid interface printing (CLIP). The basic forming principle of CLIP technology is the same as that of DLP technology, with the difference being that, in addition to allowing ultraviolet light to pass through, the transparent window at the bottom of the liquid resin also allows oxygen to pass through. By controlling the amount of oxygen passing through, a region of approximately 20–30 μm thick resin near the transparent window cannot undergo photopolymerization, forming a "dead zone." The photosensitive resin in the dead zone maintains a stable liquid state, preventing the cured workpiece from adhering to the bottom transparent window (Fig. 3.7). This not only greatly reduces the risk of workpiece detachment but also allows for continuous upward movement of the platform, greatly improving printing efficiency. According to the literature, when the *z*-axis resolution is less than 100 μm, the maximum printing speed can reach 30 cm/h. For low-resolution object printing, the speed can exceed 100 cm/h.

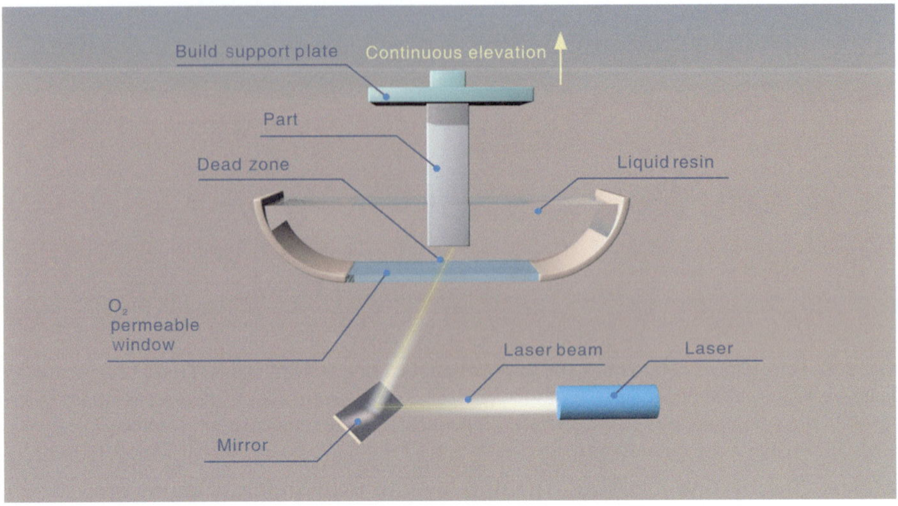

Fig. 3.7 Schematic diagram of continuous liquid interface printing (CLIP)

The main material that is used in photopolymerization molding technology is photosensitive resin, which is not suitable for long-term implantation in the body. Therefore, early photopolymerization molding technology has been mainly used to print orthopedic models and surgical guides to assist in surgical planning and precise surgical procedures. However, in recent years, photopolymerization technology has emerged as a very promising option for printing bioceramic implants that are suitable for long-term implantation.

To print bioceramics, a certain volume fraction of ceramic particles needs to be added to the photosensitive resin, and under the action of surfactants and other additives, a uniformly dispersed and stable ceramic suspension is formed. After the photosensitive resin is cured, the ceramic powder is bonded together to form a green body, which is then sintered at high temperatures. The ceramic powder is bonded together through the diffusion of molecules at high temperatures to form the final workpiece, while the photosensitive resin and other additive agents are removed during the sintering process. Based on the DLP process, it is possible to manufacture alumina and zirconia structural components with Vickers hardnesses exceeding 13 GPa and densities ranging from 97% to 99% (He et al. 2018; Zhou et al. 2016), comparable to those of components made by traditional methods. Alumina and zirconia are the main materials that are used for manufacturing joint friction components (such as hip joint ceramic heads and ceramic liners). This means that in the future, it may be possible to directly prepare a complete set of customized joint replacement prostheses through 3D printing processes. DLP can also be used to print porous and biologically active artificial bone implants, such as porous hydroxyapatite artificial bones (Xue et al. 2024) and β-tricalcium phosphate artificial bones (Liu et al. 2021), which are expected to be used for the structural repair of bone defects (Fig. 3.8).

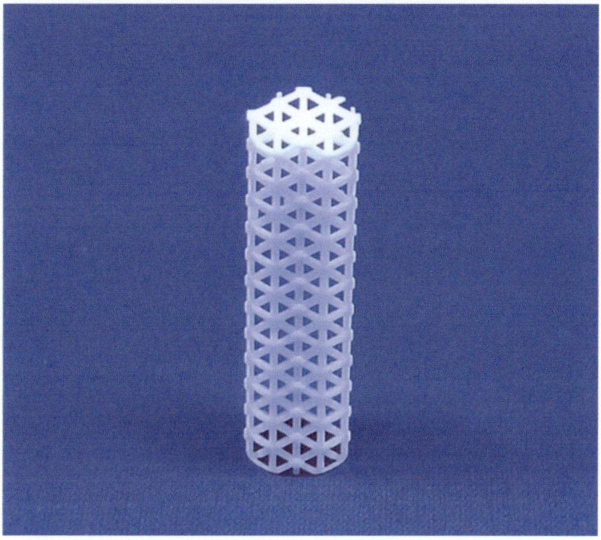

Fig. 3.8 Artificial hydroxyapatite bone with a porous structure printed by the DLP process

3.1.2 Postprocessing Techniques for 3D-Printed Custom Prostheses

The postprocessing procedures for implants made from different materials or using different techniques vary. The typical postprocessing procedure for 3D-printed implants is shown in Fig. 3.9.

3.1.2.1 Removing Residual Powder

Metal implants that are printed using SLM or EBM processes, as well as polymer material implants that are printed using SLS processes, may have residual free powder on their surfaces, internal channels, or porous structures. These powders are not chemically bonded to the printed product but instead remain on the product through physical locking. During the subsequent processing of these implants, the residual powder may affect product quality. Moreover, residual powder can enter the bodies of processing personnel through the respiratory system and mucous membranes, leading to acute or chronic respiratory or mucosal diseases. Therefore, regardless of product quality control or occupational health considerations, it is necessary to thoroughly remove residual free powder from 3D-printed implants.

Common cleaning methods currently used include vibration powder removal, gas blowing, and ultrasonic cleaning. Vibration powder removal involves fixing the parts along with the substrate on a vibrating table, using high-frequency vibration and positional changes to remove the powder, and this process is generally suitable for the initial removal of powder from large parts (Fig. 3.10). For smaller parts, residual powder can also be removed by tapping the substrate. Gas blowing typically refers to the use of high-pressure gas (such as compressed air, nitrogen, or argon) to blow away the powder on the surface and in the cavities of the parts.

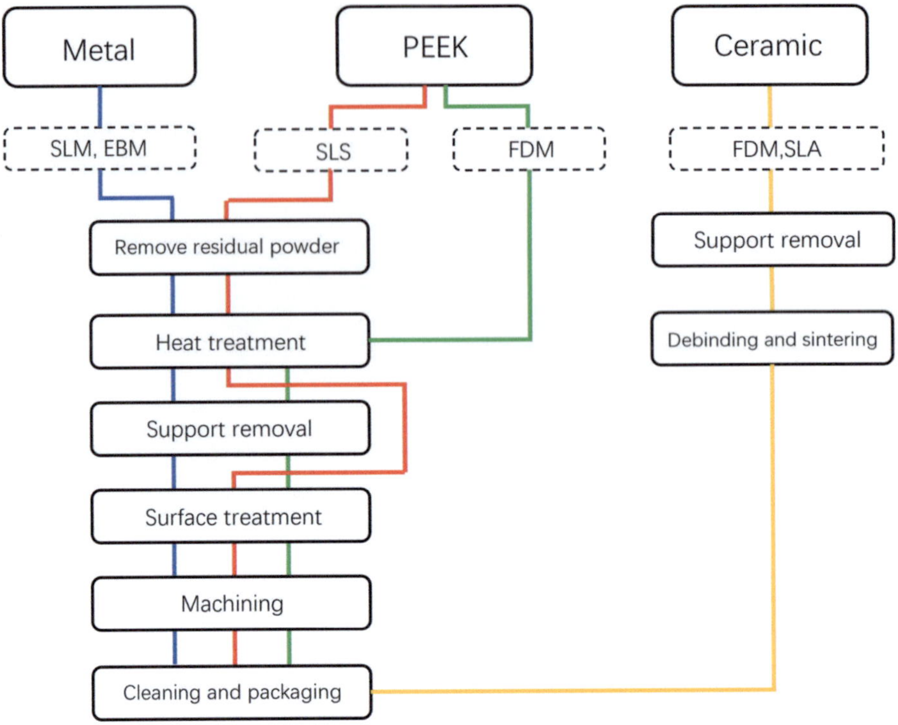

Fig. 3.9 General postprocessing pipeline for 3D-printed prostheses

Vibration powder removal or gas blowing is suitable for the initial removal of the powder, and the cleaned powder can be recycled through a vacuum material recovery system. It is important to note that both vibration and high-pressure gas blowing can easily cause a large amount of powder to float in space, so operations generally require a closed space to achieve complete isolation between personnel and powder. The removal of flammable and explosive metal powders (such as aluminum alloy powder and titanium alloy powder) should be carried out under inert gas protection. After the initial removal of powder, the implants also need to undergo ultrasonic cleaning, and the frequency, number of cleaning cycles, power, and cleaning time should be determined based on the structural characteristics of different implants.

3.1.2.2 Heat Treatment

Heat treatment is an indispensable postprocessing step in various 3D printing processes, but the parameters and purposes of heat treatment vary for different materials and different 3D printing processes.

(a) Heat Treatment for Titanium Alloy Prostheses

During SLM, the solid titanium powder is irradiated by a laser beam and rapidly melts into a liquid alloy, followed by quick cooling and solidification, which results in the formation of a fine needle-like martensitic structure inside the

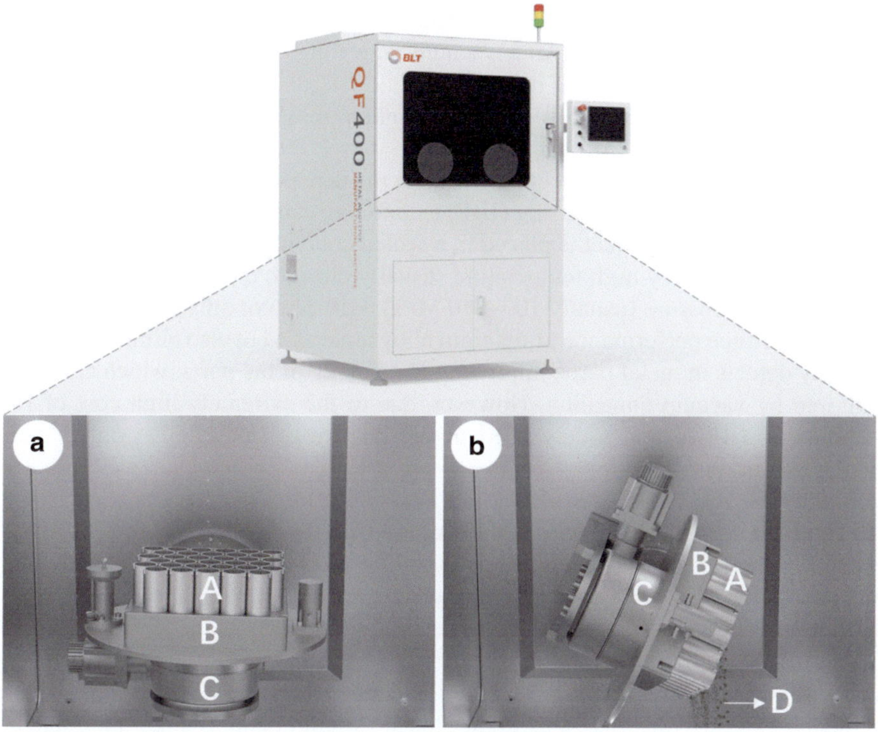

Fig. 3.10 Equipment and principle of rotary vibration powder cleaning; During powder removal, part (A) was fixed together with the substrate (B) on the vibrating table (C), and the residual powder in the part was removed by vibration and rotation (D) The powder removal process was performed under the protection of inert gas

titanium alloy. This microstructure increases the tensile strength of titanium alloys compared with that of traditionally forged titanium alloys but decreases their plasticity and fatigue performance. Therefore, heat treatment is required to improve the plasticity and fatigue performance of these materials. In addition, thermal expansion and contraction during the printing process can result in local internal stresses, which may lead to cracks or warping, and these stresses also need to be eliminated through heat treatment. When EBM is used to print titanium alloy parts, the electron beam rapidly scans the powder layer to preheat it, and the preheating temperature can reach 600–1200 °C. The liquid alloy melted by the electron beam during the printing process is cooled relatively slowly and is not easily stressed internally. Therefore, titanium alloy parts that are printed by EBM generally do not require heat treatment.

The heat treatment method that is commonly used for titanium alloy parts is vacuum annealing. A titanium alloy part is placed in a vacuum furnace, slowly heated to a certain temperature that is maintained for a period of time, and then slowly cooled. Because titanium alloys are prone to oxidation at high temperatures, the vacuum level required for heat treatment is less than 10^{-3} Pa, and the holding temperature is generally approximately 800–850 °C; then, the alloy is cooled in the furnace after heat treatment. After vacuum annealing, the tensile strength of the titanium alloy decreases, while its plasticity and fatigue performance increase, and the surface of the titanium alloy becomes brighter, making vacuum annealing also known as bright annealing.

If there are more stringent requirements for the density or fatigue performance of the implants, hot isostatic pressing (HIP) technology can be used for heat treatment as needed. In HIP, a product is placed in a sealed container filled with inert gas and then subjected to very high temperature (usually close to the forging temperature) and very high pressure (usually 100–140 MPa). HIP can not only improve the plasticity and fatigue performance of titanium alloy materials but also eliminate internal porosity defects in metal parts, improving the density of the parts, which cannot be achieved by vacuum annealing. However, due to the extremely high cost of HIP technology, HIP is not widely used in the heat treatment of 3D-printed metal implants at present.

(b) Heat Treatment of Polyetheretherketone Prostheses

Polyetheretherketone (PEEK) is a semicrystalline thermoplastic material with a certain proportion of crystalline and amorphous regions when the polymer is in a solid state. The amount of the crystalline region can be indicated by its degree of crystallinity. PEEK with low-crystallinity exhibits lower Young's modulus and tensile strength but higher elongation at break and good toughness. Conversely, high-crystallinity PEEK demonstrates higher tensile strength and Young's modulus but lower toughness. The crystallinity of low-crystallinity PEEK implants produced using FDM can be locally or globally enhanced through subsequent heat treatment methods, resulting in differences in crystallinity and mechanical properties in different structural regions of an implant. The heat treatment method that is commonly used involves heating the implants locally or globally to 150–300 °C for a certain duration, followed by rapid cooling, thereby creating implants with more biomimetic mechanical properties (Fig. 3.11).

(c) Debinding and Sintering of Ceramics

Debinding and sintering are specific heat treatment processes that are used for 3D-printed ceramic materials. Unlike metals and polymer materials, ceramic materials do not form direct bonds between the particles when initially printed; instead, these particles are bound together to form a green body by polymeric organic binders such as photosensitive resins. When a green body is heated, the organic materials gradually decompose and eventually oxidize and escape between room temperature and 600 °C; a stage known as debinding, leaving the ceramic particles held together by van der Waals forces in their original form. Subsequently, further heating at high temperatures allows the ceramic particles to fully sinter together, forming a dense ceramic material. Compared with those of a green body, the dimensions of a sintered ceramic part noticeably decrease.

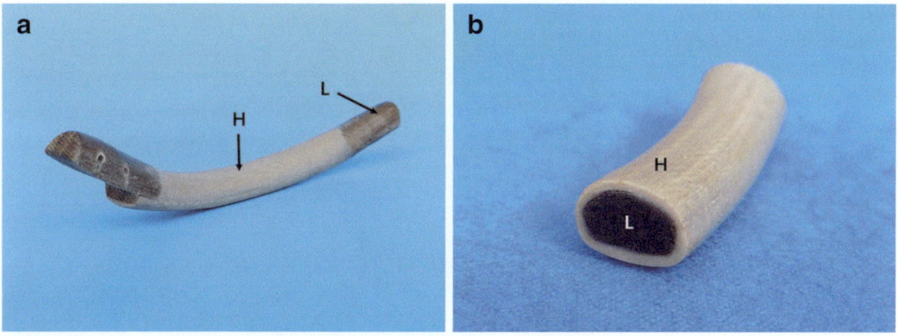

Fig. 3.11 (**a**) Variable modulus rib prosthesis, with the high modulus region in the middle section and the low modulus region in the connection structures at both ends; (**b**) Cross section of a variable modulus rib prosthesis; The simulated cortical bone region in the periphery has a high modulus and high strength, while the inner layer of the simulated cancellous bone region has a low modulus and high toughness H: Highly crystalline and high modulus region, L: Lowly crystalline and low modulus region

3.1.2.3 Support Removal

Due to the limited support capability of a powder bed, the majority of metal parts that are produced by SLM printing include support structures, particularly at the bottom of the parts and surfaces with angles less than 45° to the baseplate (Fig. 3.12). Similarly, in EBM processes, although the powder bed's supporting capability is better than that of SLM, fewer supports are used, but support structures are still necessary at the bottom of the parts, overhanging horizontal surfaces, and areas prone to overheating. These support structures enhance the stability of parts during the printing process, facilitate the timely dissipation of heat that is generated during printing, prevent warping and deformation, and reduce the risk of printing failures.

Upon completion of heat treatment (EBM processes may not require heat treatment), internal stresses within the parts are largely alleviated, allowing for the removal of support structures and the detachment of implants from the baseplate. In the case of SLM processes, parts, along with their supports, are typically detached from the baseplate using wire cutting or other physical cutting methods, followed by the meticulous removal of remaining support structures using appropriate tools such as pliers or pneumatic or electric grinding tools. Due to the complexity of 3D-printed custom implants, support removal is primarily carried out manually, which not only results in low removal efficiency but also poses a risk of damaging the structural integrity of the implants. While a few manufacturing companies are exploring the use of Computer Numerical Control (CNC) machine tools or industrial robotic arms to automatically remove support structures based on 3D models of implants, to improve support removal efficiency and to avoid damage to the implant structure, these methods still face challenges related to high costs, difficulties in clamping, and initial positioning, and these methods have not been widely adopted.

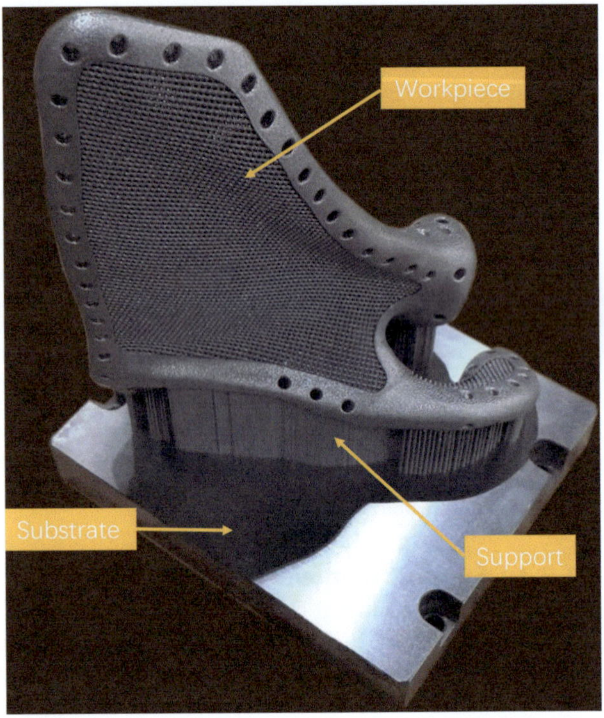

Fig. 3.12 SLM-printed titanium alloy workpiece, support, and substrate

The removal of supports for polymer and ceramic materials is relatively simpler than that for metal materials, and manual removal remains the mainstream approach. Generally, for FDM and photopolymerization processes, complex parts with overhanging structures require more support during printing and are more cumbersome to remove. However, SLS processes, due to the powder bed's ability to provide good support, can achieve support-free printing, thereby avoiding the laborious support removal process.

3.1.2.4 Surface Treatment

(a) Surface Treatment of Titanium Alloy Prostheses

Common surface treatment methods for 3D-printed titanium alloy implants include acid etching, alkali corrosion, sandblasting, abrasive flow machining, and surface coating. During the 3D printing process, metal is melted by a laser or electron beam, forming a molten pool that bonds metal powder particles to the surface. These metal powder particles form a metallurgical bond with the implant surface, making them difficult to remove through simple vibration or ultrasonic cleaning methods. Sandblasting can be used to remove metal powder particles that are partially melted to the external surface, while for internal channel surfaces, sandblasting may not be effective. In such cases, abrasive flow machining can be considered for the removal of these powder particles. For microporous structures with pore sizes in the hundred-micrometer range, acid etching can be used to remove powder particles that are partially melted to internal surfaces. It is important to note that due to the high hydrogen absorption of titanium alloys, which leads to hydrogen embrittlement, an appropriate process should be employed after acid etching to ensure that the hydrogen mass fraction in the titanium alloy remains below 0.008%.

The main components of the commonly used medical titanium alloy (TC4) are titanium, aluminum, and vanadium, with aluminum being relatively active and prone to leaching, resulting in a certain level of toxicity to the human body. Implants with a significant amount of porous structures increase the risk of aluminum ion leaching due to their larger surface area. Research indicates that applying a pure tantalum coating to the inside and outside surfaces of an implant via a vapor deposition method can, to some extent, reduce the risk of ion leaching and enhance the biocompatibility of the implant (Li et al. 2013).

Alkali corrosion can introduce hydroxyl groups on the surface of titanium alloys, promoting the natural formation of nanosized hydroxyapatite layers in bodily fluid environments (Heinl et al. 2008), thereby improving their biological performance. Additionally, hydroxyapatite coatings can be directly prepared on titanium alloy surfaces through processes such as vacuum plasma spraying (Huang et al. 2015), enhancing the osseointegration performance of implants (Fig. 3.13).

(b) Surface Treatment of PEEK Prostheses

PEEK itself is an inert and highly hydrophobic material, resulting in poor osseointegration performance. Various surface treatment techniques have been used to modify the surface of PEEK to enhance its osseointegration performance; these techniques include physical surface modification and coating techniques, including sandblasting, surface etching to increase surface roughness, and plasma spraying to prepare coatings such as titanium (Walsh et al. 2015), titanium oxide, or hydroxyapatite (Sargin et al. 2021). However, these processes are not entirely suitable for 3D-printed PEEK implants with complex structures, especially those with microporous structures. Chemical modification of PEEK surfaces, such as introducing

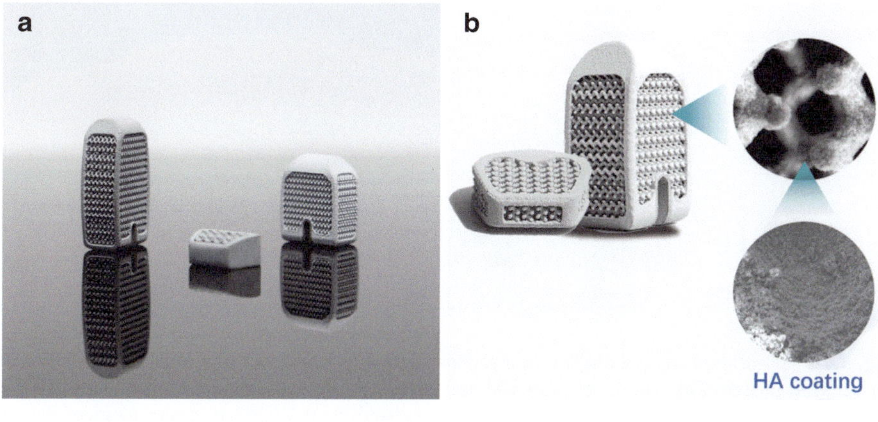

Fig. 3.13 Porous titanium alloy intervertebral fusion cage with an HA coating

hydrophilic groups through sulfonation, has been explored to improve its hydrophilicity and enhance cell adhesion (Su et al. 2020). Surface biofunctionalization, involving the introduction of highly adhesive polydopamine (PDA) on the surface of PEEK materials, followed by the attachment of functional groups such as peptides (Meng et al. 2020), antibiotics (Sun et al. 2021), or biologically active metal ions (Wei et al. 2023), has also been considered for complex porous structures. For more discussion on the surface treatment of prostheses, refer to Chap. 12.

3.1.2.5 Machining

Due to limitations in the precision and surface quality of the 3D printing process, it is not possible to directly fabricate structures on implants that require precise assembly, such as intricate threaded structures or Morse taper structures. Additionally, it is not feasible to directly create smooth friction surfaces on implants. Therefore, for certain implants, specific mechanical processing after 3D printing is required to obtain the final product. Common mechanical processing methods include tapping, polishing, and milling (Fig. 3.14). The primary challenge in postprinting mechanical processing is precise positioning, which should be thoroughly considered during the implant design phase.

3.1.2.6 Cleaning and Packaging

Before the use of implants, strict cleaning is required to remove various processing aids that are introduced during the aforementioned manufacturing processes, such as cutting fluids, machine oils, acid or alkali residues, metal debris, and other contaminants.

The cleaning of medical implants typically involves the use of purified water or ethanol as cleaning agents, employing a combination of rinsing and ultrasonic cleaning. Cleaning parameters that are tailored to each implant's characteristics, including cleaning agents, rinsing water pressure, ultrasonic frequency, power, cleaning time, and number of cycles, need to be established. If special contaminants

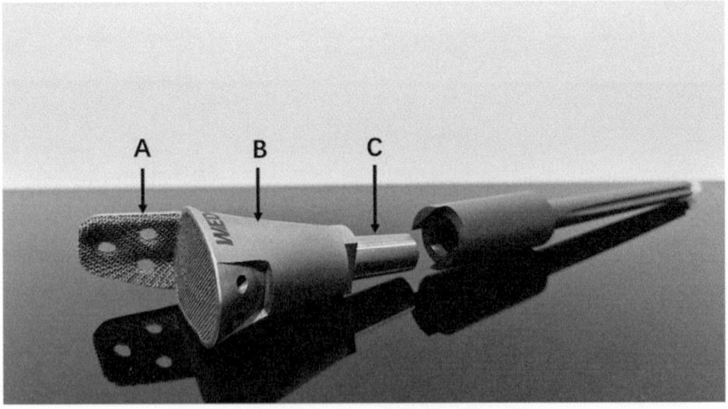

Fig. 3.14 3D-printed custom distal femur reconstruction prosthesis The prosthesis was prepared by the SLM process The porous structure (A) and the surface (B) were sandblasted, and the assembled connection structure (C) was secondarily processed by the CNC machine to meet the fit accuracy requirements

are introduced during implant production, suitable alternative cleaning agents (such as organic solvents) and detergents (generally surfactants and enzymes) should be chosen based on the characteristics of the contaminants, ensuring that the residual levels of cleaning agents and detergents on the final product meet the requirements for biocompatibility.

After cleaning, the efficacy of the cleaning process should be verified. The structure and manufacturing process used for each custom prosthesis differ, impacting the cleanliness of the implants. However, it is difficult to verify the cleanliness of each implant during actual production. Therefore, the concept of a "cleaning family" should be introduced during verification. A cleaning family refers to a series of implants that undergo similar or identical cleaning processes. By verifying the cleanliness of the most challenging implants within the cleaning family (worst-case specimens), the suitability of the cleaning process for all implants within the same cleaning family can be ensured. Methods for assessing implant cleanliness during cleaning verification include measuring the electrical conductivity and pH of the final rinse water, measuring insoluble particles, and measuring residual total hydrocarbon and total organic carbon. For more information on cleaning verification, refer to ISO 19227: General Requirements for Cleanliness of Orthopedic Implants.

After cleaning, implants should be appropriately packaged to meet the implant protection requirements during transportation and temporary storage. For implant-grade products, it is recommended to perform final rinsing and inner packaging of implants in a clean environment with a cleanliness level of at least 100,000.

3.1.3 Sterilization of Custom-Made Prostheses

Sterilization refers to the use of physical or chemical methods to permanently eliminate the ability of all microorganisms in a product to grow and reproduce. Microorganisms include both pathogenic and nonpathogenic microorganisms, as well as bacterial spores and fungal spores. After the sterilization process, the probability of individual viable microorganisms remaining on the implant is referred to as the sterility assurance level (SAL). The typical concept of "sterile" indicates an SAL of 10^{-6}, meaning that there may be one viable microorganism per million products. Common methods for sterilizing implantable devices include radiation, ethylene oxide, and high-pressure steam sterilization.

3.1.3.1 Radiation Sterilization

The main principle of radiation sterilization involves the use of high-energy rays such as γ-rays or electron beams to directly or indirectly damage genetic material (DNA or RNA), structural proteins, and enzymes in microorganisms.

The primary indicator for radiation sterilization is the radiation dose, which refers to the total amount of radiation absorbed by a unit mass of material, measured in "gray" (Gy). 1 Gy is defined as the absorption of 1 J of energy per kilogram of material.

The selection of radiation dose is closely related to the types and quantities of microorganisms on the product, as well as the characteristics of the product itself. Different types of microorganisms have varying degrees of resistance to radiation, and the resistance of the same microorganism may vary at different stages of development. Generally, the reproductive and vegetative forms of microorganisms are less resistant to radiation, while spores are more resistant. The resistance of the same strain of microorganism in different media also varies, with stronger resistance inside metal products and weaker resistance inside nonmetal products. Additionally, the tolerance to radiation varies for different types of implants and packaging materials, as excessive doses may lead to decreased material strength, material denaturation, aging of packaging materials, and reduced legibility of labels. Therefore, strict validation and confirmation procedures are required to determine the necessary radiation dose for a specific type of implant.

The advantages of radiation sterilization include strong penetration, high sterilization efficiency, and the absence of chemical residues in the sterilization process. Products can be directly used without the need for additional processes such as drying or aeration. This method is suitable for the sterilization of metal implants, especially those containing a large number of microporous structures, and for the sterilization of certain polymer materials. However, the limitations of radiation sterilization lie in its dependence on radiation sources or specialized equipment, high initial investment, and certain risks associated with operation and maintenance, which often necessitate outsourcing to qualified third parties.

3.1.3.2 Ethylene Oxide Sterilization

Ethylene oxide (EO) has strong penetration potential. The principle of EO sterilization involves interaction with the amino, hydroxyl, and carboxyl groups in microbial protein molecules, enzymes, and nucleic acids, resulting in alkylation. This process causes irreversible damage to the metabolic processes of microbial cells, resulting in sterilization.

When using EO for sterilization, the temperature, humidity, sterilization gas concentration, and sterilization time within the sterilization cabinet are all important parameters that affect sterilization effectiveness. These parameters are interrelated, and any failure to meet the requirements of any parameter can affect the overall sterilization effectiveness. Therefore, strict validation and confirmation procedures are necessary to determine the appropriate sterilization parameters for a specific type of product.

Implants that are sterilized with EO must be packaged in breathable packaging to allow EO to enter and take effect. EO is toxic to the human body, and products that are sterilized with EO should be placed in a ventilated area for aeration. The effects of ventilation and the duration and temperature of aeration on residual EO need to be evaluated with corresponding validation and confirmation procedures.

The advantage of EO sterilization lies in the minimal damage it causes to items, as sterilization occurs through alkylation rather than oxidation. This approach is widely used for heat-sensitive or radiation-unstable materials and equipment. However, this approach is limited to use with breathable packaging and poststerilization, and there is residual EO that requires a designated aeration time. For implants with a significant number of microporous structures, the aeration time may be prolonged, potentially affecting the timely delivery of customized implants.

3.1.3.3 High-Pressure Steam Sterilization

High-pressure steam sterilization involves the use of high-temperature, high-pressure steam to disrupt microbial proteins, enzymes, and nucleic acids, leading to microbial death. This is the most commonly used physical sterilization method in medical institutions.

The temperature, steam pressure, and sterilization time are important parameters that affect the effectiveness of high-pressure steam sterilization. Although classic sterilization parameters are available for general medical devices, rigorously validating and confirming the sterilization effectiveness of 3D-printed customized implants, especially large and complex implants containing a significant number of microporous structures, is recommended to ensure the expected sterilization effectiveness.

The advantage of high-pressure steam sterilization lies in its low cost, simplicity, and reliable sterilization effectiveness. However, its use is limited to materials that are capable of withstanding high-temperature steam. If a manufacturer provides customized implants to medical institutions in a clean form, such implants are typically sterilized using high-pressure steam sterilization at the hospital.

3.2 Quality Control in the Process of Producing 3D-Printed Custom Prostheses

Quality control in the process of producing customized prostheses using 3D printing has always been a focal point. Manufacturers, regulatory authorities, and clinicians hope to have a systematic, efficient, and feasible system to ensure the quality of 3D-printed customized prostheses. However, despite the rapid development of 3D printing technology, there is still no broad consensus on quality control methods for 3D-printed medical implants. This section briefly introduces the quality control of 3D-printed customized prostheses from two perspectives: the key steps in quality control and printing quality assessment methods. It should be noted that this section only lists general quality control methods for 3D-printed customized prostheses. Due to variations in the printing processes and design concepts of prostheses, each type of 3D-printed customized prosthesis has a unique quality control system. Designers and manufacturers should develop appropriate and feasible quality control systems based on factors such as product processes, structural characteristics, intended use, and potential failure risks.

3.2.1 Key Links of Quality Control in the Production Process of Custom Prostheses

3.2.1.1 Quality Control of the Raw Materials

First, it is necessary to establish quality standards and methods for testing raw materials based on relevant national and industry standards combined with actual production requirements. The quality standards for raw materials should include key indicators that are directly related to the performance of the final printed products. For instance, in powder bed fusion processes, the chemical composition, particle size distribution, and flowability of raw materials can significantly impact the performance of the final products. Interstitial solute elements such as oxygen and hydrogen in titanium alloy powders can affect the mechanical properties, such as strength, hardness, and ductility, of the final product. The particle size distribution of powders can influence indicators such as density, dimensional accuracy, and surface quality of the final product. Flowability also plays a crucial role in layer thickness and uniformity, thereby affecting the printing accuracy of the product. Therefore, establishing quality standards for raw materials is essential for controlling printing quality.

Second, for recyclable printing materials, standards for material recycling should be established. After each recycling cycle, the chemical composition and physical properties of the raw materials may undergo slight changes due to the printing process and the surrounding environment. Studies have shown that the chemical composition (such as oxygen content), sphericity, particle size distribution, and flowability of titanium alloy powders can change after multiple recycling cycles. To prevent the cumulative effects of these changes on material performance, it is necessary to thoroughly assess the impact of the printing environment and process on the raw materials and determine the number of times the raw materials can be reused through process validation.

3.2.1.2 Control of the Printing Device

Complete installation, operation, and performance verification of the 3D printing and postprocessing equipment used should be carried out.

The purpose of installation and operation verification is to ensure the quality of the equipment. When developing verification plans, it is recommended to consider the following aspects. First, all components of the equipment must be correctly installed, and any missing or damaged parts, especially critical components that have a significant impact on the safe use of the equipment, such as lasers, cooling pipelines, and filtration systems, must be identified. Second, the facilities supporting the equipment (such as voltage stabilizers, cooling devices, and inert gas supply devices) must meet the requirements and be installed correctly. Third, the equipment must start up and run normally, and attention must be given to any warning messages that may appear during operation. Fourth, the equipment must be tested under extreme conditions during operation, such as the platform's maximum lifting height and precision, the limits of the scraper's left and right positions, and the scanning range and accuracy of the laser. Smooth operation of the equipment must be ensured to meet the requirements of the printing process.

Performance verification of the equipment should focus on the printing accuracy, surface quality, microscopic structure of the printed products, mechanical properties, etc. Due to the anisotropic nature of 3D printing, these parameters need to be tested separately in the *X–Y* and *X–Z* directions to determine if the equipment performance meets the production requirements of the product. Additionally, it is advisable to use appropriate methods to verify the stability of equipment operation to demonstrate that performance parameters, such as printing accuracy, remain stable within the equipment maintenance cycle.

3.2.1.3 Process Control During Printing

In terms of the printing process, it is essential to understand the impact of various printing parameters on product quality. For specific performance requirements and intended use of the product, optimal parameters should be identified and validated. Common parameters in the 3D printing processes that may affect the quality of the final product include product orientation and printing direction, types and positions of supports, and the layer thickness. Additionally, the impacts of unique parameters that are specific to different 3D printing processes on product quality should be considered. For example, for powder bed fusion processes, parameters such as the chamber environment, preheating temperature, scanning paths, scanning speed, and power should be considered. In contrast, for fused deposition modeling processes, parameters such as the nozzle diameter and extrusion temperature should be considered. After process validation, it is crucial to maintain the stability of the printing process during product production and to strictly control the key printing parameters. If key process parameters change, revalidation should be conducted to demonstrate that the performance meets or exceeds the original requirements.

The validation of printing equipment performance, printing process, and product performance is closely intertwined. When developing corresponding plans, comprehensive consideration should be given to avoid redundant validation, enhance validation efficiency, and reduce costs and time.

3.2.1.4 Operator Control

Quality control in printing is closely linked to the knowledge and skill levels of operators. Operators of 3D printing equipment should have relevant professional backgrounds and undergo specialized operational training and assessment. A suitable professional background enables operators to better understand the basic structure and printing principles of the equipment, to promptly identify problems during the printing process, and to take appropriate measures. Specialized training familiarizes operators with the operation of 3D printing equipment (e.g., powder addition, scraper installation and leveling, air washing/vacuuming operations, powder recovery, etc.), provides information about key parameters during the printing process (such as oxygen content, airflow, torque, and filter pressure drop), and ensures an understanding of various equipment warning messages during printing. Operators should be capable of handling common printing faults (e.g., excessive torque and high filter pressure drops). Additionally, safety awareness training is essential, especially when using potentially hazardous materials (such as titanium alloy powders), to address potential safety risks and appropriate responses.

3.2.2 Methods for Evaluating the Print Quality of Custom Prostheses

3.2.2.1 Evaluation of the Overall Structure

For implants that are manufactured using 3D printing processes, the overall structure includes both the macrostructure and microporous structure of the implant. Attention should be focused on whether these structures exhibit deformations or any other defects. Common structural defects include deformations or cracks caused by part stress issues (Fig. 3.15a), lattice distortions in the porous structure due to printing anisotropy (Fig. 3.15b), and structural deformations or defects caused by part placement or support design issues.

The presence of structural defects does not necessarily mean that the product is unusable. The impact of defects on the mechanical and biological performance of the implant should be thoroughly evaluated. For example, deformations in the primary load-bearing structure of the implant may be unacceptable, but currently, there is no evidence to suggest that slight lattice distortions in the porous structure significantly affect its biological properties for bone ingrowth. Designers and manufacturers can establish an acceptable range of deformations based on actual requirements and sufficient experimental data.

Methods for evaluating overall structural quality include visual inspection, optical or electron microscopy, X-ray examination, micro-CT scanning, and ultrasonic probing, which sometimes require surface scan reconstruction methods depending on the situation. Typically, most structural defects can be detected using visual

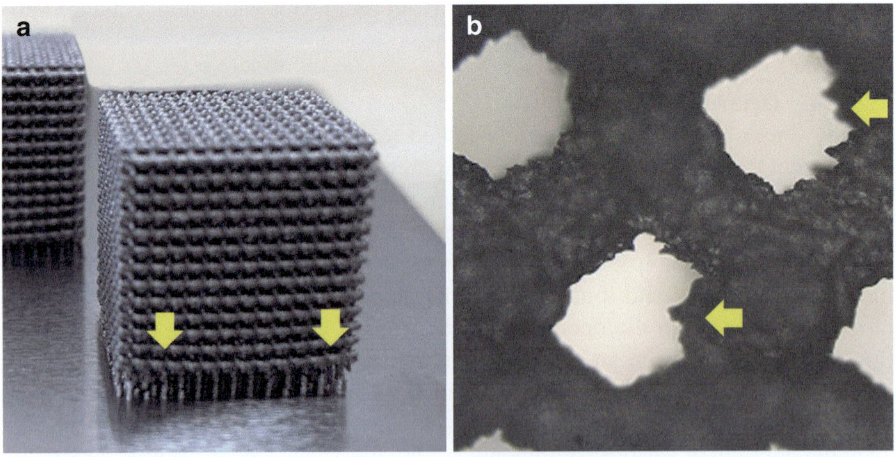

Fig. 3.15 (**a**) Structural deformation caused by stress (**b**) lattice distortion

inspection and microscopy, but for some internal and special structures, as well as porous structures, detection methods such as X-ray or CT scans are necessary.

3.2.2.2 Evaluation of Printing Accuracy

Manufacturers should clearly define the printing accuracy of the equipment that is used in different printing directions, scales, and modes as the basis for evaluating the product's printing accuracy. Assessment of the accuracy of the implant's external structure can involve measuring the geometric dimensions of key areas, while evaluating the accuracy of porous structures requires measuring parameters such as porosity, pore size, and filament diameter. When assessing product printing accuracy, particular attention should be given to potential printing quality issues that are hidden by abnormal changes in printing accuracy. For example, a shift from positive to negative tolerance in a specific dimension of a printed product may indicate material or equipment quality issues that should be promptly investigated and corrected. However, stable and predictable deviations in accuracy during the printing process do not require excessive attention and can typically be corrected through design-time allowances or postprocessing methods.

Common methods for evaluating printing accuracy include general tool measurements, laser measurements, optical or electron microscopy measurements, and sometimes micro-CT scanning to measure the parameters of porous structures.

3.2.2.3 Evaluation of Surface Quality

The evaluation of surface quality generally includes the evaluation of surface defects and the evaluation of surface roughness. Common surface defects include burrs, sharp edges, and dents. In very rare cases, defects such as surface discoloration may occur due to excessive oxygen levels in the build chamber. The occurrence of such defects may mean that the printed products have serious quality problems. The surface of products that are prepared by the powder bed fusion molding process usually consists of a layer of partially melted metal powder particles bonded to the surface. This layer of metal powder particles may obscure the true surface quality of the product, especially the surface quality of the trabecula inside the porous. The quality of the surface often has a major impact on posttreatment processes such as acid etching. Therefore, to better evaluate the surface quality of the porous trabeculae, a cross section of the porous structure can be prepared to observe the surface conditions (Fig. 3.16). When applicable, surface roughness can also be used to evaluate the surface quality of products, but this is not required. In most cases, it is necessary to perform secondary treatment on the implant surface to achieve the desired surface roughness.

Common methods for evaluating surface quality include visual inspection, optical or electron microscopy measurements, and roughness measurements. Similar to printing accuracy, surface quality is closely related to factors such as printing direction and support design, which should be carefully considered during the printing process.

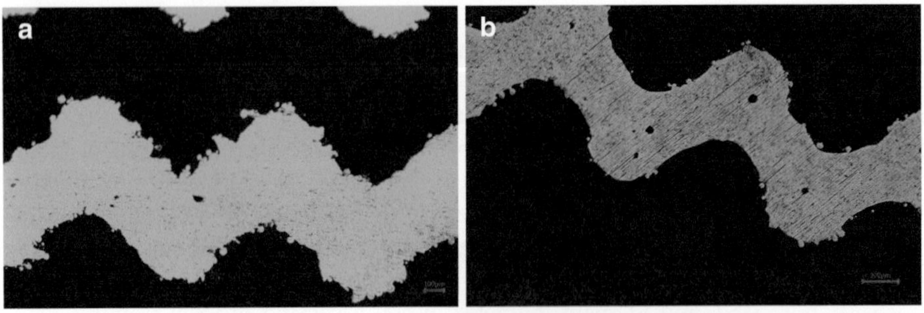

Fig. 3.16 Cross-sections of the trabeculae in the two different SLM printing modes (**a**) There were more burrs on the trabecular surface (**b**) The trabecular surface was smoother

3.2.2.4 Assessment of Internal Quality

The characteristics of the microstructure (metallography) of metal materials are directly related to their preparation process. Different preparation processes typically result in different microstructures, and we can predict their mechanical properties by observing the characteristics of the microstructure. For example, using the selective laser melting (SLM) process to prepare Ti-6Al-4V results in a microstructure that is mainly composed of needle-like martensite (α'), with a small amount of β phase (Fig. 3.17a), and this structure exhibits high hardness and tensile strength but poor ductility. However, after vacuum annealing, a basket-weave structure with interlaced needle-like or lamellar $\alpha + \beta$ phases can be obtained (Fig. 3.17b), leading to a decrease in hardness and tensile strength but a significant increase in ductility compared to martensite. The preparation of Ti-6Al-4V using electron beam melting (EBM) directly yields a basket-weave structure (Murr et al. 2009). Additionally, by observing the microstructure, internal material defects, such as pores, microcracks, delamination, and unmelted powder particles, can be identified, which may affect the material's mechanical or corrosion resistance properties.

Microstructures are typically observed using a metallographic microscope, and sample preparation and observation should adhere to relevant standards, with the recommended standard in China being GB/T 5168. Microstructural analysis is a destructive testing method that can indirectly assess the microstructural characteristics of printed products by testing samples from the same batch.

3.2.2.5 Evaluation of the Chemical Composition

The chemical composition of each batch of raw materials used in the 3D printing process must be tested and approved. Furthermore, the chemical composition of 3D-printed products should also be analyzed to evaluate whether harmful contaminating elements are introduced during the printing process. For instance, for titanium alloy implants, the content of elements such as hydrogen and oxygen in the finished product is typically checked for compliance, as even slight increases in these interstitial solute element concentrations can lead to a decrease in the

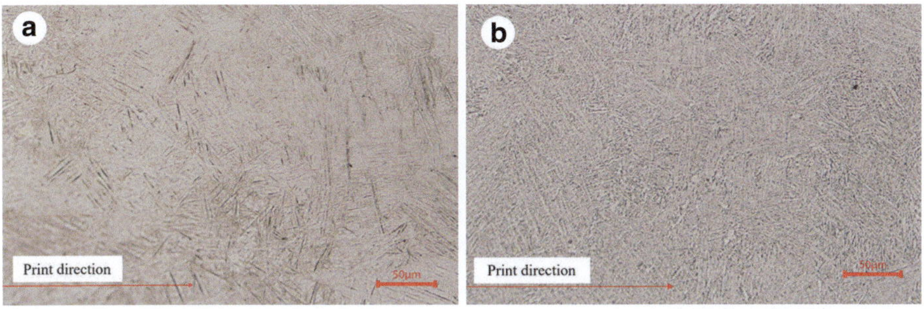

Fig. 3.17 (**a**) Microstructure of Ti-6Al-4V prepared by the SLM printing process mainly composed of needle-like martensite with a small amount of β-phase (**b**) Ti-6Al-4V prepared by the EBM printing process with a needle-like $\alpha + \beta$ interlaced basket microstructure

mechanical properties of the final product. If there is a risk of introducing other harmful elements during the printing process, the contents of these elements in the finished product should also be analyzed. It is important to note that measuring chemical composition is not a routine test for personalized 3D-printed implants but rather a part of the validation process for 3D printing technology.

The methods for measuring the chemical compositions vary depending on the specific elements that are tested. Currently, there are mature testing methods for common elements that can be referenced against relevant national and industry standards.

3.2.2.6 Evaluation of Mechanical Properties

The evaluation of mechanical properties can be divided into material mechanical property evaluation and implant mechanical property evaluation. Indicators that are commonly used for evaluating the mechanical properties of metal materials include strength indicators (tensile strength, yield strength), plasticity indicators (elongation at break, reduction of area), and hardness indicators (Brinell hardness, Rockwell hardness). For porous metal materials, compression strength, elastic modulus, and other evaluation indicators are also commonly used. Material mechanical property evaluation is not specific to a particular 3D-printed implant, but rather, it is an assessment of the 3D printing process itself. Standardized test samples need to be prepared for evaluation, which is often conducted as a part of the validation process for the 3D printing equipment or processes.

The evaluation of the mechanical properties of orthopedic implants is often complex, and in orthopedics, the specific evaluation methods and standards are closely related to the implant's intended site and design type. Implants that are intended for different sites (spines or joints) and different types of implants (fusion or nonfusion) typically require different evaluation methods and standards. Once the intended site and type of personalized 3D-printed orthopedic implant are determined, relevant testing can be carried out in accordance with international, national, and industry standards for similar types of implants.

The evaluation of mechanical properties, particularly for implants, reflects the overall quality of implant preparation. It is closely related to the implant's structure, microstructure, chemical composition, and even surface quality. Mechanical properties are crucial indicators for ensuring that orthopedic implants function as expected within the body, making them a key performance metric for implant quality. However, mechanical property testing is often destructive, making it impractical to conduct mechanical testing on every personalized 3D-printed implant. Instead, systematic mechanical testing can be performed on the worst-case model of implants designed with the same structural type to demonstrate the mechanical performance of that implant category.

References

Gao C, Yang B, Hu H, et al. Enhanced sintering ability of biphasic calcium phosphate by polymers used for bone scaffold fabrication. Mater Sci Eng C Mater Biol Appl. 2013;33(7):3802–10.

He R, Liu W, Wu Z, et al. Fabrication of complex-shaped zirconia ceramic parts via a DLP- stereolithography-based 3D printing method. Ceram Int. 2018;44(3):3412–6.

Heinl P, Muller L, Korner C, et al. Cellular Ti-6Al-4V structures with interconnected macro porosity for bone implants fabricated by selective electron beam melting. Acta Biomater. 2008;4(5):1536–44.

Huang H, Lan P-H, Zhang Y-Q, et al. Surface characterization and in vivo performance of plasma-sprayed hydroxyapatite-coated porous Ti-6Al-4V implants generated by electron beam melting. Surf Coat Technol. 2015;283:80–8.

Li X, Wang L, Yu X, et al. Tantalum coating on porous Ti-6Al-4V scaffold using chemical vapor deposition and preliminary biological evaluation. Mater Sci Eng C Mater Biol Appl. 2013;33(5):2987–94.

Liu S, Mo L, Bi G, et al. DLP 3D printing porous β-tricalcium phosphate scaffold by the use of acrylate/ceramic composite slurry. Ceram Int. 2021;47(15):21108–16.

Lorrison JC, Dalgarno KW, Wood DJ. Processing of an apatite-mullite glass-ceramic and an hydroxyapatite/phosphate glass composite by selective laser sintering. J Mater Sci Mater Med. 2005;16(8):775–81.

Meng X, Zhang J, Chen J, et al. KR-12 coating of polyetheretherketone (PEEK) surface via polydopamine improves osteointegration and antibacterial activity in vivo. J Mater Chem B. 2020;8(44):10190–204.

Murr LE, Quinones SA, Gaytan SM, et al. Microstructure and mechanical behavior of Ti-6Al-4V produced by rapid-layer manufacturing, for biomedical applications. J Mech Behav Biomed Mater. 2009;2(1):20–32.

Sargin F, Erdogan G, Kanbur K, et al. Investigation of in vitro behavior of plasma sprayed Ti, TiO2 and HA coatings on PEEK. Surf Coat Technol. 2021;411:126965.

Su Y, He J, Jiang N, et al. Additively-manufactured poly-ether-ether-ketone (PEEK) lattice scaffolds with uniform microporous architectures for enhanced cellular response and soft tissue adhesion. Mater Des. 2020;191:108671.

Sun A, Lin X, Xue Z, et al. Facile surface functional polyetheretherketone with antibacterial and immunoregulatory activities for enhanced regeneration toward bacterium-infected bone destruction. Drug Deliv. 2021;28(1):1649–63.

Walsh WR, Bertollo N, Christou C, et al. Plasma-sprayed titanium coating to polyetheretherketone improves the bone-implant interface. Spine J. 2015;15(5):1041–9.

Wei X, Zhou W, Tang Z, et al. Magnesium surface-activated 3D printed porous PEEK scaffolds for in vivo osseointegration by promoting angiogenesis and osteogenesis. Bioact Mater. 2023;20:16–28.

Wu H, Wei X, Liu Y, et al. Dynamic degradation patterns of porous polycaprolactone/beta-tricalcium phosphate composites orchestrate macrophage responses and immunoregulatory bone regeneration. Bioact Mater. 2023;21:595–611.

Xue R, Yuan P, Zhao B, et al. DLP printing of BT/HA nanocomposite ceramic scaffolds using low refractive index BT crystals. J Materiomics. 2024;10:1036–48.

Zhou M, Liu W, Wu H, et al. Preparation of a defect-free alumina cutting tool via additive manufacturing based on stereolithography – optimization of the drying and debinding processes. Ceram Int. 2016;42(10):11598–602.

Part II

Clinical Applications of 3D-Printed Custom-Made Prostheses

4 Different Types of 3D-Printed Custom-Made Prostheses

Hai Huang, Jun Fu, Wenwen Liu, and Zheng Guo

4.1 Artificial Vertebral Bodies for Spinal Applications

4.1.1 Advantages of 3D-Printed Artificial Vertebral Body

Spinal vertebral lesions (tumors, trauma, inflammation, deformity, etc.) often require resection of the affected vertebral body and restoration of spinal stability via bone grafting or artificial vertebral body implantation. Artificial vertebral bodies are currently the primary products that are used to restore spinal stability; these products include titanium mesh and adjustable artificial vertebral bodies. For malignant or highly aggressive tumors of the spine, total en bloc spondylectomy (TES) is often required to control the tumor (Fig. 4.1), but this approach is associated with more difficult reconstruction techniques and higher rates of postoperative complications (Tomita et al. 1997, 2006).

Clinical studies have reported that the incidence of titanium mesh subsidence after multivertebral en bloc resection with titanium mesh reconstruction is approximately 90% (Matsumoto et al. 2011; Yoshioka et al. 2013), leading to spinal instability after reconstruction (Fig. 4.2). For some unique parts (such as axis) or in the resection and reconstruction of superlong vertebral segments, it is difficult to achieve effective reconstruction with traditional titanium mesh artificial vertebral bodies.

There are several reasons for the failure of artificial vertebral body reconstruction with titanium mesh: (1) Poor local blood supply affects the healing of the bone graft in the titanium mesh. (2) Destruction of the adjacent vertebral endplate that was implanted during resection results in insufficient interface support. (3) Spinal osteoporosis leads to insufficient support strength of adjacent vertebral bodies. (4) The

H. Huang · J. Fu · W. Liu · Z. Guo (✉)
Department of Orthopedics, Tangdu Hospital, Xi'an, China
e-mail: fmmufujun@263.net; guozheng@fmmu.edu.cn

Z. Guo et al. (eds.), *3D-Printed Prosthesis in Orthopedic Oncology*,
https://doi.org/10.1007/978-981-95-1454-0_4

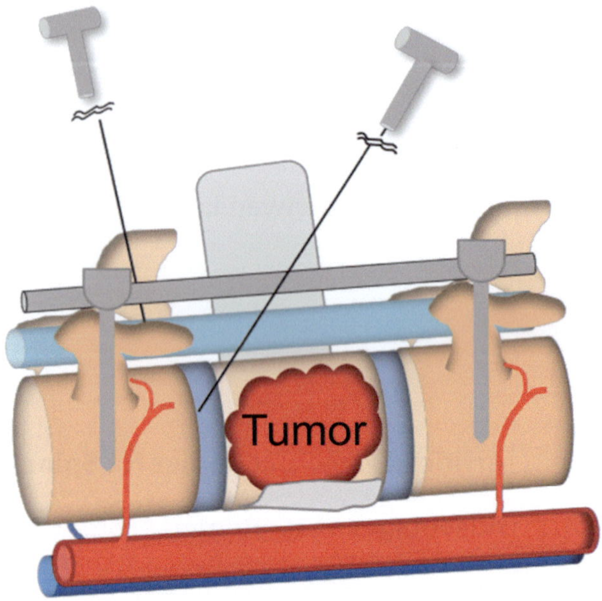

Fig. 4.1 Schematic diagram of posterior total en bloc spondylectomy (TES)

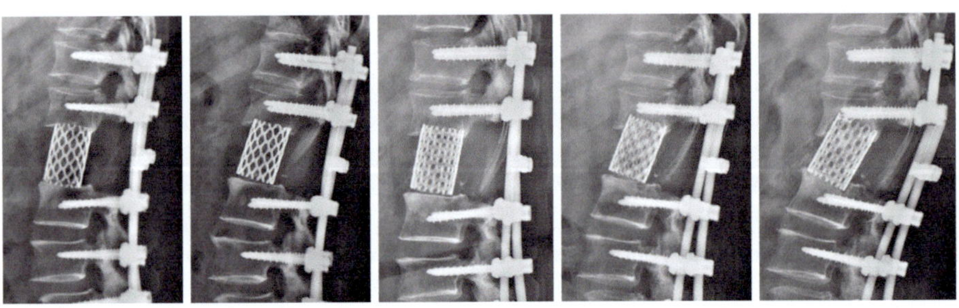

Fig. 4.2 Total vertebral resection of an L1 tumor with titanium mesh combined with bone grafting reconstruction; titanium mesh subsidence occurred with time, and the posterior fixation rod broke

titanium mesh and bone interface cannot form support for osseointegration. (5) The top of the titanium mesh does not match the morphology of the vertebral endplate, and the stress at the serrated interface of the titanium mesh is too concentrated, resulting in stress-induced cutting, which may be the main reason for titanium mesh subsidence.

3D printing can be used to prepare personalized artificial vertebral bodies to meet the different needs of spinal reconstruction. The advantages of this approach are as follows: (1) Vertebral bodies that are prepared with 3D printing are more compatible with the anatomical morphology of the upper and lower vertebral endplates. (2) The interface stress is dispersed, reducing cutting. (3) The porous structure is conducive to bone ingrowth and achieves more lasting biological stability. (4) A self-locking structure or locking parts combined with a posterior fixation system can be designed to improve the immediate stability of the artificial vertebral body. (5) 3D-printed artificial vertebral bodies can better restore the physiological curvature of the spine. (6) 3D-printed artificial vertebral bodies can meet the requirements of accurate reconstruction without pruning. (7) The porous surface can be combined with induced osteogenic materials to accelerate osseointegration. The main characteristics of 3D-printed personalized artificial vertebral bodies and traditional titanium mesh artificial vertebral bodies are compared in Table 4.1.

Due to advances in spinal surgery technology, the traditional titanium mesh artificial vertebral body no longer meets the requirements of the reconstruction of unique anatomical sites and repair of large-scale loss of spinal structure. 3D-printed customized artificial vertebral bodies can facilitate accurate spinal reconstruction through precise surgical design to achieve optimal functional recovery and long-term spinal stability. The following section describes the reconstruction of the lumbar spine after tumor resection as an example to illustrate the advantages of 3D-printed customized artificial vertebral bodies in clinical applications (Fig. 4.3 & Fig. 4.4).

Compared with the traditional titanium mesh artificial vertebral bodies, 3D-printed personalized artificial vertebral bodies can be designed to meet the anatomical and mechanical requirements of vertebral reconstruction, effectively overcome postoperative spinal instability, and restore the physiological curvature of the spine. The porous surface and the endplate-bone interface of these bodies can support good bone fusion, achieve long-term biological stability, and restore spinal

Table 4.1 Comparison of characteristics of 3D-printed, customized artificial vertebrae and traditional titanium mesh artificial vertebrae

Key features	3D-printed personalized customized artificial vertebral body	Traditional titanium mesh artificial vertebral body
Selected materials	Porous titanium alloy	Solid titanium alloy
Processing technique	3D printing (additive manufacturing)	Machining (subtractive manufacturing)
Anatomical matching	Exact match	Mismatch
New bone ingrowth	Porous internal bone ingrowth (biological stability)	No osseointegration at the interface (combined bone grafting is required)
Distribution of stress	Stress at the interface is uniformly distributed	Stress at the interface is concentrated and easily causes subsidence
Mechanical properties	Structurally optimized design that meets the mechanical requirements	Difficult to adjust to meet local demand
Locking device	Self-locking to increase stability	Cannot self-lock; auxiliary fixation is needed
Intraoperative procedures	Must be placed in one step, cannot be cut or easily adjusted	Can be cut, size can be adjusted
Technical requirements	Preoperative design and surgical accuracy high demand	Low surgical accuracy is required

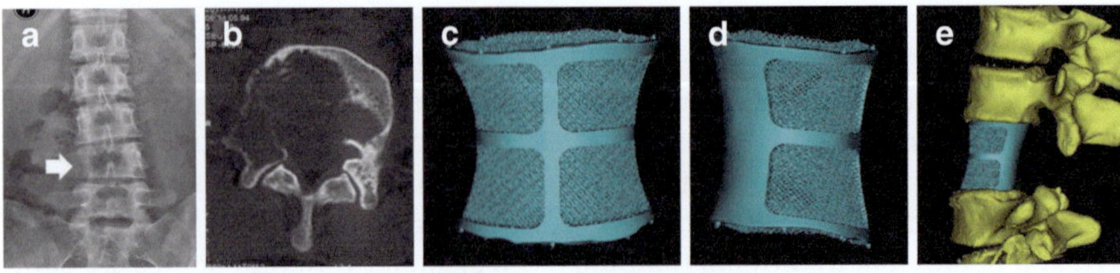

Fig. 4.3 Model of a 3D-printed artificial vertebral body for the reconstruction of the L4 vertebra body after giant cell tumor resection: (**a**) X-ray film of lumbar spine tumor: L4 bone destruction as indicated by the arrow. (**b**) Axial view of L4 bone tumor. (**c**) Anterior view of artificial vertebral body design drawing. (**d**) Lateral view of artificial vertebral body design drawing. (**e**) Simulation diagram of lumbar spine tumor resection and reconstruction

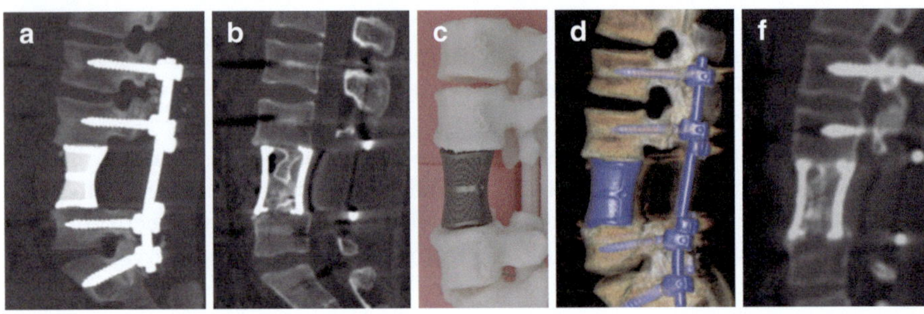

Fig. 4.4 Effect of a 3D-printed artificial vertebral body on the reconstruction of the L4 vertebra after giant cell tumor resection: (**a**) CT image captured 2 months after total vertebral resection of a giant cell tumor in the L4 vertebra and 3D-printed personalized artificial vertebral reconstruction. (**b**) CT image (sagittal section) captured 2 months after the operation showing that the artificial vertebral body and the upper and lower endplates matched well, the physiological curvature of the lumbar spine was restored, and the bone graft had preliminarily healed. (**c**) Preoperative physical model of the effect of the installation of the 3D-printed personalized L4 artificial vertebral body. (**d**) Follow-up CT 14 months after the operation revealed a three-dimensional reconstruction effect, and artificial vertebral reconstruction was satisfactory (**e**) CT (sagittal section) 14 months after the operation revealed satisfactory osseointegration between the artificial vertebral body and the upper and lower endplates

function to the greatest extent. However, personalized artificial vertebral bodies have higher requirements in terms of Surgical precision.

4.1.2 Types of 3D-Printed Artificial Vertebral Body

At present, the 3D-printed artificial vertebral bodies that are used in clinical practice can be divided into two main categories: standardized artificial vertebral bodies and individualized artificial vertebral bodies (Fig. 4.5).

The 3D-printed standardized artificial vertebral body was first registered by the Aikang Company in 2016 with the China Food and Drug Administration. This model was the first 3D-printed artificial vertebral body that was registered worldwide. Currently, this artificial vertebral body has been officially used in

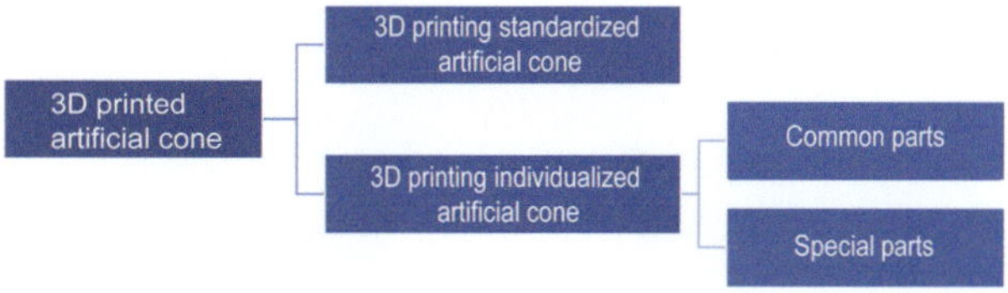

Fig. 4.5 Classification of 3D-printed artificial vertebral bodies

clinical practice. The design of this artificial body is based on a unified design standard and has the same configuration as traditional titanium mesh. It has different diameters and lengths, which allow it to meet the needs of different parts of the spine so that the surgeon can select the appropriate model for use during the operation. The advantages of this artificial body are that it is convenient to use, it is flexible and can be adjusted according to the intraoperative condition of the spinal defect, and the configuration is determined, which is easy to promote. The disadvantage of this artificial body is that, for postoperative spinal defects, individualized matching for spinal defect reconstruction has not been achieved; rather, implantation of these bodies is an empirical surgical reconstruction method that still fails to fully exploit the advantages of 3D-printing technology. In particular, this standardized artificial vertebral body cannot be used for the reconstruction of spinal defects in some unique anatomical parts, such as those in the upper cervical vertebra and the sacrum.

In addition to 3D-printed standardized artificial vertebral bodies, the remaining 3D-printed artificial vertebral bodies used in clinical practice are basically individualized ones, but these are still in clinical trials. According to the different parts of the spine, 3D-printed individualized artificial vertebral bodies can be further divided into two types: the individualized artificial vertebral body for use in ordinary parts and individualized artifical vertebral body for use in special parts.

The design of individualized artificial vertebral bodies for use in ordinary parts is based on the needs of spinal reconstruction. The basic design framework remains unchanged, but individualized modifications are made to match the vertebral body that needs to be reconstructed in each patient to achieve an individualized and accurate intraoperative spinal reconstruction. To facilitate the placement of the prosthesis, the author's team designed an individualized artificial vertebral body with a "waist-receiving" structure and successfully applied this body to the reconstruction of cervical, thoracic and lumbar vertebrae, achieving satisfactory clinical results (Fig. 4.6). Such artificial vertebral bodies are designed based on the individual spinal structure of each patient, simulating the reconstruction of normal spinal morphology, through the three-dimensional finite element topology optimization design, the final individualized artificial vertebral body that accurately matches the patient is generated. According to the actual requirements for the artificial vertebral body during spinal reconstruction, the ventral surface of the artificial vertebral body that is adjacent to the spinal cord is smoothed to reduce the interference of scars on the ventral surface and prevent the ingrowth of large amounts of soft tissue into the spinal cord. The other surfaces of the artificial vertebral body are designed to be porous to

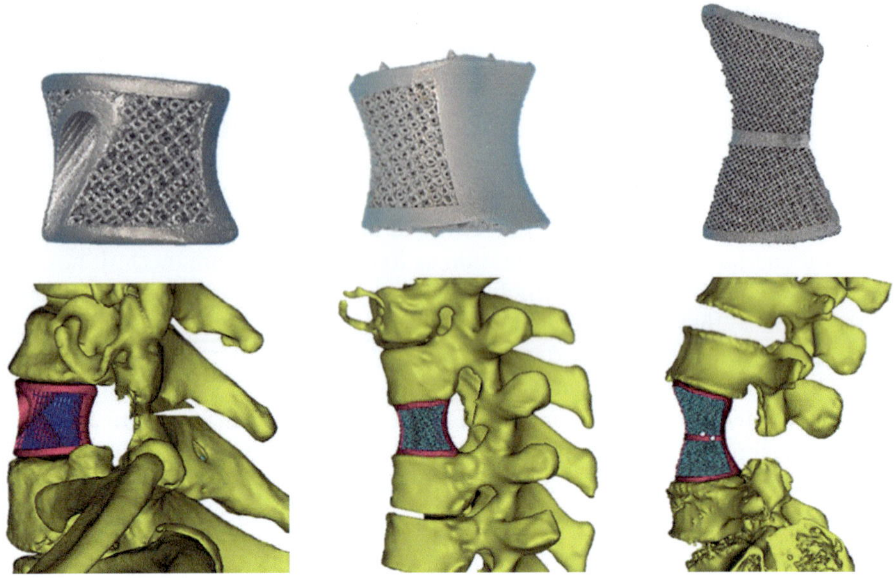

Fig. 4.6 3D-printed individualized artificial vertebral body in the cervical, thoracic, and lumbar regions

facilitate the bone ingrowth of adjacent vertebral bodies and promote early fracture integration.

The artificial vertebral bodies that are used in special parts of the spine are related to those that are used in ordinary parts. This kind of artificial vertebral body did not exist before the emergence of 3D-printing technology, and similar products have never been used clinically. This kind of artificial vertebral body was invented with the continuous improvement of 3D-printing technology. The most important parts of the spine that have been reconstructed with this kind of artificial vertebral body are the upper cervical spine and the sacrum. In these special parts of the spine, different types of artificial vertebral bodies with different shapes are personalized to match individual patients and can be designed according to the actual surgical design and the surgical resection range of the patients. The design of these artificial bodies is based on actual clinical needs and is closely related to the surgeon's own surgical experience. Therefore, there is currently no unified design standard, and the design of each artificial body is extremely specialized. The author's team designed a "fox head" type of 3D-printed individualized artificial vertebral body for use in cervical vertebra 2. Based on the theory of triangular stability, two screws were C1 vertebra C2 vertebra C3 vertebra artificial vertebral body. The patient recovered well after the operation, and the artificial vertebral body showed no loose displacement (Fig. 4.7). Wei et al. also used 3D-printing technology to prepare porous titanium alloy artificial vertebral bodies for vertebral reconstruction in nine patients who underwent C2 tumor resection (Wei et al. 2020). In addition to the wing plate screw groove, the prosthesis also had an internal screw groove. During the

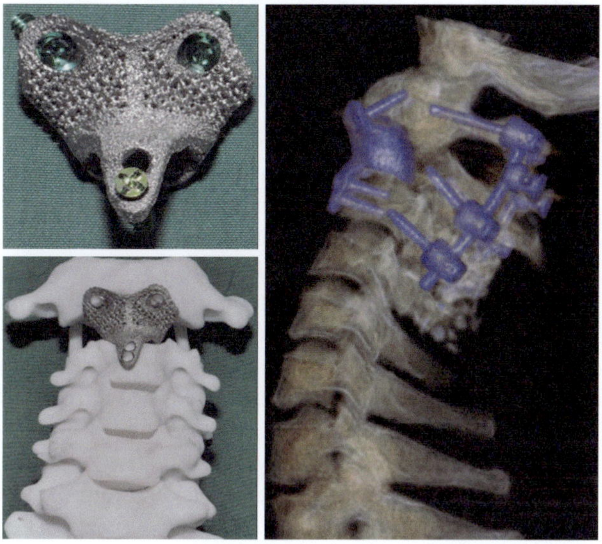

Fig. 4.7 3D-printed individualized cervical artificial vertebral body

operation, the appropriate screw groove can be selected according to the actual exposure situation to facilitate placement and fixation and reduce the size of the anterior notch of the prosthesis.

Currently, the standardized 3D-printed artificial vertebral body has been approved for clinical applications, but its application range is limited, and it cannot completely solve the problem of precise spinal reconstruction. As a supplement, 3D-printed individualized artificial vertebral bodies can achieve accurate matching and precise reconstruction of special parts, and these are indispensable characteristics of 3D-printed artificial vertebral bodies.

4.1.3 Details of 3D-Printed Individualized Artificial Vertebral Body Design

The stability of 3D-printed individualized artificial vertebral bodies is the key to successful spinal reconstruction surgery. There are various methods to ensure the stability of artificial vertebral bodies that are used for spinal reconstruction, and each method has its own advantages and disadvantages. The appropriate fixation method should be chosen based on the particular patient's condition, surgical method, artificial vertebral body design, and other factors.

At present, there are a few main fixation methods that are used with 3D-printed individualized artificial vertebral bodies: (1) Compression fixation of the artificial vertebral body by a steel plate or screw rod system, (2) Self-locking fixation of the artificial vertebral body and adjacent vertebral body and (3) Connection fixation of the artificial vertebral body and a posterior screw rod system.

Currently, compression fixation of 3D-printed individual artificial vertebral bodies by a plate and screw rod system is the most conventional and commonly used fixation method. Compression fixation is mainly achieved by the following three approaches (Fig. 4.8).

1. Anterior rod fixation of the cervical spine is the fixation method that is most commonly used during anterior cervical spine surgery. This approach is advantageous because it is easy to implement, it is associated with reduced intraoperative bleeding, and it can achieve artificial cervical vertebral body compression.
2. Lateral screw rod or plate fixation of the thoracolumbar vertebral body is the conventional fixation method for the anterior approach of the thoracolumbar vertebral body lesion side. The advantages of this method are that the artificial vertebral body can be directly observed, which makes it easy to adjust the position of the artificial vertebral body, and the artificial vertebral body can be compressed and fixed by a screw rod or plate.
3. Conventional posterior rod and screw system fixation is the fixation method that is typically used for posterior spinal surgery. The advantages of this method include the ability to relatively fix the artificial vertebral body to the posterior anatomy, reduced risk during surgery, and the fact that it is the most widely used technique. This method can be used alone for posterior vertebrectomy and compression fixation after artificial vertebral body implantation, and it can also be used for anterior or lateral anterior surgery and enhanced fixation of artificial vertebral bodies.

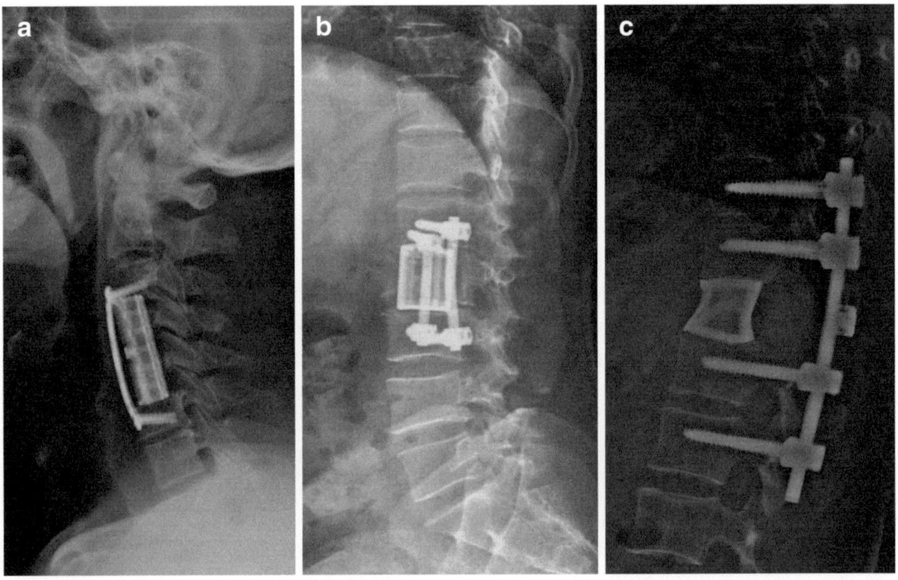

Fig. 4.8 Compression fixation of 3D-printed individualized artificial vertebral bodies by plate and screw rod system. (**a**) Anterior plate fixation. (**b**) Lateral screw rod fixation. (**c**) Posterior screw rod fixation

Self-locking fixation of the artificial vertebral body and adjacent vertebral body is based on the individualized design of 3D-printed artificial vertebral bodies. Through the locking of the artificial vertebral body and adjacent vertebral body, the artificial vertebral body is fixed. This approach can be divided into the following two main approaches (Fig. 4.9):

1. Self-locking screw fixation: Prefabricated screw holes are included in an artificial vertebral body during the printing process. The length of the angle between the fixation screw and the adjacent vertebral body is determined according to the anatomy of the particular patient. The artificial vertebral body and adjacent vertebral body are fixed by inserting screws into the artificial vertebral body. The advantage of this fixation method is that, as long as the artificial vertebral body is placed in the correct position, there is no need to worry about the direction and length of the screw, which is beneficial during the surgical operation.
2. Mixed fixation of self-locking screws and wing plates: In unique anatomical positions (upper cervical vertebra, cervicothoracic segment, and lower lumbar vertebra), it is difficult to fix artificial vertebral bodies with adjacent vertebral bodies via simple self-locking screws. In these cases, the design of a wing plates for the artificial vertebral body allows surgeons to use small-angle screws and vertebral bodies instead of large-angle screws, thus reducing the difficulty of the operation; this is especially beneficial in the design and placement of artificial vertebral bodies in some anatomically complex regions. The self-locking fixa-

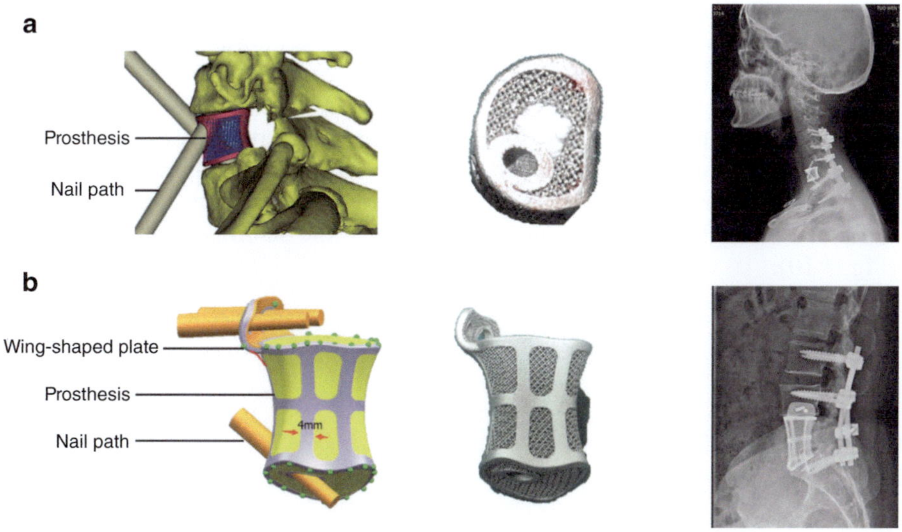

Fig. 4.9 Self-locking fixation of an artificial vertebral body and adjacent vertebral body. (**a**) Self-locking screw fixation. (**b**) Self-locking screw and wing plate mixed fixation

tion method for artificial vertebral bodies is based on the correct placement of the artificial prosthesis. Thus, there are greater requirements associated with the surgical operation.

Artificial vertebral body and posterior nail and rod system connection fixation is a unique fixation method that is used specifically for 3D-printed individualized artificial vertebral bodies (Choy et al. 2017; Girolami et al. 2018), and this method can be divided into two main cases:

1. Screw fixation with a posterior internal fixation system typically involves driving a screw through an artificial vertebral pedicle screw connection hole and through the posterior internal fixation system to connect the artificial vertebral body to the vertebral pedicle screw and the rod, forming a complete frame structure in this space.
2. Connecting rod fixation with a posterior internal fixation system, which is typically designed on an artificial vertebral body special connection device, is used to connect the artificial vertebral body to a posterior connecting rod. Thus, the final integrated frame structure is composed of the artificial vertebral body, the connecting device, and the connecting rod.

The advantages of this artificial vertebral body and posterior nail and rod system connection fixation are that the isolated artificial vertebral body anterior column fixation structure is replaced with a three-column space stereo fixation structure, which is, in theory, more conducive to promoting the stability of the artificial vertebral body. Additionally, due to the unique properties of the nail hole in the artificial vertebral body that is used during the fixation process, the artificial vertebral body must be placed in the correct position in order to ensure proper screw placement; this also ensures the correct placement of the artificial vertebral body during the operation. The author's team performed the world's first seven-vertebral resection and artificial vertebral reconstruction. Because of the large size of the artificial vertebral body, the stability of the simple posterior rod fixation was poor. Thus, the artificial vertebral body was connected to the posterior rod through the connecting rod to enhance the stability of the prosthesis (Fig. 4.10).

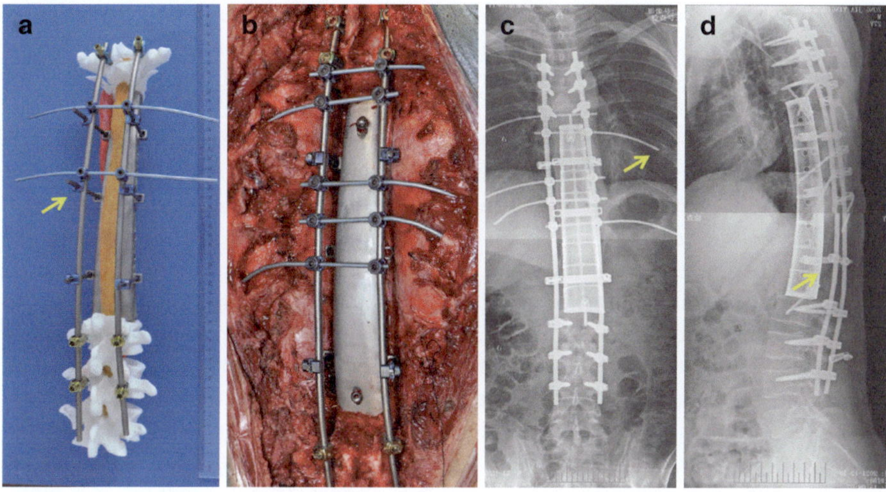

Fig. 4.10 (**a**) Model of artificial vertebral body installation. The yellow arrow indicates the connection device between the artificial vertebral body and the posterior connecting rod. (**b**) Intraoperative artificial vertebral body placement. (**c**) Postoperative anteroposterior radiograph. The yellow arrow indicates that the lateral connecting rod was inserted into the rib stump to restore the integrity of the chest wall. (**d**) Postoperative lateral radiograph. The yellow arrow indicates that a complete frame structure was formed via the combination of the artificial vertebral body with the connecting rod and the spinal connecting rod

4.2 Pelvic and Sacral Prostheses

4.2.1 Key Points for the Design and Application of 3D-Printed Pelvic Prosthesis

The pelvis is an important structure in the body, and it is formed by the sacral and coccygeal bones in the back and the iliac, ischial, and pubic bones on both sides. The pelvis transfers the weight of the trunk to the lower limbs and uses the acetabulum as the basis of lower limb activity, while supporting and protecting the organs in the abdomen and pelvis.

Because the pelvis has an irregular shape, complex anatomical relationships, and high requirements for mechanical performance, the repair of pelvic defects and reconstruction of the pelvic bone are difficult. The history of pelvic bone defect repair can be divided into nonprosthetic reconstruction and prosthetic reconstruction. Nonprosthetic reconstruction methods include the Harrington method, autologous bone grafting, inactivated replantation, and allogeneic bone grafting, but these methods are associated with problems such as nonunion, low functional scores after surgery, long immobilization time after surgery, and many complications. Prosthetic reconstruction methods include the implantation of saddle-type prostheses, ice cream handle/iliac handle prostheses, assembled hemipelvic prostheses, and customized hemipelvic prostheses. The last two types of prosthesis require retaining most of the iliac bone, and the possibility of prosthesis loosening is high. Even though an assembled hemipelvic prosthesis improves the mesh structure of the bone interface, problems such as poor interface matching, easy mechanical failure of the prosthesis joint, and difficulty in grasping the hip rotation center during surgery remain. Moreover, treatment with customized hemipelvic prostheses and bone interfaces is still not ideal. However, customized 3D-printed pelvic prostheses have gradually become the preferred choice for pelvic defect repair in many bone tumor centers in China due to the advantages of these prostheses, such as conformal matching, three-dimensional pelvic ring reconstruction, biological fixation, and good bone integration at the prosthesis-bone interface. The design of 3D-printed pelvic prostheses generally meets the composite requirements of bone defect repair, soft tissue repair, and mechanical conduction. Following the premise of conformal matching, the integrity of the pelvic ring is reconstructed according to the actual condition of the patient. The prosthesis consists of a solid structure and a trabecular-like porous structure. The solid structure includes the arc support structure that extends along the arch edge, screw hole, acetabulum, and pubic branch, and it ensures that the weight of the prosthesis is within an appropriate range. In addition, appropriately removing or reducing the volume of the prosthesis in unnecessary regions is conducive to placement and coverage, such as reducing the size of the iliac wing and removing the posterior iliac spine and the ischial spine. Numerous suture holes are distributed along the prosthesis crest to reconstruct the gluteus muscle and iliacus muscle, resulting in a streamlined design.

According to different anatomical sites of pelvic bone damage, Enneking and Dunham et al. classified pelvic bone defects into types I–IV. Type I refers to defects that involve all or part of the iliac bone, ranging from the ipsilateral sacroiliac joint to the top of the acetabulum. Type II refers to defects that involve the periphery of the acetabulum, ranging from the top of the acetabulum to the superior branch of the pubis and the lateral edge of the ischial branch. Type III refers to defects that involve the pubis and the obturator ring of the ischial. Type IV refers to defects that involve iliac lesions involving the sacrum. Customized 3D-printed prostheses can be designed specifically to treat pelvic bone defects that involve different regions. (1) In Zone I, the iliac bone—the medial iliac bone along the arc edge of the greater sciatic foramen—is an important path for the mechanical conduction of the sacrum to the acetabulum, so prostheses that are placed in this area must have a solid, high-strength structure, while prostheses that are used to treat simple iliac wing lesions must have a trabecular-like, porous, low-strength structure. (2) In Zone II, prostheses that are placed in the acetabulum must have an overall solid, high-strength structure, a trabecular-like, porous bone interface, and a standard acetabular prosthesis. (3) In Zone III, the obturator ring is formed by the pubic and ischial bones, and it is controversial whether pelvic Zone III defects should be reconstructed. Maintaining the integrity of the pelvic ring is beneficial for long-term functional rehabilitation, but reconstruction of Zone III is likely to lead to mechanical complications such as internal fixation fracture and loosening. If reconstruction is chosen, especially reconstruction of the upper and lower branches of the pubis or the upper branches of the pubis and the ischial branches, the prosthesis may have an entirely solid, high-strength structure with a trabecular, porous bone interface. For reconstruction of the symphysis pubis, insertion fixation or suture reconstruction of the fibrous joint can be chosen. The reconstruction of the ischial branches is determined by the preservation of the ischial tuber. (4) In Zones I + IV, if the iliac lesions involve the midline of the sacrum or the contralateral sacral foramen, the support of a solid, high-strength structure on the L5 vertebral body and a trabecular, porous structure to achieve osseointegration with the L5 and the contralateral sacral iliac bone should be considered. These types of prostheses need to be supplemented by the use of a pedicle screw rod system. (5) In Zone II zone, including Zones II + I, Zones II + I + III, Zones II + III, Zones II + I + IV, and Zones II + I + III + IV, the design requirements are mainly a trabecular, porous structure supplemented by a solid, high-strength structure to meet the requirements of mechanical conduction and stability, with a standard acetabular prosthesis supplemented by a pedicle screw rod system if necessary. Of course, in some specific cases, such as revision of a pelvic prosthesis and treatment of severe infection, the design of the Zone III prosthesis can be avoided due to the shielding of fibrous scar tissue.

Consider pelvic bone defects after unilateral iliac en bloc resection as an example, prosthesis design needs to functionally address the three problems described above. First, the integrity of the pelvic ring must be restored. Second, the mechanical and motor structure of the lower limb must be rebuilt. Third, the abdominal organs must be protected. After hemipelvic resection, the remaining bone structures are the sacroiliac joint surface, the contralateral symphysis pubis, and the free femur. From the perspective of structure, the pelvic prosthesis needs to connect the sacroiliac joint and the symphysis pubis, provide support for the free femur, and restore the movement of the hip joint.

Due to these functional and structural requirements of pelvic prostheses, as well as the special requirements of pelvic prostheses, it is difficult to produce a satisfactory pelvic prosthesis via traditional processes. Using 3D-printing technology, these requirements can be easily met (Figs. 4.11 and 4.12). In the sacroiliac joint surface, a pelvic prosthesis and the sacral articular surface are in close contact, and the contact surface can be designed to have a porous structure. A screw hole can be designed in the prosthesis, and the screw can be driven into the prosthesis and into the sacral bone; thus, early fixation can be achieved. In the pubic symphysis, prostheses are designed to closely fit the contralateral pubic bone, and the contact surface is designed to have a porous structure. Nail holes are added in the prosthesis, and screws are inserted into the contralateral superior and inferior ramus of the pubis. In terms of hip joint reconstruction, according to the experience of the author's team, after hemipelvectomy, it is often necessary to replace the entire hip joint. Therefore, the size of the acetabular prosthesis should include the acetabulum of the entire hip joint. The acetabular angle needs to be restored to the anatomical anteversion angle and abduction angle. From the sacroiliac joint surface to the acetabulum, the connection structure needs more strength. However, from the acetabulum to the pubic symphysis, the connection site needs less strength.

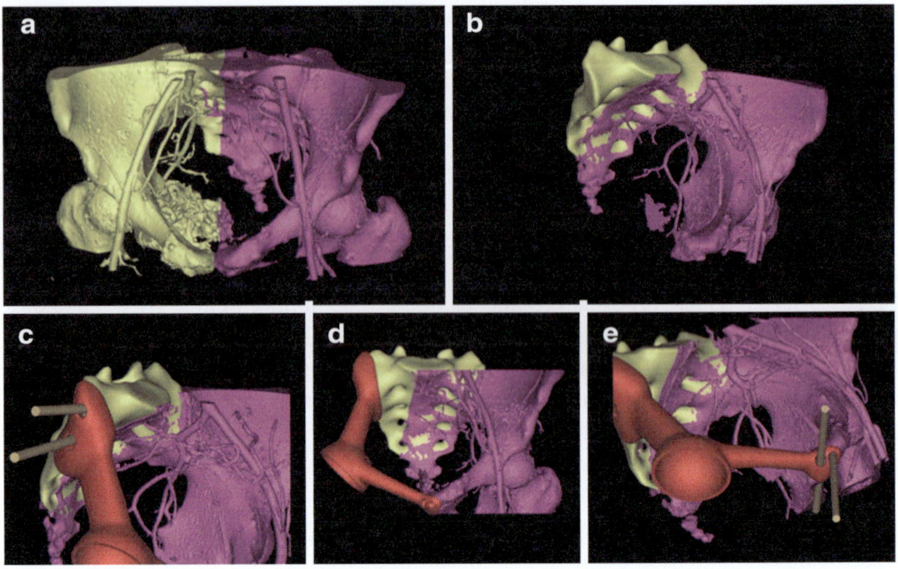

Fig. 4.11 Process of designing 3D-printed customized hemipelvic prostheses: (**a**) Enhanced CT scanning was used to scan the lesion site of a pelvic tumor patient. After obtaining the data, the morphology of the tumor site and the relationships between important blood vessels were reconstructed. (**b**) The residual bone was simulated after tumor resection. (**c**) The combination and fixation method of the hemipelvic prosthesis and the iliac bone. (**d**) Front view of the simulated installation of the prosthesis. (**e**) Side view of the simulated installation of the prosthesis

Fig. 4.12 The appearance of the prosthesis after 3D printing

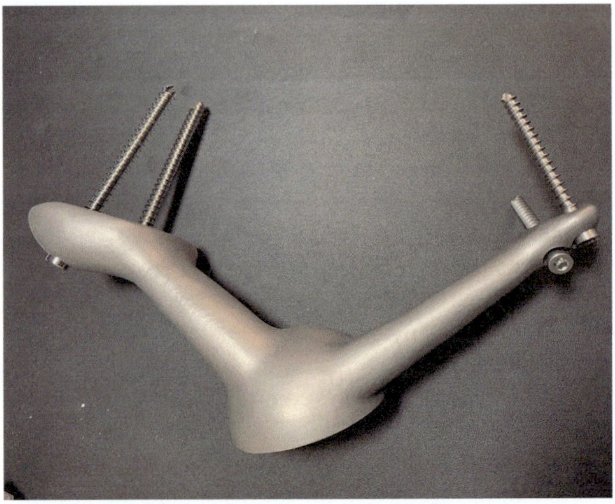

4.2.2 Key Points in the Design and Application of Sacral Prosthesis

As an important component of the pelvic ring, the sacrum is responsible for stress transfer of the trunk and stability of the pelvis (Fig. 4.13). When the sacrum, especially the high sacral region, is damaged by tumors and needs to be removed, the stability of the pelvis is affected. Clinically, lumbar-pelvic fixation reconstruction is used according to the range of sacrectomy to restore the structure and stability of the pelvic ring.

Total sacrectomy is the main method used to treat high sacral malignant tumors. Because the anatomical structure of the pelvic ring is damaged by total sacrectomy, the continuity of the lumbar spine and the pelvis is interrupted. If not reconstructed, lumbar subsidence occurs, seriously affecting the appearance and function of this region. Previously used reconstruction methods mainly include modified Galveston technology, anterior and posterior joint stabilization, customized prosthesis, and autologous bone or allogeneic bone transplantation. Although different methods can achieve certain degrees of reconstruction, the main problems associated with these methods include internal fixation loosening and fracture, prosthesis displacement, nonunion, infection, wounds, and complex reconstruction techniques.

The development of 3D-printed personalized sacral prostheses has overcome the technical bottleneck of traditional sacral reconstruction. The main advantages of these prostheses include the following: (1) The personalized customized prosthesis is well matched to the defect area, such a prosthesis meets the requirements of mechanical support, making the force transfer more aligned with physiological requirements. (2) The support interface of the spine and pelvis is porous and can meet the requirements of interface bone integration and maintain long-term biological stability. (3) The intraoperative operation is simpler, shortening the operation

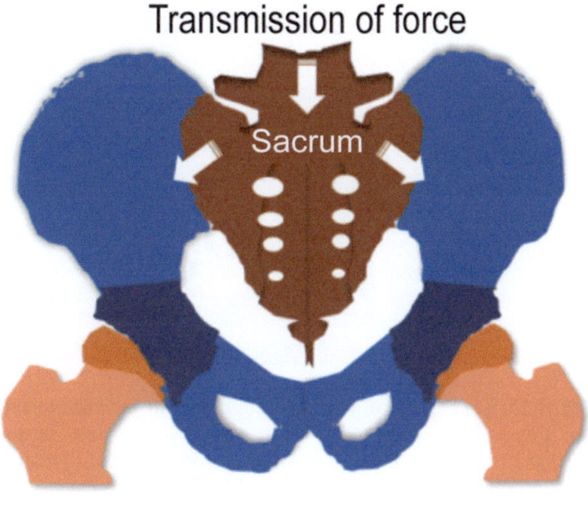

Fig. 4.13 Anatomical position and force transfer function of the sacrum in the pelvic ring

time. (4) The risk of postoperative complications is reduced compared with that of traditional reconstruction methods.

In light of the technical characteristics of total sacrectomy and reconstruction, some domestic scholars have used 3D-printing technology to prepare customized sacral prostheses and applied these prostheses in clinical practice. Professor Guo Wei, Department of Bone Oncology, Peking University People's Hospital, designed a 3D-printed customized total sacral artificial prosthesis. The characteristics of this prosthesis included a defect body connected between the vertebral osteotomy end and the left and right iliac osteotomy ends. The defective body had three contact surfaces, among which the vertebral contact surface was in contact with the vertebral osteotomy end, and the bilateral iliac osteotomy ends were in contact with the left and right iliac osteotomy ends, respectively. The vertebral contact surface and the left and right iliac osteotomy surfaces were porous. A hollow "herringbone" soft tissue attachment region, which was also porous, was situated between the vertebral contact surface and the left and right iliac osteotomy surfaces of the defect body. A number of fixation holes were also made in the defect body, and the defect body was fixed between the vertebral osteotomy end and the left and right iliac osteotomy ends via fixation. Relying on the characteristics of 3D-printing technology, this method used a herringbone design similar to the structure of the human sacral bone, achieved the fusion and stability of the three dimensions of the lumbar-iliac, posterior pelvic ring and anterior vertebral body, and achieved "triangle" support, which improved the restoration of mechanical support (Fig. 4.14). Professor Li Jianmin from the Department of Bone Oncology, Qilu Hospital of Shandong University designed another hanging support sacral prosthesis structure, the "H-shaped" assembly type, and the preliminary clinical application effect was satisfactory (Fig. 4.15).

However, most total sacral prostheses that are currently used encompass the entire structure, rendering these prostheses large and difficult to place. During surgery, the range of exposure needs to be expanded, increasing surgical trauma. Second, the shape and size of these prostheses are fixed. If the surgical accuracy is

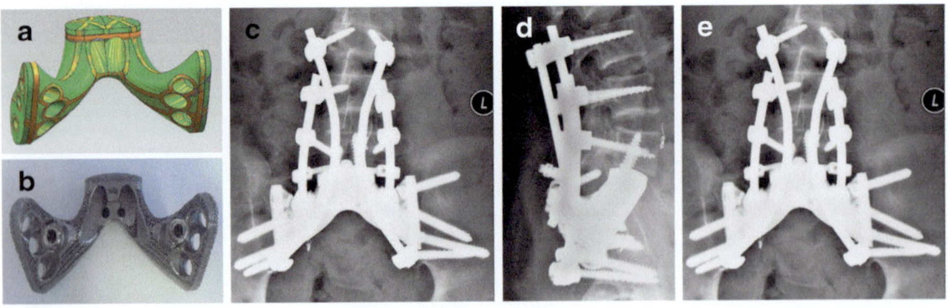

Fig. 4.14 (**a**) Design of a 3D-printed, personalized, customized "herringbone" sacral prosthesis. (**b**) Physical drawing of a 3D-printed, personalized, customized sacral prosthesis. (**c, d**) Reconstruction with the personalized customized sacral prosthesis after total sacral tumor resection (postoperative anteroposterior and lateral X-ray views)

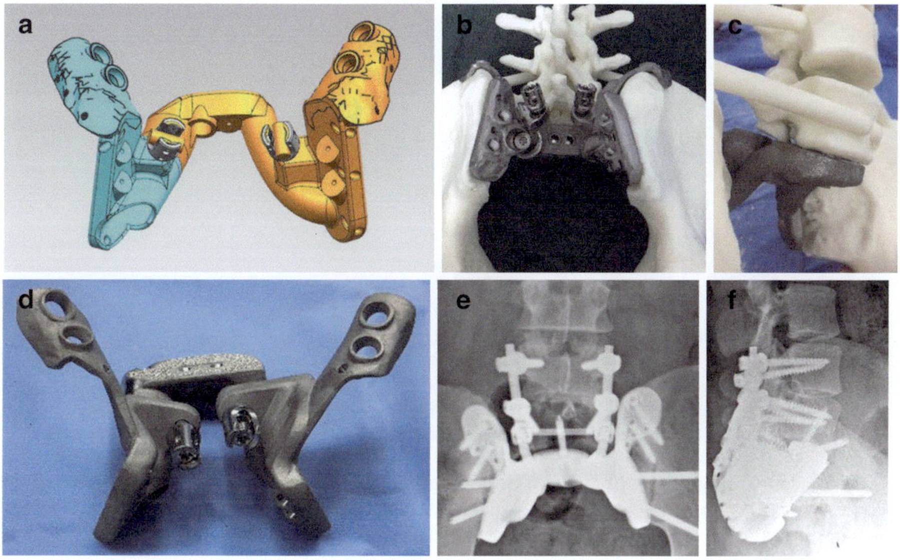

Fig. 4.15 (**a**) Design of a 3D-printed, personalized, customized “H-shaped” sacral prosthesis. (**b**) Physical drawing of a 3D-printed, personalized, customized sacral prosthesis. (**c**, **d**) Preinstalled prosthesis on a three-dimensional solid model of the pelvis (anteroposterior and lateral view). (**e**, **f**) Reconstruction with the personalized, customized sacral prosthesis after total sacral tumor resection (postoperative anteroposterior and lateral X-ray views)

insufficient or the actual range of resection differs from the preoperative design, poor matching of the prosthesis may occur, or it may be difficult to place the prosthesis and restore the pelvic structure. To improve the convenience of prosthesis installation and provide a new option for partial sacrectomy reconstruction, the author’s team designed a 3D-printed split artificial sacral prosthesis (Fig. 4.16), which can be placed between the lumbar spine and the iliac bone, to restore the integrity of the pelvic ring after partial or total sacrectomy.

As a unique anatomical site in the human body, the sacrum has its own particular shape, structure, and function. The operation of traditional sacral reconstruction methods is complicated, and it is difficult to consider the dual role of support and fusion stability. The development of 3D-printed, personalized, customized prostheses has overcome the shortcomings of traditional technology. However, the design of these prostheses still needs to be optimized, and their effect needs to be evaluated in the long term.

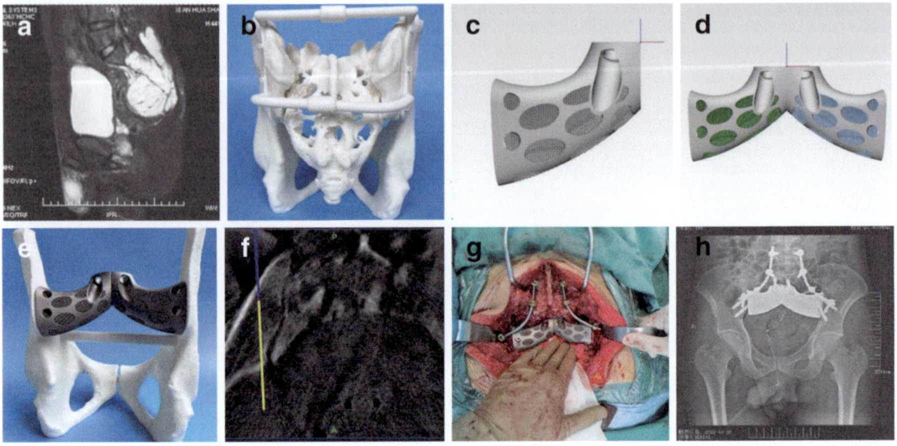

Fig. 4.16 (**a**) Chordoma involving the whole sacrum. (**b**) Model and guide plate of the sacral chordoma. (**c**) Design of a 3D-printed split artificial sacral prosthesis. (**d**) Model showing the combination of the 3D-printed split artificial sacral prosthesis. (**e**) Pre-installed prosthesis on a three-dimensional solid model of the pelvis. (**f**) Navigation verification of the osteotomy plane. (**g**) Reconstruction with the 3D-printed split artificial sacral combination after resection of the sacral chordoma. (**h**) Reconstruction with the 3D-printed split artificial sacral prosthesis (postoperative anteroposterior and lateral X-ray images)

4.3 Prostheses Designed for the Replacement of Long Bone Segments

Long bones, which are long and tubular and can be divided into two ends, mainly exist in the limbs. The bodies of long bones are called bone stems; of the bone stem, the peripheral part is dense, the central part is the bone marrow cavity that contains bone marrow, and the two ends are enlarged, called the epiphysis. The surface of the epiphysis is attached via articular cartilage, forming an articular surface, which forms a flexible joint with the articular surface of the adjacent bone to complete a larger range of motion. Long bone defects are mainly caused by trauma, infection, bone nonunion, bone resorption, congenital disease, bone tumor resection, secondary injury, etc. In addition to bone loss, long bone defects also lead to the loss of limb function, loss of adjacent joint function, and even secondary infection of surrounding soft tissues and bone tissues, which are often difficult to treat and seriously affect the quality of life and survival of patients (Abudu et al. 1997).

4.3.1 Advantages and Disadvantages of Methods for Repairing Long Bone Defects

The repair of long bone defects, especially large bone defects, has always been a major problem in the clinical treatment of traumatic orthopedics. Currently, there are various approaches for treating large bone defects in clinical practice, such as autologous bone, allogeneic bone, heterogeneous bone grafting, artificial bone grafting, Masquelet technology, Ilizarov technology (bone transport technology), and 3D-printed metal prostheses. Each of these different methods has its own advantages and disadvantages.

4.3.1.1 Bone Grafting Technology

Bone transplantation is the most traditional method used to repair bone defects. Bone grafting materials can be chosen from among autologous bone, allogeneic bone, or xenogeneic bone. Autologous bone is the most economical and effective material for bone transplantation. Autologous bone mainly comes from the host itself, has high histocompatibility and does not trigger rejection reactions, retains active components such as osteoblasts and cytokines of the host, and has strong bone induction activity. However, when the bone defect is large, autologous bone transplantation is limited by bone mass, which makes it difficult to fully meet the bone repair needs with this approach. In addition, the use of autologous bone can cause new bone defects when autologous bone is harvested, inevitably increasing the operation time and donor site trauma. Although allogeneic bone transplantation is not limited by bone mass and does not cause secondary trauma, it is associated with low bone histocompatibility and increased rejection. To reduce the rejection of allogeneic bone, a variety of physical methods are often used to prepare allogeneic bone, such as frozen or freeze-dried bone samples. Although this preparation reduces the antigenicity of bone tissue, it also inactivates osteoblasts and cytokines, reducing the ability of allogeneic bone to induce bone regeneration.

4.3.1.2 Masquelet Technology

In recent years, Masquelet technology has been increasingly applied to the repair of bone defects, especially the repair of defects of large segments of long bones. This technology includes two stages. In the first stage, the formation of a membrene is induced in the body, and the bone cement is thoroughly debrided, fixed, and filled. In the second stage, bone grafting is induced. That is, 6–8 weeks after Polymethyl Methacrylate (PMMA) implantation, infection control is confirmed, bone cement is removed, and bone grafting is performed. Masquelet technology is simple, effective, and widely used, and it can improve infection resistance to a certain extent. Therefore, for patients with osteomyelitis complicated by large bone defects, Masquelet technology has clear advantages. However, this technology requires two operations, which increases the risk of trauma and surgery at both the defect site and the bone removal site. For patients with large bone defects, bone grafting is also needed, which can lead to more complications. Additionally, the inducer that is used in this technology is not sufficiently well developed, and further research and development are still needed.

4.3.1.3 Ilizarov Technology

Ilizarov technology exposes living tissues to a continuous and stable slow stretch, stimulating or activating the regeneration and active growth of some tissue cells whose mode of growth involves the same cell division. This technology has been successfully used in the repair of severe defects in limb tissues by relying on the self-repair and self-regeneration processes of tissues. Promoting osteogenesis via this technology has many advantages. (1) Osteogenesis is not limited by the length of the bone defect. (2) This process is simple and involves less trauma. (3) This approach is a dynamic treatment, and the adjustment speed of the external fixator can be changed at any time according to the degree of osteogenesis, achieving the external control of bone repair. (4) This approach relies on autologous bone transport, without issues related to biological contamination or biocompatibility, and it does not require the removal of bone from other areas. (5) The new bone segment that forms is normal bone tissue, and its thickness is consistent with that of the surrounding healthy bone. (6) The process of distraction osteogenesis also has a reparative effect on the surrounding soft tissue, and no additional surgical repair of soft tissue is needed. However, this treatment method requires a long treatment time, involves inconvenient activities during treatment, and is associated with poor patient compliance. Moreover, the needle path of the external fixator can provide a channel for bacterial infection, which seriously affects the promotion and use of this technology.

4.3.1.4 3D-Printed Metal Prosthesis

With the development of 3D-printing technology in the medical field, the use of 3D printing to produce metal prostheses has allowed the personalized customization of prostheses as well as the preparation of porous titanium alloy prostheses with accurate spatial configurations, allowing both the shape and elastic modulus of these prostheses to match those of the bone defect site in the patient. Additionally, the controllable porosity, pore size, and pore structure not only reduce the elastic modulus of the metal prosthesis so that it is compatible with natural bone but also provide space for the growth of bone and blood vessels. The locking structure that is formed between the bone tissue and the metal prosthesis further strengthens the stability of the prosthesis. Therefore, 3D-printed metal prostheses have been recognized by an increasing number of orthopedic surgeons. Titanium alloy (generally Ti-6Al-4V) is relatively easy to obtain, and its elastic modulus is similar to that of bone tissue; therefore, it is often used for the preparation of bone tissue prostheses. Therefore, 3D-printed, porous titanium alloy prostheses match the shape and mechanical properties of bone tissue defects. However, the bioactivity of the titanium alloy is poor. To date, many scholars have enhanced the bioactivity of titanium alloy by surface modification and achieved good results.

In summary, there are many methods for repairing bone defects in long bones, but they all have certain advantages and disadvantages. The use of 3D-printed metal prostheses can avoid many of the disadvantages of other methods. The operation is simple, and the bone repair effect is good. Therefore, how orthopedic surgeons design and use 3D-printed metal prostheses is the main obstacle restricting the use of this technology. It is urgent to develop reasonable designs and use specifications for 3D-printed metal prostheses for long bone defects.

4.3.2 Ideas for the Design of 3D-Printed Prostheses for Long Bone Defects in Different Stress Environments

Long bones are tubular bones that are characterized by a relatively simple morphology and structure, high stress, and a small contact area between the bone defect section and the prosthesis. In the design of segmental prostheses for long bone defects, stress and long-term bone growth should be emphasized. Because they are implanted in different stress environments, segmental prostheses for long bone defects can be divided into high-stress prostheses and low-stress prostheses.

4.3.2.1 High-Stress Segmental Prosthesis for Long Bone

(a) Design and Application of 3D-Printed Titanium Alloy Segmental Prosthesis

Long bones in high-stress environments, including the femur, tibia, and humerus, that are either located in the lower limbs or independently support the limbs, need to bear high stress in their anatomical environment. When bone defects in this region are repaired with a 3D-printed customized prosthesis, the prosthesis will also be subjected to high stress. When designing prostheses for these bones, the stress conditions of the prosthesis need to be fully considered, and the design should include a porous structure on the surface where the prosthesis and the bone are in contact to facilitate the long-term stability of the prosthesis. During the design of the prosthesis, it is necessary to distinguish between solid structures and porous structures. In theory, simple solid structures need to meet the stress requirements of long bones, and finite element biomechanical analysis should be performed. For segmental prostheses of these parts, it is also possible to consider designing a cavity in which to place the fibular flap with blood vessels. Such a design and operation will better support the long-term stability of the prosthesis (Fig. 4.17). In addition, and most importantly, the 3D-printed customized prosthesis of the femur, tibia, and humerus must be used together with standard internal fixation, and it is necessary to avoid using 3D-printed prostheses alone on these bones (Fan et al. 2015; Mayfield et al. 2022).

(b) Application of 3D-Printed Metal Hot Dogs for Large Segmental Defects in Long Bones

In a high-stress environment, the prosthesis needs to have greater mechanical strength. 3D-printed metal hot dog technology can provide better mechanical support, which is conducive to the long-term stability of the prosthesis. Hot dog technology was proposed by Capanna, an Italian scholar, in 1993 (Capanna et al. 1993). In brief, this method uses large segmental allograft bone combined with a vascularized fibula to repair segmental bone defects in long bones caused by the resection of bone tumors (Fig. 4.18). The advantages of this approach are that it can improve the

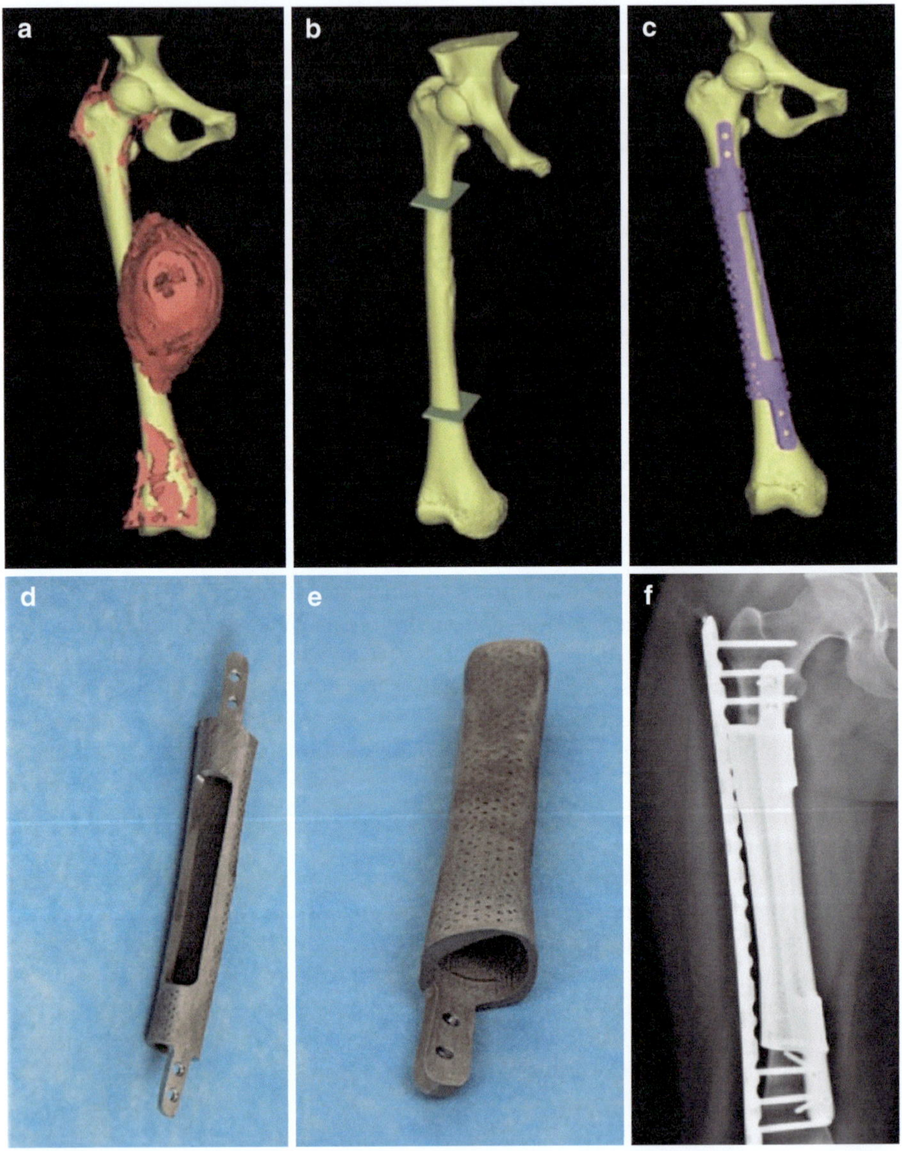

Fig. 4.17 After resection of the ultralong segment of femoral osteosarcoma, a segmental, 3D-printed customized prosthesis was designed for repair, the internal space of the prosthesis was designed to hold the vascularized fibular flap, and the bone plate was used for auxiliary fixation in clinical application. (**a**) After the patient's CT and MRI images were merged before the operation, the position and range of the simulated lesion was reconstructed in three dimensions. (**b**) According to the preoperative image, the range of the proximal and distal osteotomy was determined. (**c**) According to the range of the femoral defect, the appearance of the prosthesis was determined. (**d, e**) The appearance of the femoral prosthesis after 3D printing was completed. (**f**) Anteroposterior X-ray film of the surgical area after the implantation operation

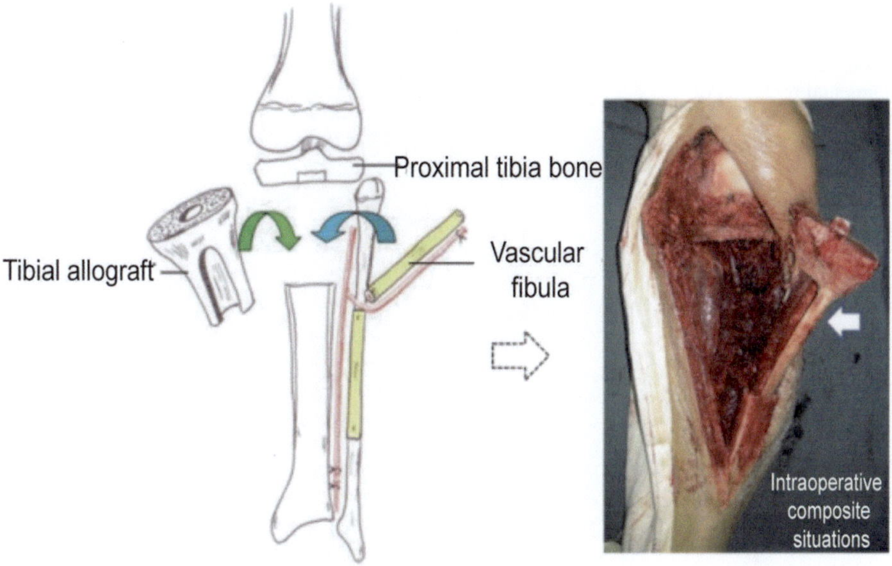

Fig. 4.18 Tibial allograft combined with a vascularized fibula (hot dog technique) to repair segmental bone defects caused by the resection of an upper tibial bone tumor while retaining the proximal tibial epiphysis

mechanical strength of the bone, reduce the occurrence of nonunion and infection, and achieve long-term biological stability, especially in adolescent patients.

However, this traditionally advantageous technique has problems, such as insufficient allograft sources, risk of cross infection, mismatch of the anatomical morphology of the donor and recipient bone, and a technically difficult operation. Currently, intercalary prostheses are also customized by machining methods and used to repair bone defects in the clinic, but long-term biological stability is difficult to achieve at the prosthesis-bone interface, and prosthesis failure due to loosening is likely (Fig. 4.19). This traditional metal prosthesis is difficult to combine with bone transplantation technology to improve the long-term survival of the prosthesis.

3D-printing technology can overcome the shortcomings of traditional prosthesis structures because it can generate individualized, customized prostheses (metal shells) that can be combined with vascularized fibulae; this approach is called the metal hot dog technique (Figs. 4.20 and 4.21), and it avoids the problems of material and application bottlenecks that are associated with the traditional hot dog technique. The characteristics of 3D-printed prostheses that are produced with the metal hot dog technique are as follows: (1) The shape of the metal support is consistent with the anatomical morphology of the bone defect. (2) Physicians can customize the fixation method according to the needs of local bone reconstruction to improve the stability of the prosthesis. (3) The porous structure of the prosthesis interface plays a role in bone conduction so that the prosthesis-bone interface has good osseointegration to maintain the long-term biological stability of the prosthesis. (4) The

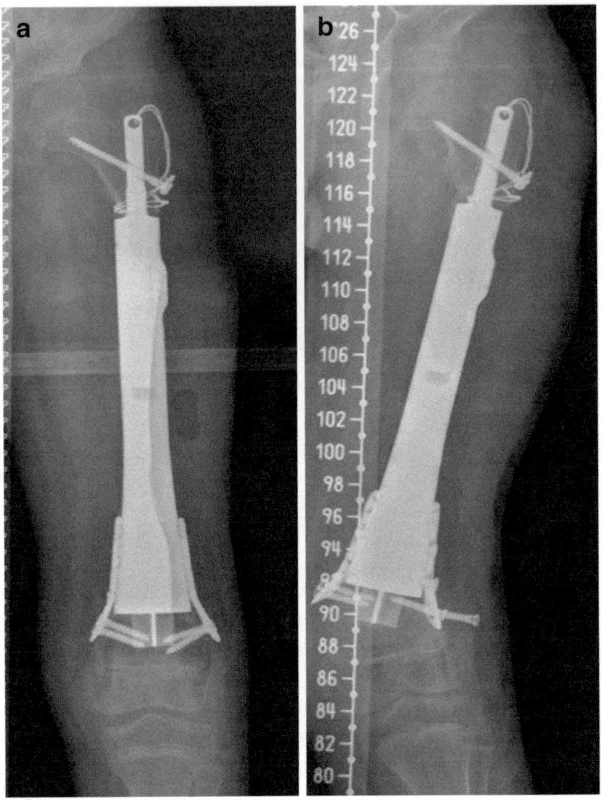

Fig. 4.19 Individualized segmental prosthesis reconstruction after segmental resection of femoral osteosarcoma in children. (**a**) One year after the operation, the prosthesis position was satisfactory. (**b**) Five years after the operation, the distal prosthesis was loose, and angular displacement occurred

porous structure of the prosthesis surface allows soft tissues to attach more closely, reducing the size of the effective cavity and reducing the occurrence of infection. (5) According to the mechanical limb load-bearing requirements, the topology of the prosthesis can be optimized, not only improving the strength of the prosthesis but also preventing bone resorption caused by stress shielding. (6) The porous structure of the prosthesis increases the flow of nutrients within the prosthesis, which allows the prosthesis and bone graft to achieve more effective bone healing.

3D-printed metal hot dog technology can fully exploit the advantages of 3D-printed customized prostheses and vascularized fibular grafts, meet the mechanical requirements of segmental bone defect repair, achieve the fine matching of anatomical structures, accelerate bone healing, and achieve rapid and lasting biological reconstruction. By optimizing the structure and mechanics of 3D-printed, customized segmental prostheses, with improvements in 3D-printed technology, the use of 3D-printed metal prostheses alone may achieve the same therapeutic effect.

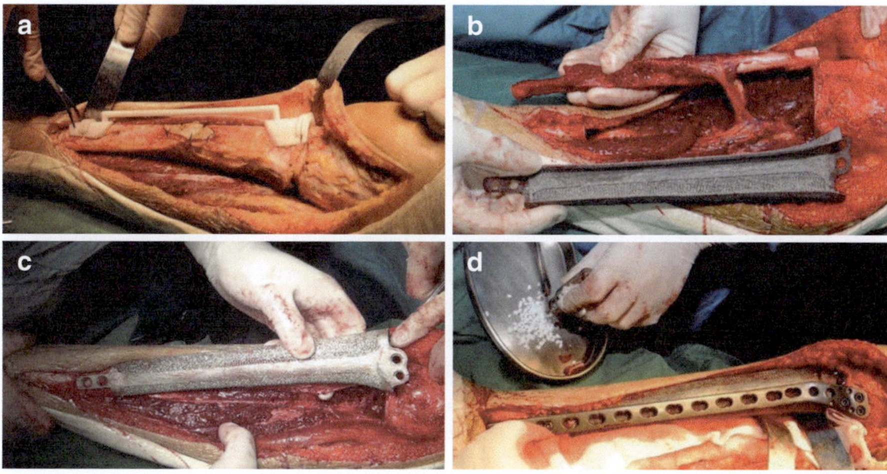

Fig. 4.20 Diagram of a surgical operation with 3D-printed metal hot dog technology. (**a**) Precise resection of tibial osteosarcoma with the assistance of a 3D-printed, customized surgical osteotomy guide plate. (**b**) Reconstruction with a 3D-printed customized prosthesis combined with a vascularized fibular graft (metal hot dog) after tibial tumor resection. (**c**) The metal hot dog complex was precisely installed in the bone defect area. (**d**) The metal hot dog complex with lateral auxiliary plate support fixation was used to improve the stability of the prosthesis

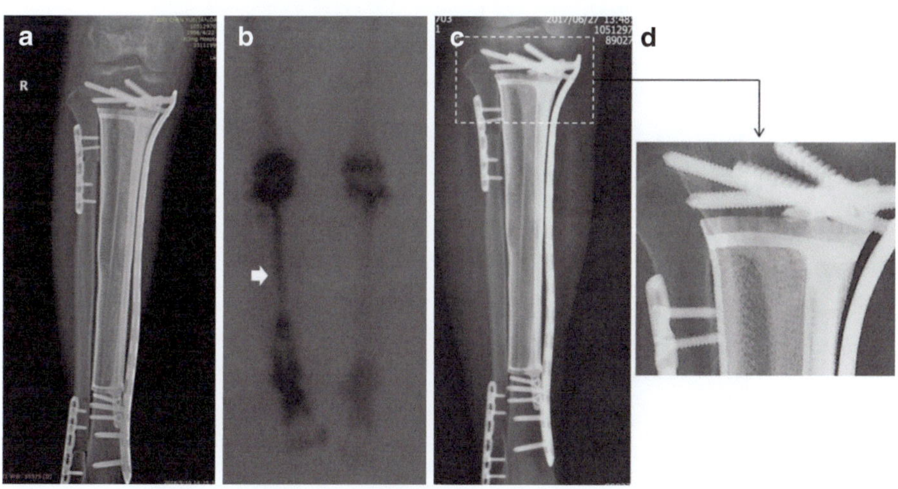

Fig. 4.21 Evaluation of reconstruction with a 3D-printed metal hot dog after tibial tumor resection. (**a**) Postoperative X-ray images showing that the 3D-printed metal hot dog accurately reconstructed the segmental tibial bone. (**b**) Radionuclide bone scan at 6 months after the operation, showing osteogenic activation of the fibula in the hot dog compound (white arrow indicates the zone with concentrated active bone metabolism). (**c**) At 21 months after the operation, the imaging showed that the hot dog complex was stable and that the surrounding bone had healed. (**d**) At 21 months after the operation, local magnification of the upper tibial end of the hot dog complex showed that the prosthetic-bone interface was accurately matched, the osseointegration was satisfactory, the fibular bone end had healed, and the patient's lower limb function had recovered completely

4.3.2.2 Low-Stress Long Bone Prostheses for Defects of Different Lengths

Some long bones, including the ulna, radius, and fibula, are subjected to a low-stress environment, but the low stress described here, in relative terms, should depend on the length of the bone defect. The contact surface between a prosthesis and bone should be designed to be anatomical, and the prosthesis should have good contact with the bone surface. Porous structures are recommended for these contact surfaces, and the use of solid structures in bone contact surfaces should be avoided as much as possible. Between the contact surfaces on the two sides of a prosthesis, the use of a long, regular, cylindrical structure is recommended for extension; however, this does not necessarily restore the anatomical form (Fig. 4.22). For short bone defects, no internal fixation material can be used. However, even in these three bones, if the extent of the bone defect is large, the use of a prosthesis with standard internal fixation is recommended to reduce stress on the prosthesis (Krishna et al. 2022).

In conclusion, the use of metal 3D-printing technology to design and prepare customized prostheses has great advantages for the repair of segmental long bone defects, and the local stress environment and long-term osseointegration should be considered during the design process.

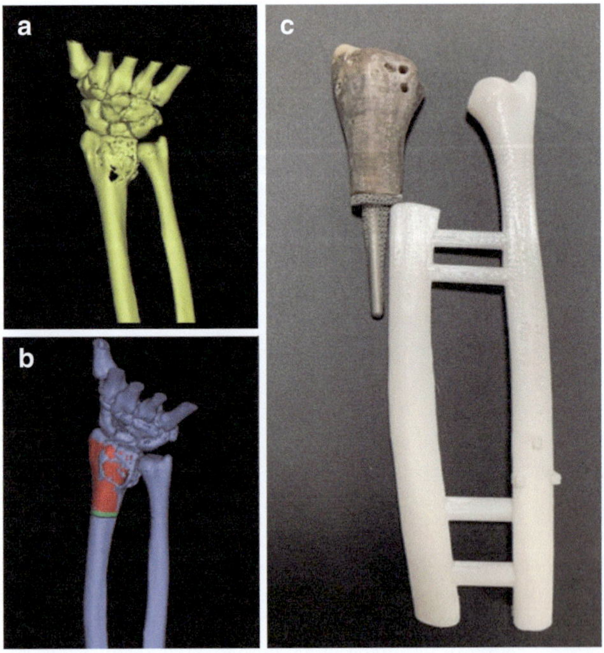

Fig. 4.22 Clinical process of reconstruction of a segmental defect of the distal radius after tumor resection using 3D-printed, customized prosthesis technology. (**a**) 3D visualization of the distal radius lesion. (**b**) The extent of distal radius tumor resection and the appearance of the prosthesis. (**c**) Finished 3D-printed customized distal radius prosthesis

4.4 Prostheses of Other Types

Bone defects at special sites are different from ordinary simple bone defects because of the complex anatomical structure and geometry of these sites, which greatly increase the difficulty of intraoperative anatomical reduction and rigid fixation. In addition to bone defects at special sites, malunion often occurs due to changes in bone morphology during remodeling, resulting in limitations in limb appearance and function. Due to intraoperative complexity and the lack of detailed preoperative planning, traditional surgical methods not only prolong the operation time and increase the amount of bleeding but also often cause problems such as poor fracture reduction and poor postoperative functional recovery. 3D-printing technology can be used to tailor the production of a prosthesis according to a particular patient's bone defect, to retain the patient's original bone, simplify the surgical process, shorten the operation time, and reduce the risk of surgery as much as possible. This section describes 3D-printed, custom-made prostheses for the scapula, clavicle, calcaneus, and ribs.

4.4.1 Design and Application of 3D-Printed Scapular Prosthesis

4.4.1.1 The Anatomy and Function of the Scapula

The scapula is a triangular flat bone that connects the torso and the upper limbs of the human body. The scapula is located between the second and seventh ribs and can be divided into two faces, three edges, two joint connections, and one ligament connection. Functionally, the scapula is an important structure for the transmission of force from the extremities. The glenohumeral joint is tightly connected with the humerus and provides the shoulder joint with abduction, adduction, forward flexion, and back extension. Additionally, the scapula is also the start and end point of many muscles around the shoulder joint. Structurally, the scapula is an important structure that connects the trunk and limbs, and it is united with the clavicle to maintain the integrity of the shoulder joint. In patients with malignant tumors of the scapula, complete resection of the scapula is often needed. After the scapula is removed, it is difficult to maintain the structure and function of the shoulder joint. Additionally, it was difficult to design and produce a suitable scapular prosthesis with previously available prosthesis technology. Therefore, shoulder suspension or exclusion was often performed to treat scapular defects in the past. However, this approach causes asymmetry and an unaesthetic appearance of the bilateral shoulder joints, affecting the activity of the shoulder joints and causing inconvenience to the patients.

4.4.1.2 3D-Printed Individualized Prosthesis Based on Anatomical Structure of the Scapula

3D-printing technology can be used to design prostheses with anatomical structures that match the appearance of the patient. These scapular prostheses are almost the same as the original scapula; they have two faces, three margins, an acromion, a coracoid process, a glenoid, and other important anatomical structures. In contrast to other 3D-printed prostheses, scapular prostheses have no bony connection structure; rather, all the structures are soft connections, which requires that the attachment of soft tissue should be considered in the design of the prosthesis (Fig. 4.23).

These soft tissue attachment connections can be divided into three types: joint structure, ligament structure, and muscle structure. The joint structures included mainly the glenoid and acromioclavicular joints. Holes around these two structures need to be designed to suture the joint capsule. The ligament structure is mainly used for the reconstruction of the coracoclavicular ligament. The base part of the coracoid process can be retained, and the pinhole on the surface is designed for ligament suture (Fig. 4.24). The muscular junction structure mainly includes the three edges of the main scapula, the lateral acromion, and the scapular spine.

Because the scapula is a structure of the upper limb, the stress it experiences is low. In addition, there is no bony connection around the scapula. Therefore, metal materials or non-metallic materials, such as polyether ether ketone (PEEK), can be selected for prosthesis design. In the design stage, the choice of printing material should be clear. If a metal material is selected, a structural design that reduces the weight can be chosen, and if a PEEK material is selected, the structure should be solid (Fig. 4.25).

In conclusion, the scapula belongs to the girdle bone of the upper limb. Due to its irregular shape, it is difficult to effectively reconstruct the scapula using traditional technology. The advantages of 3D printing can be fully exploited in such cases (Streck et al. 2023). When designing the scapular prosthesis, it is necessary to consider the suturing of each joint capsule during reconstruction as well as the suturing of the soft tissue around the scapula.

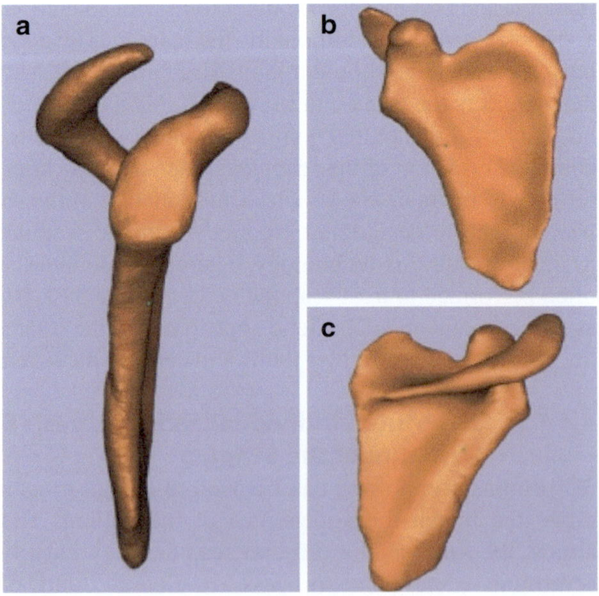

Fig. 4.23 Contour design of a 3D-printed customized scapular prosthesis. (**a**) The outer surface of the prosthesis. (**b**) Costal surface (anterior) of the prosthesis. (**c**) Dorsal surface (posterior) of the prosthesis

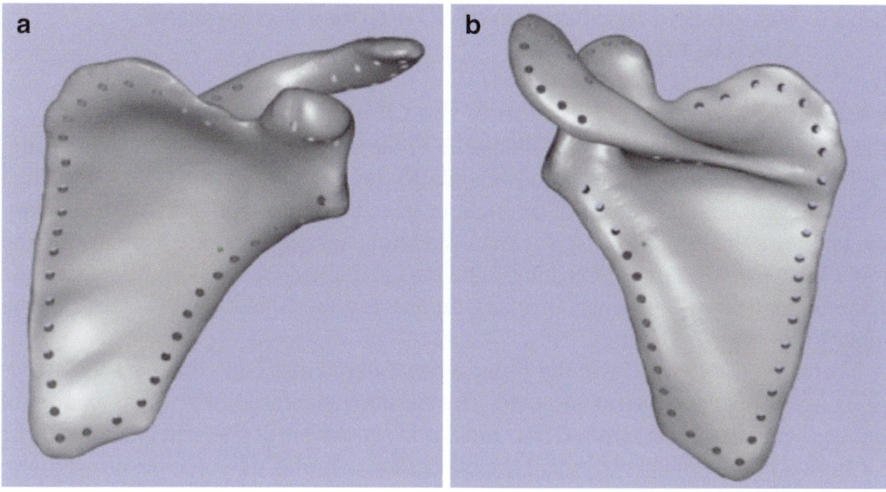

Fig. 4.24 Planning and design of the suture hole for a 3D-printed custom-made scapular prosthesis. (**a**) Ventral view of the planned suture hole. (**b**) Dorsal view of the planned suture hole

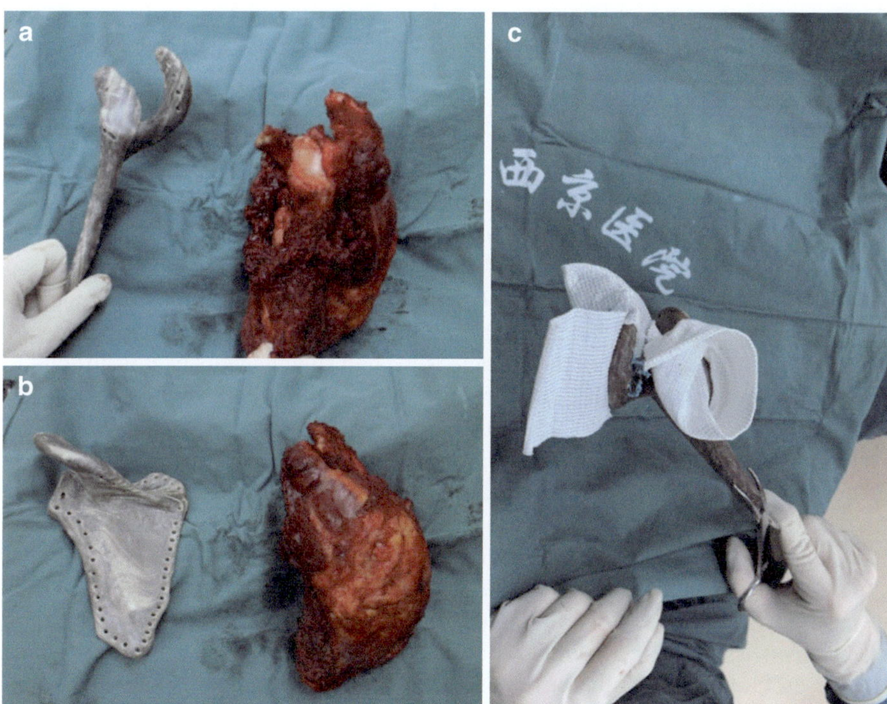

Fig. 4.25 Surgical procedure for the clinical application of a PEEK 3D-printed, customized scapular prosthesis. (**a**) Comparison of the scapular prosthesis and the resected tumor showing the lateral face ratio. (**b**) Dorsal contrast. (**c**) The joints that need to be sutured are shown

4.4.2 Design and Application of 3D-Printed Customized Clavicle Prosthesis

4.4.2.1 Anatomy and Function of the Clavicle

The clavicle is an integral part of the girdle of the upper limb. The clavicle is a long, "S"-shaped bone that connects the scapula to the sternum. The clavicle is located under the skin, and it can be felt throughout its entire length. Functionally, the clavicle connects the upper limb to the axial skeleton, serving as a pole, supporting the upper limb from the trunk, expanding the range of a person's vision, increasing the range of motion of the upper limb, and improving the functional efficiency of the upper limb.

Normally, the sternoclavicular joint, acromioclavicular joint, and coracoclavicular ligament need to be reconstructed. The sternoclavicular joint is a polyaxial joint that connects the upper limb to the trunk, and it consists of the articular surface of the sternal end of the clavicle and the clavicular notch of the manubrium sternum. The acromioclavicular joint consists of the articular surface medial to the acromion of the scapula and the articular surface at the acromion end of the clavicle. The coracoclavicular ligament is connected to the coracoid process of the scapula and the clavicle. This ligament connects the clavicle and the coracoid process of the scapula. It starts at the coracoid process, extends posteriorly to the upper part, and ends at the lower edge of the outer end of the clavicle. The coracoclavicular ligament plays a unique and important role in maintaining the stability of the acromioclavicular joint, so it must be repaired to maintain reduction during clavicle reconstruction.

4.4.2.2 3D Printing of Customized Prosthesis Based on Collarbone Anatomy

For patients with malignant tumors of the clavicle, complete resection of the clavicle is often needed. After the clavicle is removed, the shoulder joint becomes cohesive, and its structure and function, as well as its shape in particular, are affected. Because the entire segment of the clavicle is located subcutaneously, it is difficult to design and produce appropriate clavicle prostheses with previously available prosthesis technology. Therefore, in the past, patients with clavicular defects were often excluded from receiving prostheses. However, the lack of a prosthesis results in asymmetry and an unaesthetic appearance of the bilateral shoulder joints, affecting the function of the upper limbs and causing inconvenience for patients.

Using 3D-printing technology, a clavicular prosthesis with a structure and function that meet the needs of patients can be designed (Chen et al. 2021). In appearance, a clavicle prosthesis is almost the same as the original clavicle; it has two articular surfaces and a ligament connection structure. Unlike other 3D-printed prostheses, clavicular prostheses have no bony connection structure, and all the connection structures are soft connections, which requires that the attachment of soft tissue be considered during prosthesis design. The attachment and connection of these soft tissues can be divided into two types: joint structure and ligament structure. The joint structure mainly includes the sternoclavicular joint and acromioclavicular joint. These two structures need to be polished, and the surrounding holes need to be designed to suture the joint capsule. The ligament structure is mainly used for the reconstruction of the coracoclavicular ligament, and the surface has a pinhole that is used to suture the ligament. Because the clavicle is a structure of the upper limb, the stress it experiences under some specific circumstances (such as upper limb support) is greater; therefore, the use of metal materials can be recommended. However, because of its subcutaneous location, a porous structure should be used as much as possible while also ensuring the strength of the prosthesis (Fig. 4.26).

Prosthetic reconstruction has not generally been performed after clavicle resection in clinical practice because the anatomy of this site is complex, the surface soft tissue coverage is poor, and postoperative complications are likely to occur. However, with the help of 3D-printing technology, prostheses can be fabricated with a porous structure. Therefore, when designing a clavicular prosthesis, the prosthesis should be fully porous, and attention should be given to the suturing and reconstruction of each joint capsule.

4.4.3 Clinical Application and Risk of 3D-Printed Customized Calcaneal Prostheses

The calcaneus is the largest tarsal bone in the sole of the foot; it has an irregular shape and forms a joint with the talus and cuboid. The calcaneus is the main weight-bearing bone structure in the human body. When a person walks normally, the calcaneus can bear more than 50% of the body weight (Fig. 4.27).

Calcaneal lesions (tumor, trauma, infection, etc.) can lead to calcaneal defects. If not reconstructed, the appearance and function of this area could be seriously affected. The purpose of calcaneal reconstruction is to optimally restore the local anatomical morphology, stability, and function of this site while considering the shape and abrasion resistance of the heel skin. The reconstruction methods that are

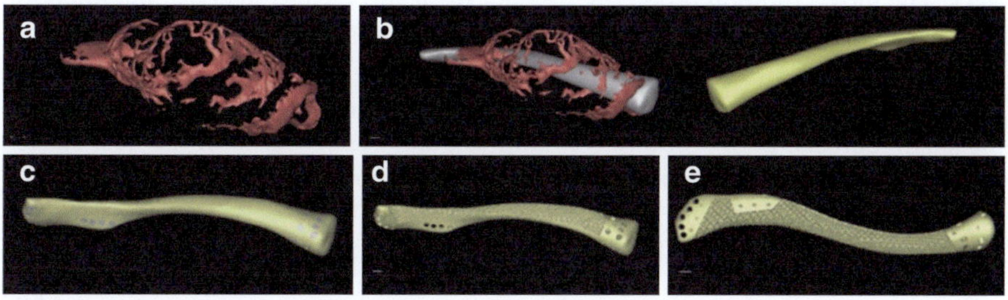

Fig. 4.26 Process of designing a 3D-printed customized clavicular prosthesis. (**a**) The 3D structure of the clavicular tumor on the affected side. (**b**) The appearance of the clavicle prosthesis was designed to mirror the anatomical morphology of the contralateral clavicle. (**c**) The location of the suture hole was determined according to the needs of each joint reconstruction. (**d**) The anterior view of the overall design of the prosthesis. (**e**) Bottom view

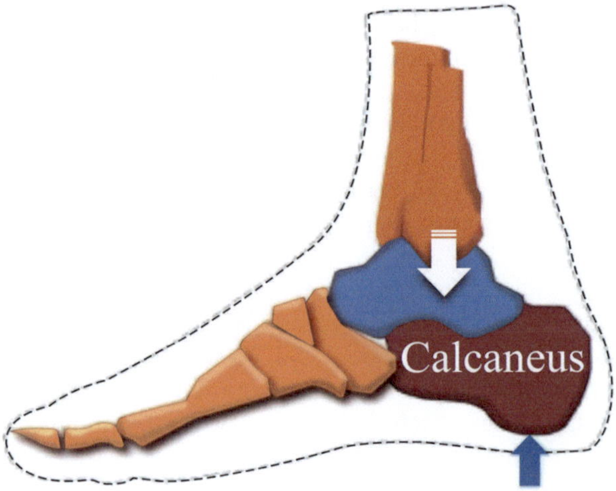

Fig. 4.27 Anatomical location and bearing function of the calcaneus

used after calcaneal malignant tumor resection mainly include autogenous fibular grafting, tumor bone inactivation, and reconstruction with allogeneic bone grafting. Autogenous fibular grafting can cause new trauma, and the probability of infection, fracture, nonunion, and wound dehiscence of the inactivated bone and allogeneic bone is high. Previous case reports have described custom-made calcaneal prostheses that cause moderate weight-bearing pain despite satisfactory appearance and function (Chou and Malawer 2007).

The advent of 3D-printing technology provides new options for reconstructing the complex morphology of the calcaneus. In 2014, for the first time, a medical and engineering interaction team in Australia reconstructed a calcaneus after tumor resection in an elderly patient with a calcaneal tumor using a 3D-printed individualized prosthesis, and the shape and weight-bearing function of the heel were restored after the operation (Imanishi and Choong 2015).

However, 3D-printed customized calcaneal prostheses are also associated with risks. The most common problems are poor local soft tissue coverage and infection (Fig. 4.28), because with current 3D-printed metal prostheses, the plantar skin experiences too much stress during weight-bearing while walking, which often causes unbearable pain and eventually leads to prosthesis removal (Fig. 4.29). Therefore, local skin defects, poor soft tissue conditions, and hypoesthesia of the heel caused by diabetes or neurological diseases are contraindications for prosthetic reconstruction.

The heel is the main load-bearing part of the human body. The local soft tissue coverage is relatively thin, and surgery further damages the local blood supply, which causes pain while weight bearing and the risk of infection after calcaneal prosthesis implantation. Therefore, more caution should be taken when using 3D-printed metal prostheses to reconstruct weight-bearing body parts with poor soft tissue conditions (Zhao et al. 2023).

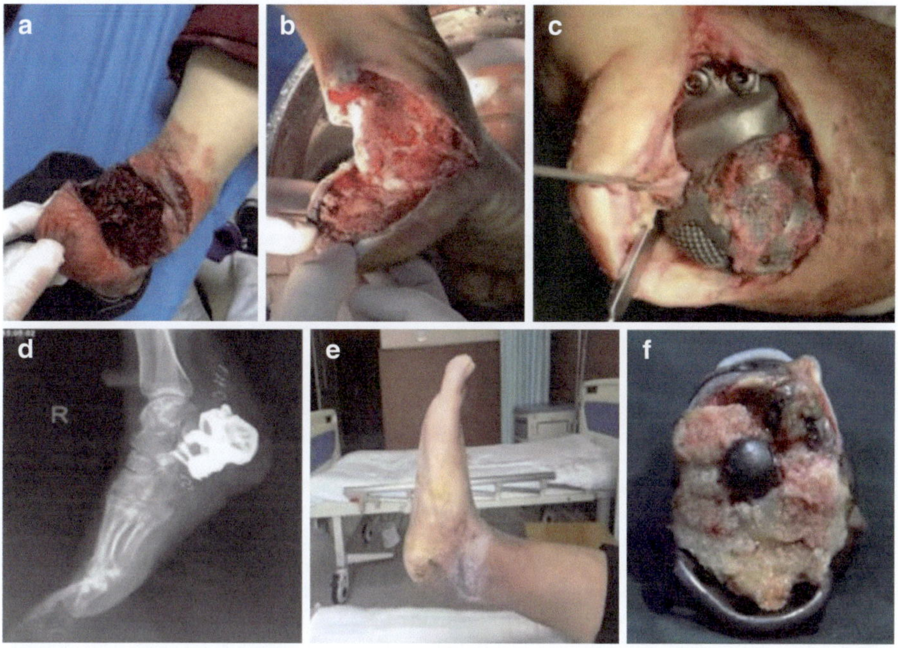

Fig. 4.28 3D-printed customized calcaneal prosthesis implantation with infection and removal. (**a**) Heel avulsion injury and calcaneal comminuted fracture. (**b**) Calcaneal defect after local debridement. (**c**) The calcaneal defect was repaired with a 3D-printed customized calcaneal prosthesis combined with autologous bone 6 months after one-stage debridement. (**d**) X-ray image after calcaneal reconstruction showing that the position of the prosthesis was satisfactory. (**e**) The shape of the heel was good 3 months after calcaneal reconstruction. (**f**) The calcaneal prosthesis was removed because infection could not be controlled 6 months after calcaneal reconstruction

4.4.4 Design and Application of 3D-Printed Customized Rib Prosthesis

The ribs are small, flat, curved bones, one end of each rib is attached to both sides of the thoracic vertebra in the trunk, the rib curves and extends anteriorly along the chest wall, and the other end is attached to the sternum in the center of the chest or to the sternum by cartilage (Fig. 4.30). The ribs and the bones to which they are attached form the rib cage. The chest can protect the heart and lungs and strengthen respiratory function by combining the muscles between the ribs. Rib defects are caused by various factors. When a single rib defect occurs, reconstruction is not necessary because a single rib defect does not affect the patient's appearance or respiratory function. However, tumors, trauma, and other factors can often cause multiple rib defects at the same time, and multiple rib defects can affect respiratory function, decreasing the ability of the rib cage to protect the heart, lungs, and other important organs. Therefore, it is necessary to reconstruct the ribs after multiple rib

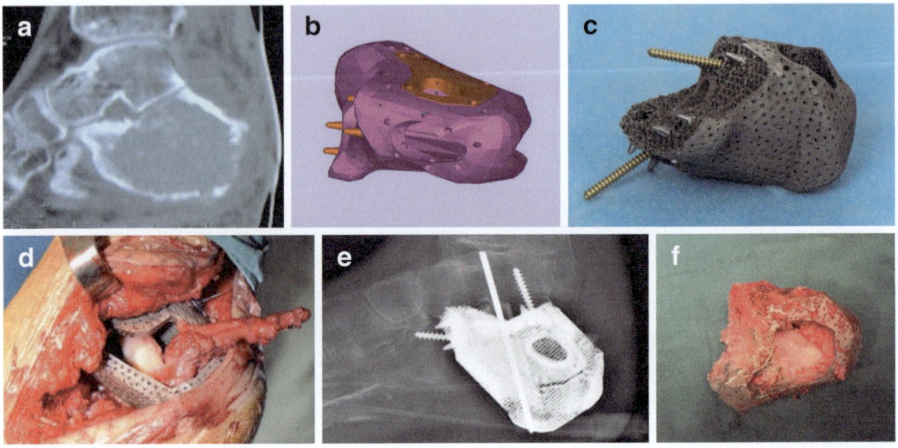

Fig. 4.29 Intractable pain and removal of a 3D-printed, personalized, customized calcaneal prosthesis after implantation. (**a**) Calcaneal invasive tumors with radiographic findings of bone destruction. (**b**) Design of an individualized calcaneal prosthesis. (**c**) 3D-printed customized calcaneal prosthesis. (**d**) Intraoperative tumor resection and reconstruction with a calcaneal prosthesis combined with a free vascularized fibula. (**e**) X-ray images at 3 months after the operation showed that the calcaneal prosthesis was in a good position and was stably fixed (**f**) The calcaneal prosthesis, which was removed one year postoperatively due to intractable heel load-bearing pain, showed evidence of robust osseointegration at its interface with the talus

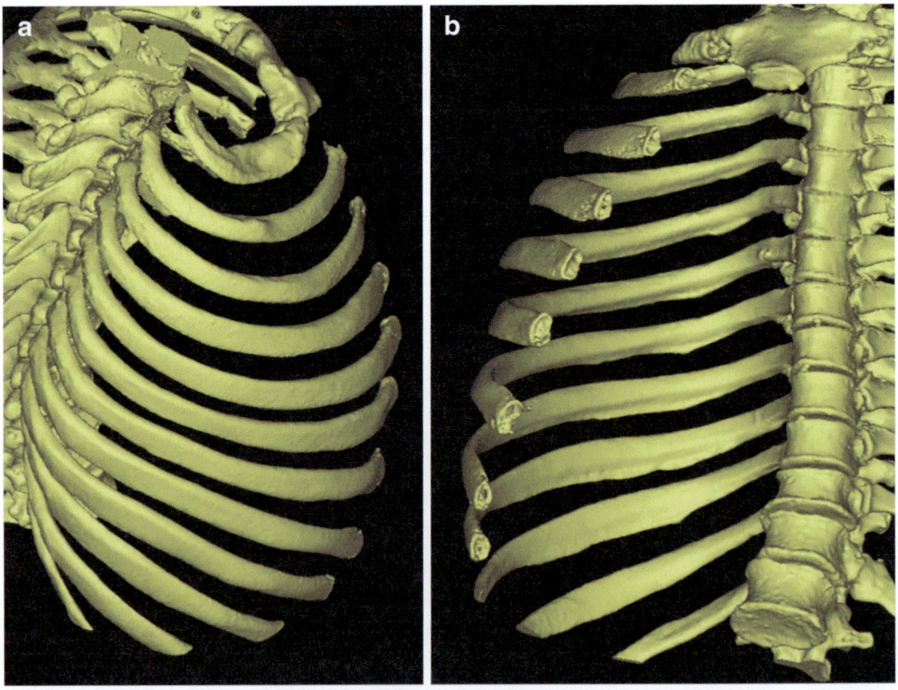

Fig. 4.30 Anatomical structure and shape of ribs. (**a**) Lateral view of the thorax and ribs. (**b**) Medial view of the thorax and ribs

defects occur. With previously available processing technology, it was rare for mature standard rib prostheses to be available on the market. Individualized customization through 3D printing is a good solution.

When designing a rib prosthesis, the unique anatomy of the rib should be considered first (Fig. 4.31). The ribs are flat and thin, so it is difficult to use screws to fix the remaining ribs and the prosthesis, and the ribs need to be sutured with nonabsorbable sutures or wire sutures. The shape of the rib prosthesis should be based on the original shape of the rib, which is flat and curved.

Second, the unique mode by which the ribs move should be considered. As the thorax moves during respiration, the ribs mainly exhibit pump handle movement and bucket-handle movement. Pump handle movement involves rotation of the head end of the rib, similar to the rotation of a fixed shaft, thus driving the up and down movement of the other end. This movement leads to an increase in the chest anteroposterior diameter. "Bucket-handle motion, in which the rib ends are fixed and serve as the axes of rotation, allows only the middle region to move between these two points along a fixed rotation axis, resulting in an increase in the left and right diameter of the thorax." This requires a certain bonding strength between the prosthesis and the rib. The contact points between the two ends and the rib can be designed as flat supports, which are convenient for fitting the rib. Additionally, at least three suture holes are recommended to help firmly fix the rib and the prosthesis.

During prosthesis installation, it should be noted that the ribs are in a relatively superficial position, and it is preferable to be able to use the surrounding muscles to provide good soft tissue coverage of the prosthesis.

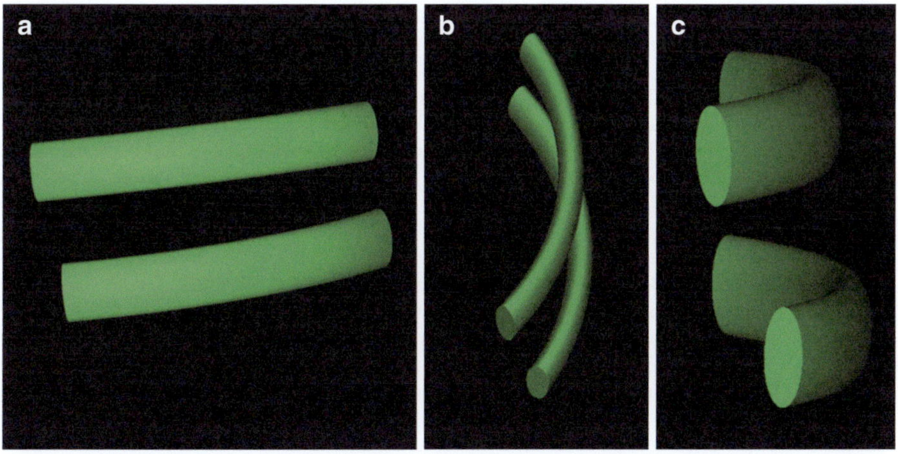

Fig. 4.31 During the design of 3D-printed customized prostheses for ribs, the anatomical morphology of the ribs and the combination of the rib prosthesis and remaining ribs should be fully considered. (**a**) Lateral view of rib prosthesis structure design. (**b**) Top view of a rib prosthesis structure design. (**c**) Lateral design of the rib prosthesis structure

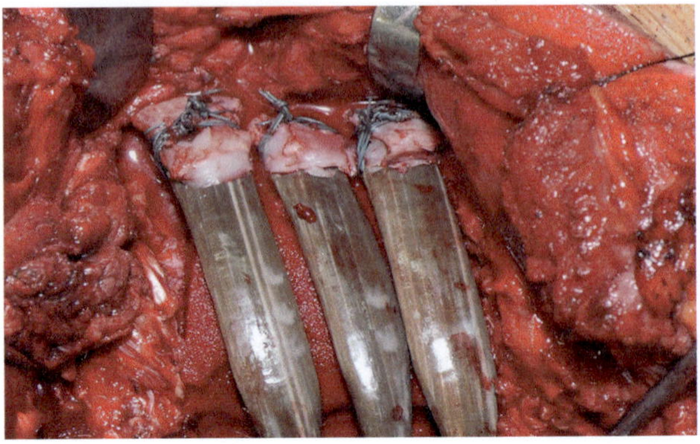

Fig. 4.32 During a surgical operation, a 3D-printed PEEK custom rib prosthesis for the repair of rib defects was fixed between the prosthesis and the rib using soft sutures

In addition, there are many other 3D printing materials that can satisfactorily meet the anatomical and mechanical requirements of rib reconstruction, such as PEEK material (Fig. 4.32) (Zhang et al. 2020).

References

Abudu A, Grimer RJ, Cannon SR, et al. Reconstruction of the hemipelvis after the excision of malignant tumours. Complications and functional outcome of prostheses. J Bone Joint Surg Br. 1997;79(5):773–9.

Capanna R, Bufalini C, Campanacci M. A new technique for reconstructions of large metadiaphiseal bone defects. Orthop Traumatol 1993;3:159–77.

Chen C, Yin Y, Xu H, et al. Personalized three-dimensional printed polyether-ether-ketone prosthesis for reconstruction after subtotal removal of chronic clavicle osteomyelitis: a case report. Medicine (Baltimore). 2021;100(17):e25703.

Chou LB, Malawer MM. Osteosarcoma of the calcaneus treated with prosthetic replacement with twelve years of followup: a case report. Foot Ankle Int. 2007;28(7):841–4.

Choy WJ, Mobbs RJ, Wilcox B, et al. Reconstruction of thoracic spine using a personalized 3D-printed vertebral body in adolescent with T9 primary bone tumor. World Neurosurg. 2017;105:1032.e1013–7.

Fan H, Fu J, Li X, et al. Implantation of customized 3-D printed titanium prosthesis in limb salvage surgery: a case series and review of the literature. World J Surg Oncol. 2015;13:308.

Girolami M, Boriani S, Bandiera S, et al. Biomimetic 3D-printed custom-made prosthesis for anterior column reconstruction in the thoracolumbar spine: a tailored option following en bloc resection for spinal tumors: preliminary results on a case-series of 13 patients. Eur Spine J. 2018;27(12):3073–83.

Imanishi J, Choong PF. Three-dimensional printed calcaneal prosthesis following total calcanectomy. Int J Surg Case Rep. 2015;10:83–7.

Krishna SV, Gupta SK, Holla N, et al. Resection of osteoid osteoma using three-dimensional (3D) printing. Indian J Orthop. 2022;56(9):1657–61.

Matsumoto M, Watanabe K, Tsuji T, et al. Late instrumentation failure after total en bloc spondylectomy. J Neurosurg Spine. 2011;15(3):320–7.

Mayfield CK, Ayad M, Lechtholz-Zey E, et al. 3D-printing for critical sized bone defects: current concepts and future directions. Bioengineering (Basel). 2022;9(11):680.

Streck LE, Straub A, Boettner F, et al. Treatment of symptomatic pseudarthrosis following acromion fracture with a patient-specific implant customized on a 3D-printed scapula. Oper Orthop Traumatol. 2023;35(5):270–7.

Tomita K, Kawahara N, Baba H, et al. Total en bloc spondylectomy. A new surgical technique for primary malignant vertebral tumors. Spine (Phila Pa 1976). 1997;22(3):324–33.

Tomita K, Kawahara N, Murakami H, et al. Total en bloc spondylectomy for spinal tumors: improvement of the technique and its associated basic background. J Orthop Sci. 2006;11(1):3–12.

Wei F, Xu N, Li Z, et al. A prospective randomized cohort study on 3D-printed artificial vertebral body in single-level anterior cervical corpectomy for cervical spondylotic myelopathy. Ann Transl Med. 2020;8(17):1070.

Yoshioka K, Murakami H, Demura S, et al. Clinical outcome of spinal reconstruction after total en bloc spondylectomy at 3 or more levels. Spine (Phila Pa 1976). 2013;38(24):E1511–6.

Zhang C, Wang L, Kang J, et al. Bionic design and verification of 3D printed PEEK costal cartilage prosthesis. J Mech Behav Biomed Mater. 2020;103:103561.

Zhao J, Wang Z, Long C, et al. Using 3D printing-assisted shaping titanium cages and Masquelet techniques to reconstruct calcaneal osteomyelitis complicated by extensive soft tissue and uncontrolled defects. Injury. 2023;54(10):110977.

Evaluation of 3D-Printed Custom-Made Prostheses Applications

5

Shuo Guo, Yanjun Pei, and Xiaokang Li

5.1 Preoperative Assessment of customized Prostheses Produced Via 3D Printing

Preoperative assessments are a crucial part of clinical investigation before surgery and significantly influence the anesthesia method that is chosen, surgical planning, and intraoperative decision-making. A thorough and detailed preoperative evaluation can notably reduce surgery duration and decrease both the surgeon's and patient's exposure to X-rays during the procedure. Preoperative evaluation also plays a pivotal role in accurately identifying surgical risks for the patient. Among surgical procedures, preoperative assessments for orthopedic surgery have unique tendencies and focus areas. These will be introduced one by one below.

Orthopedic surgery is a common surgical procedure that aims to treat diseases and injuries of the skeletal system. Preoperative assessment for orthopedic surgery is vital for ensuring the safety and success rate of the procedure. Given that orthopedic surgery involves critical structures and functions of the skeletal system, evaluating the patient's physical condition, disease characteristics, and complexity of the surgery is essential for predicting surgical risks and implementing measures to mitigate them.

The use of 3D-printing technology to produce customized prosthetic implants for use during orthopedic surgery introduces unique requirements into the

S. Guo
Department of Orthopedics, Tangdu Hospital, Xi'an, China

Department of Radiology, Functional and Molecular Imaging Key Lab of Shaanxi Province, Tangdu Hospital, Xi'an, China

Y. Pei
Department of Orthopedics, People's Hospital of Shenzhen Baoan District, Shenzhen, China

X. Li (✉)
Department of Orthopedics, Tangdu Hospital, Xi'an, China

Z. Guo et al. (eds.), *3D-Printed Prosthesis in Orthopedic Oncology*,
https://doi.org/10.1007/978-981-95-1454-0_5

preoperative assessment process. The generation of 3D-printed customized prostheses involves creating a personalized implant for a patient by using imaging data of the patient's bones and soft tissues. This process identifies the extent and shape of bone loss due to surgical removal. A digital design approach is then used to generate a three-dimensional graphic file, which can be created using 3D-printing technology. The resulting prosthetic is tailored to fit the patient perfectly, mimicking the natural structures of bone at the contact surface and offering excellent bone integration capabilities for reconstruction. It is important to note that, unlike traditional prostheses, 3D-printed prostheses are prepared based on a detailed analysis of the patient's preoperative imaging data. Therefore, the success of prosthetic implantation relies heavily on accurately assessing the anticipated defect size during the preoperative assessment phase and potentially modifying the plan during the intraoperative phase. Thus, the preoperative evaluation of customized prostheses produced by 3D printing is an integral part of the surgical planning process.

5.1.1 Orthopedic Surgery Risk Assessment Methods

(1) Clinical Evaluation This initial step involves a thorough physical examination and medical history review by the surgeon to determine the patient's overall health status, medical history, and symptoms. The evaluation extends to assessing the health of the patient's cardiovascular system, respiratory system, and kidney function to determine surgical risks. For surgeries that involve 3D-printed customized prostheses, identifying the appropriate indications and contraindications is crucial.

Indications for using 3D-printed customized prostheses:

1. The general and local conditions of the patient are conducive to undergoing surgery.
2. Bone defects that have occurred due to any cause need to be repaired.
3. Conventional prostheses cannot meet the requirements for bone defect repair, or the repair process will be challenging.
4. In accordance with standard treatment principles, tumor patients should comply with the principles of surgical treatment for tumors.

Contraindications:

1. The patient cannot undergo surgery due to their overall and local conditions, such as active infections, inability to achieve optimal surgical margins for tumor removal, inability to ensure adequate soft tissue coverage, or the function cannot be restored after primary tumor resection, or the function would be inferior compared to that achieved by prosthetic alternatives.
2. The bone defects can be repaired using conventional prostheses or other methods and, in some cases, may not require repair at all. Compared with these methods,

the use of customized 3D-printed tumor prostheses does not significantly improve limb function.
3. The patient and their family may not want to use such treatments or may not be able to afford the associated medical costs.

(2) Laboratory Tests Routine laboratory tests, such as complete blood counts, biochemical markers, and coagulation profiles, are conducted to gauge the patient's physiological condition and identify potential surgical risk factors.

(3) Imaging Studies Imaging techniques, such as X-rays, CT scans, and MRIs, are crucial for evaluating the patient's bone structure, the extent of the injury, and the condition of surrounding tissues. These tests help determine the complexity and risks of surgery. For a precise assessment, imaging studies might include X-rays of the pelvis, three-dimensional CT, MRI, standing X-rays of both lower limbs, whole-body bone scans, or PET-CT. For a CT scan to meet the necessary standards, the following conditions should be satisfied:

1. Multislice spiral CT with a small pitch is recommended.
2. The scan range should be determined based on the requirements for prosthesis design and clinical needs.
3. A scan interval of 1 mm or less is recommended.
4. Scan parameters should be set according to the needs of the prosthesis design and clinical requirements.
5. A CT device that offers a resolution with a pixel matrix of 512 × 512 and a pixel size range of 0.1~0.5 mm is recommended.
6. Proper positioning during scanning, ensuring that the long axis of the limb aligns with the scanning direction and that both limbs are symmetrically placed, is beneficial for preoperative planning and measurement.
7. The removal of metal artifacts should meet clinical needs.
8. Vascular enhancement is useful for elucidating the relationship between blood vessels and lesions. MRI offers excellent resolution for soft tissues.

Among MRI techniques, T1 images reveal clear anatomical structures, and this approach is suitable for 3D modeling of bone joints and for guiding prosthesis design. Enhanced MR 2D images are useful for marking tumors and their infiltration range, including the surrounding reaction zone. MRI of water content is particularly helpful for visualizing the lumbar and sacral plexus nerves.

The final step involves creating a visual 3D-image model through medical image fusion. This process combines images from different radiological examinations (such as CT or MRI) of the same patient and the same body part. By integrating the strengths and details of various imaging techniques, a richer image can be produced. This allows for the creation of a 3D digital model that visualizes the patient's radiological data. Surgeons can use this model for preoperative assessment to determine the tumor's location, depth, and blood supply, aiding in the development of a preoperative plan to improve surgical outcomes. For bone tumors, this method can simultaneously display the bone tumor and soft tissue masses, facilitating the determination of the extent of the tumor and the proximity of important surrounding structures.

(4) Specialist Assessment Orthopedic surgeries require evaluations by specialists who consider the type of surgery and the patient's specific conditions to assess the feasibility and risks of the procedure and to provide recommendations and plans accordingly.

5.1.2 Special Assessment for Prosthetic Implantation

Overall, the preimplantation assessment of 3D-printed prostheses encompasses factors other than those that are related to the prosthetic itself. Since medical devices are used in clinical practice, the assessment also includes consideration of the material and origin of the 3D-printed prostheses, the economic and time costs they impose on patients, and their lifespan. Depending on their purpose, these assessments can be categorized as assessments of models for presurgical planning and assessments of prostheses for preimplantation assessment, and models and prostheses require different printing materials. customized, 3D-printed, implantable prostheses, which are designed based on individual patient conditions and surgical plans, are a prime example of personalized surgical solutions. For instance, titanium alloy prostheses, once designed, are processed through metal 3D-printers, resulting in ready-to-use customized implants before surgery. These customized prostheses, which are difficult to alter once created, necessitate strict adherence to the surgical plan by the operating surgeon, including the precise cutting of bone according to the plan. This technique demands high expertise of the lead surgeon, especially for those with limited experience in customized 3D-printed prostheses, as deviations can easily occur during surgery. Therefore, a comprehensive, personalized presurgical assessment is essential.

Nonmetal 3D-printing technology plays a significant role in the presurgical assessment of individualized prostheses, offering substantial assistance. Before the clinical application of customized 3D-printed prostheses, printing skeletal and tissue models of the surgical area, including models of the area before and after tumor resection, and even 3D-printed guides for precise bone cutting or screw placement, can be invaluable. These models provide the surgical team with preliminary insights into surgical approaches and the potential involvement of vessels and nerves during surgery. Postresection models allow the direct assessment of the postsurgery deficit of surrounding tissue, aiding in the prediction of postoperative tissue preservation and functional recovery and thereby optimizing the surgical plan. Moreover, 3D-printed physical models not only technically support surgeons in familiarizing themselves with the surgical plan before surgery, but also enhance doctor–patient communication throughout the clinical process and confirm the accuracy of surgical operations.

After completing the preoperative planning of a 3D-printed prosthetic model, it is typical to proceed with intraoperative planning as the basis for printing the metal prosthetic implant at the original scale. The surgical team then evaluates the prosthetic design, interface treatment, and detail processing, modeling the entire surgical process before officially printing the prosthetic.

5.2 The Installation and Evaluation of 3D-Printed prostheses During Surgery Are Pivotal for Determining the Success of Reconstructive Efforts

Surgeons must integrate surgical procedures with potential changes in the defect area to inform the design of customized prostheses, prepare alternative reconstruction plans before surgery, and adjust the approach for prosthetic installation during the operation.

5.2.1 Assistance and Operation of Precise Installation in Prosthetic Surgery with 3D Printing

The purpose of using 3D-printed customized prostheses is to accurately repair bone and joint defects. The precision of prosthetic installation during surgery is essential for ensuring the safe and effective use of the prosthetic. Clinical causes of bone defects include congenital abnormalities, infectious bone loss, traumatic bone loss, periprosthetic bone resorption, bone tumor destruction, and surgical resection. Achieving a precise match between customized prostheses and various types of complex bone defects requires thorough preoperative planning and the use of digital technology aids, such as computer-assisted navigation and customized surgical guides, to perform osteotomy and prosthetic installation.

With the aid of digital technology, customized 3D-printed prostheses are designed and prepared based on the unique bone and joint defect of the particular patient. The consistency between preoperative design planning and clinical use determines the effectiveness of prostheses. Due to the complex morphology and structure of customized prostheses, their precise installation cannot rely only on clinical experience; rather, the assistance of digital technology, including computer-assisted navigation, customized surgical guides, and customized surgical tools, is often required (Jeys et al. 2013).

Navigation technology allows surgeons to identify the relationships between tumor lesions and surrounding anatomical structures more intuitively and accurately during surgery. This real-time three-dimensional imaging feedback enables more precise tumor removal. In the absence of navigation equipment, precise osteotomy and accurate customized prosthetic installation can still be achieved through customized osteotomy guides (Fig. 5.1); this process necessitates effective interaction between medical professionals and engineers.

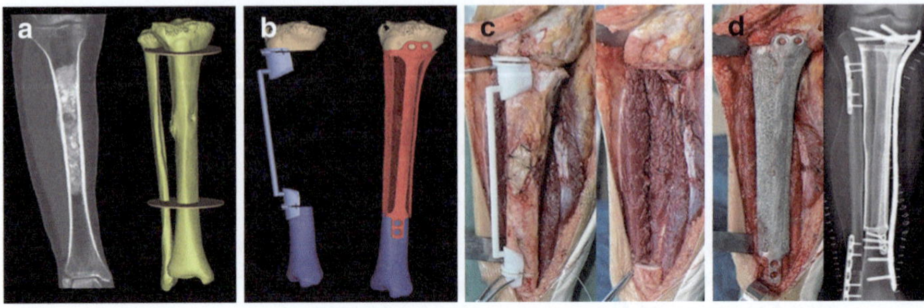

Fig. 5.1 Precision resection of osteosarcoma in the tibia assisted by a 3D-printed, individually customized osteotomy guide plate. The procedure for the personalized customization of reconstruction prostheses involves several critical steps: (**a**) Design of the osteotomy boundary for tibial tumors. (**b**) Use of personalized osteotomy guides to model precise bone cutting and prosthetic fitting. (**c**) Use of intraoperative osteotomy guides to direct the complete excision of the tumor. (**d**) Intraoperative placement of the customized prosthesis and postoperative imaging to ensure an exact fit of the prosthetic

Notably, despite the precise implementation of operational procedures to install individually customized prostheses that are produced by 3D printing, which usually ensures the execution of the installation plan, certain factors may impede the smooth placement of the prosthesis, necessitating timely modifications to the surgical plan and reconstruction strategy. These factors include the following:

1. Failure to fully consider the range of exposure in the surgical approach and the obstruction of critical tissue structures during customized prosthesis design can result in oversized prostheses that are difficult to implant. For instance, during reconstruction of a vertebral body following posterior pathological vertebral resection for a collapsed L5 vertebra, due to obstruction by nerve roots on both sides, the volume of the customized L5 artificial vertebral body was too large, making it difficult to place the implant from the back and requiring an anterior implantation approach (Fig. 5.2).
2. Intraoperative changes to the surgical plan can result in either an expansion or reduction of the bone resection area, rendering the preoperatively designed customized prosthesis unable to fully match the bone defect area. This necessitates the formulation of alternative reconstruction plans preoperatively, and traditional reconstruction methods or conventional prostheses are used in such scenarios.
3. Surgery should be terminated if no suitable replacement reconstruction material is found intraoperatively, and a second-phase implantation should be planned after a customized prosthesis is redesigned and prepared based on the range of the bone and joint defect.
4. Bone grafting is required to fill any remaining defect cavities around the implanted customized prosthesis to enhance the prosthetic-bone interface attachment and increase the stability of the prosthesis.

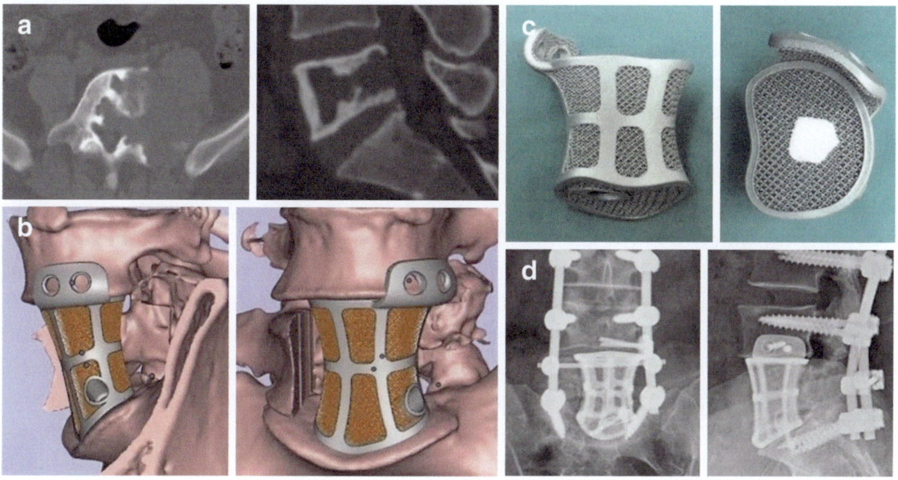

Fig. 5.2 The use of 3D printing for personalized customization to reconstruct the L5 vertebral body after tumor removal surgery. (**a**) The preoperative CT image of an L5 vertebral giant cell tumor. (**b**) The design and preoperative modeling of a personalized custom L5 artificial vertebral body. (**c**) The 3D-printed, personalized, self-locking artificial vertebral body. (**d**) The postoperative X-ray appearance following tumor resection and artificial vertebral body reconstruction of the L5 vertebra

5. When the shape or size of the customized prosthesis prevents smooth implantation, it may be necessary to appropriately adjust the defect area or increase exposure to facilitate prosthesis installation.
6. Deformations in the defect area caused by positioning or surgical maneuvers, leading to a poor match between the customized prosthesis and the original defect area, necessitate the use of auxiliary instruments to restore the original defect shape in order to ensure good matching between the defect area and the prosthesis. This often involves the use of supporting rods for personalized artificial vertebral bodies to spread, compress, or bend, thereby ensuring close attachment to the adjacent endplates and restoring the physiological curvature of the spine.

5.2.2 Key Points in Evaluating the Intraoperative Placement of 3D-Printed customized Prostheses

The precision of the intraoperative installation of 3D-printed customized prostheses is crucial for ensuring clinical efficacy. Due to their personalized nature, customized prostheses offer limited scope for adjustments during surgery, necessitating precise execution according to presurgical planning. The evaluation of prosthetic installation involves a comprehensive assessment through direct visualization, fluoroscopy, or navigation guidance, and the examination of alignment, orientation, and rotation to ensure correct placement. Depending on the application site, such as the limbs, pelvis, or spine, there are specific points of interest during the evaluation phase. For instance, the installation of artificial vertebral bodies in the spine is complicated by the fact that patients are positioned face down with their abdomen suspended, which can lead to an increased anterior curvature of the lumbar spine. The surgical procedures of stripping the posterior soft tissue and removing the posterior appendages further increase this forward curvature, making the placement and adjustment of the artificial vertebrae more challenging and complex. During surgery, accurately assessing the anterior convex angle of the sagittal plane of the spine and the compatibility of the artificial vertebrae are crucial for correct placement. For the placement of pelvic prostheses, especially the placement of acetabular prostheses in the pelvic area, it is essential to accurately evaluate the abduction angle, anteversion angle, and center of acetabular rotation of the acetabular cup. Relying solely on the surgeon's experience or intraoperative three-dimensional spatial assessments can lead to significant errors. In such cases, utilizing computer navigation technology for three-dimensional spatial positioning and assessment of acetabular placement can achieve greater accuracy.

5.3 Postoperative Evaluation of 3D-Printed customized Prostheses

5.3.1 Evaluation Indicators and Methods for Imaging 3D-Printed customized Prostheses

The evaluation of 3D-printed customized prostheses by imaging is similar to that of standard prostheses, and the methods that are used include X-rays, CT scans, bone scans, and MRI. Currently, X-rays and CT scans are the primary methods used for assessing osseointegration and implant stability. Postoperative evaluation with X-rays includes static and dynamic views to assess whether the artificial vertebral body has fused with adjacent vertebrae. Static X-ray Evaluation: Static anterolateral X-ray is the most conventional and longest-used method for assessing fusion after spinal fusion surgery. From the anterolateral view, one can determine the continuity of the bone bridge, the presence of radiolucent zones around the intervertebral fusion device and internal fixation, whether the fusion device has subsided, the position and condition of the internal fixation, and the relative displacement between vertebrae. The Brantigan and Steffee evaluation method is currently the method that is most widely used in clinical practice (Table 5.1) (Brantigan and Steffee 1993). Power Position Evaluation: In the picture archiving and communication system (PACS), a criterion for determining spinal fusion is when the interspinous motion (ISM) is less than 1 mm in a 150% magnified dynamic lateral view, and the ISM of adjacent non-fused segments is greater than 4 mm. Conversely, values outside of these criteria indicate a lack of fusion.

Unlike follow-up after the implantation of conventional prostheses, follow-up after the implantation of 3D-printed customized prostheses relies more on

Table 5.1 The spinal fusion grading system by Brantigan and Steffee

Grade	Performance
A	Pseudarthrosis leads to significant structural collapse, including loss of intervertebral disc height, vertebral slippage, broken screws, displacement of fusion devices, and bone graft resorption.
B	The formation of pseudarthrosis can result in notable bone graft resorption, with large translucent zones or cracks visible within the fusion area (all around the implant edges up to 2 mm).
C	The uncertainty of bone continuity, with the density of bone grafts in the fusion area comparable to that immediately postsurgery. At least 50% of the fusion area displays small translucent zones or cracks.
D	The entire bone graft area may show potential fusion with bone bridges of density comparable to that immediately postsurgery, with no translucent zones between vertebrae.
E	The bone density in the fusion area exceeds that observed immediately postsurgery. Even though the sclerotic lines between the implant and vertebrae suggest fusion, ideally, there should be no clear demarcation between the implant and the vertebrae. Other indications of fusion include bone bridges within the fusion area, resorption of anterior osteophytes, and fusion of the facet joints.

From Literature: Brantigan and Steffee (1993)

three-dimensional CT reconstructions. This is primarily because the follow-up after 3D-printed prosthetic reconstruction involves not only observing the position of the prosthetic but also monitoring osseointegration based on the porous structure of the prosthesis and its interaction with the adjacent bone tissue. The most critical indicator for evaluating fusion by CT is the presence of continuous bone bridges passing through the fusion segment's upper and lower endplates, with no radiolucent zones at the junctions between the implant and the vertebral body. Indicators of nonfusion include subsidence of the fusion device, cystic changes in the endplates, and the halo sign around the implant. The criteria that are most commonly used to evaluate fusion by CT (Siepe et al. 2015) (Table 5.2).

Radiostereometric analysis (RSA) has emerged as an innovative technique that is used as an alternative to traditional X-ray and CT imaging technologies (Sandberg et al. 2023). This approach enables precise measurements of bone tissue and implants marked with reference points at different time intervals using X-rays. Subsequently, with computer assistance, the positional changes of these markers can be analyzed to obtain accurate three-dimensional spatial measurements and detailed motion assessments. This has led to the widespread application of RSA in orthopedic research in recent years, including in the evaluation of joint motion and stability, prosthetic joints, and spinal fusion, among others. The measurement accuracy of RSA technology can reach 10–250 μm and 0.03–0.6°, so this approach offers a more accurate assessment of the in vivo status of implants from a three-dimensional perspective. This technique is particularly useful for the early detection of implant loosening or displacement. For instance, a study by Ryd and colleagues (Ryd et al. 1995) involving 131 patients who underwent total knee arthroplasty observed tibial components for 4 years using RSA technology. The findings indicated that a displacement of the prosthesis beyond 0.2 mm within 2 years could

Table 5.2 Metrics for fusion evaluation by CT

Grade	Integration	Performance
Level 1	Complete integration	The bone trabeculae clearly connect the superior and inferior endplates with evidence of osseous remodeling (100%)
		Continuous bone bridges have formed around the fusion device
		The interface between the fusion device and the end plate is securely connected
		The fusion device is not surrounded by a light-transmitting band
		The fusion device or vertebral body shows no visible fractures or damage
		There are no vesicular alterations adjacent to the terminal plate
		New bone formed in the center or periphery of the fusion device without linear fractures
		The fusion device remains stable without settling or shifting
Level 2	The hallmark of strong integration	Bone bridges and trabeculae constitute more than 75% of the fusion area
		Local bone trabeculae penetrate the endplate
		Elimination of any nonintegrative factors
Level 3	There may be no signs of strong integration	The terminal plate exhibits restricted bone bridging
		At the junction between the fusion device and the end plate, a robust connection is present on one side only
Level 4	Unfused	Clear indications of a lack of fusion
		Generating continuous/complete fissures
		Edge hardening of cracks
		Vacuum phenomenon
		Discontinuity in the bone bridge
		Fusion reactor's perimeter of translucent bands
		Visible fusion device damage or vertebral fracture
		Terminal plate saccular transformation
		Linear fractures or defects in the newly formed bone at the center or periphery of the fusion device
		Fusion reactor submergence and displacement
		In the fusion device, there are no continuous bone bridges either centrally or peripherally

significantly predict the likelihood of revision. With technological advancements, the RSA product line, including tantalum beads and implant devices, along with supporting computers and professional software, has matured significantly, surpassing the precision of traditional techniques and attracting the attention of those who use precision-oriented 3D-printing technology. A 2020 study by Hasan et al. applied RSA technology to assess the in vivo stability of a novel 3D-printed, nonbone cement knee prosthesis. This study utilized multiple spherical tantalum beads (φ=0.8mm; RSABiomedical, Umeå, Sweden) that were placed within the tibia and its polyethylene liner of the tibial component as markers for measurement. RSA measurements were then performed at four postoperative intervals: 2 days, 3 months, 1 year, and 2 years. The collected data were analyzed using Model-Based RSA (RSAcore, Leiden, Netherlands) software to measure the mobility of this 3D-printed, nonbone cement knee prosthesis within the body, assessing its initial stability postimplantation.

5.3.2 Metrics and Methods for the Functional Evaluation of 3D-Printed customized prostheses

The most commonly used approach for postoperative evaluation after bone tumor surgeries is the Musculoskeletal Tumor Society (MSTS) scoring system (Enneking et al. 1993), which assesses limb function after limb-sparing surgery for bone tumors. This system includes the following aspects:

1. Limb Pain: Assessed through verbal inquiries and medical records reviews, this component evaluates the patient's current pain experience, the impact of pain on activities over the past month, and the use of analgesics (Table 5.3).
2. Activity Function: The term "activity function" refers to the extent to which occupational function is lost in patients due to limited mobility, taking into account the characteristics of occupational activity levels. Typically, the volume of occupational activities and the extent of limb function application should be less than that of leisure activities. Evaluations are primarily conducted through inquiries and observation of activities (Table 5.4).
3. Self-Perception: The patient's self-perception is investigated, focusing primarily on satisfaction and emotional acceptance (Table 5.5).
4. Orthotic Usage: This study involves an investigation into patients' use of orthotics. This necessitates the preparation of canes and crutches for actual inspection at the follow-up site. Patients with intermediate scores are tested under both types of support conditions to make the choice that best suits their daily life. This selection process is documented through video recording (Table 5.6).

Table 5.3 Pain assessment

Grade	Status	Reference
5	Pain-free	No pain experienced, thus no need for any analgesics
4	Mild pain	Slight discomfort experienced, no need for medication or occasional use of nonnarcotic pain relievers
3	Moderate-light pain	Experienced pain but not debilitating pain, managed with nonnarcotic analgesics without the need for anesthetics
2	Moderate pain	A stronger sensation of pain, continuous extensive use of nonnarcotic analgesics or occasional use of anesthetics
1	Moderately severe pain	Intense pain causing disability, intermittent mobility impairment, with intermittent use of anesthetics

Table 5.4 Activity assessment

Grade	Status	Reference
5	Unrestricted	Activities are unrestricted, with leisure and professional life remaining as before the illness
4	Mild restrictions	Leisure and work are similar to preillness levels, but prolonged leisure activities may cause discomfort or a feeling of inadequacy
3	Entertainment restrictions	A minor functional disability is present, with some activities restricted. Leisure activities are limited, allowing only selective or short-term participation, and professional life is slightly affected
2	Moderate functional limitations	With a 50% functional disability, activity is notably restricted, professional life is significantly impacted, such as reduced working hours, decreased workload, or diminished efficiency, or a change in preillness profession has occurred
1	Partial occupational restrictions	The majority of functional abilities are disabled, activities are significantly limited, professional life is greatly restricted, and the patient is unable to engage in normal professional activities
0	All professions restricted	Complete disability has occurred, with all activities severely restricted, rendering any professional engagement impossible

Table 5.5 Self-perception rating score

Grade	Status	Reference
5	Extremely satisfied	The patient was very enthusiastic about undergoing the surgery, expressing gratitude and even recommending the procedure to others
4	Very satisfied	The patient was eager to undergo the operation
3	Satisfied	If given the choice again, the patient would still opt for the same surgery, indicating a level of satisfaction
2	Somewhat satisfied	The patient's attitude could be described as passable, showing some degree of acceptance
1	Acceptable	However, there was a sense of dissatisfaction, yet if faced with the same decision, the patient would reluctantly choose the same surgery again
0	Disliked	Ultimately, there was regret over choosing this type of surgery, to the extent that amputation would have been preferred

Table 5.6 Support equipment usage rating

Grade	Status	Reference
5	Unused	No support is needed for mobility
4	Occasional support use	Occasionally, or when fatigued, a cane (hand-supported) is used
3	Frequent support use	Most of the time, reliance on a cane is necessary
2	Occasional cane use	Occasionally, crutches (with underarm support) are employed
1	One cane	For the most part, crutches are essential, and without them, one can only manage minimal movement or hopping on one leg
0	Two canes	To walk, the use of two crutches is mandatory; without them, walking is not possible

5. Walking Ability: This test involves walking back and forth indoors for approximately 5 meters and outdoors for 25 meters without the use of aids. The process is recorded by video (Table 5.7).
6. Gait Changes: Changes in gait during the walking ability test are observed and recorded with video documentation (Table 5.8).

The criteria for evaluating the main joints of the body are described, and these criteria are not significantly different from those used for conventional joint assessments.

For the knee joint, the American Knee Society (AKS) scoring system, which was introduced in 1989, is primarily used. This comprehensive standard evaluates the overall function and morphology of the knee, offering a precise assessment of the joint's condition. Since its introduction, this scoring system has been widely applied in the preoperative and postoperative evaluation of total knee replacement patients.

The hip joint is most commonly assessed using the Harris score, which is a method that is widely used to evaluate hip joint function. This score is frequently used to assess the outcomes of hip preservation and joint replacement, and it includes aspects such as pain, function, deformity, and range of motion, thereby providing a comprehensive evaluation system.

Table 5.7 Walking ability score

Grade	Status	Reference
5	Unrestricted	The ability to walk is similar to that before illness
4	Occasionally restricted	There are minimal restrictions when walking, allowing for unaffected outings
3	Restricted	The ability to walk is now significantly reduced, making it unsuitable for long distances, such as more than one bus stop
2	Significantly limited	Going for walks has become risky and is not recommended
1	Able to walk indoors only	Movement is only possible with the support of fixed objects, and going outdoors is not an option
0	Unable to walk independently	Mobility now requires the use of a wheelchair or complete dependence on others

Table 5.8 Gait assessment score

Grade	Status	Reference
5	Normal	No changes, no need for concealment
4	Slight changes	The change in gait is subtle, not causing any surprise
3	Mild changes	There is a slight change in gait appearance, requiring concealment
2	Moderate changes	The gait is abnormal, necessitating an effort to disguise
1	Significant changes	The gait is clearly abnormal, with partial loss of function
0	Severe disability	The gait is severely impaired, with significant functional loss

The ankle joint is often evaluated with the America Orthopedic Foot & Ankle Society (AOFAS) score, which measures pain, walking ability, gait, range of motion in the lower leg joints, ankle stability, and joint alignment.

The wrist joint is assessed using the Cooney score, which measures pain, functional status, range of motion, and grip strength across four main areas.

For the shoulder joint, the University of California, Los Angeles (UCLA) system, which is designed to assess the effectiveness of total shoulder arthroplasty and to supplementarily evaluate the outcomes of rotator cuff repairs, is used. This system pays detailed attention to the range of motion and shoulder strength, increasing the ease of use.

Seven aspects of follow-up after reconstruction with 3D-printed customized prostheses are indispensable: time, imaging, positioning, secondary injuries, pathology, functional assessment, and survival rates:

1. Timing: Follow-up visits should occur in the 1st month, 3rd month, 6th month, and 12th month postsurgery and then annually thereafter.
2. Imaging: Routine examinations include X-rays and 3D CT scans, as well as color ultrasound of the surgical area. Based on specific needs, regular follow-ups with chest CT scans and whole-body bone scans using single-photon emission computed tomography (SPECT)/CT are conducted. When there is a suspicion of local recurrence or metastasis, further investigations, such as MRI or PET scans, are also performed.
3. Implant Position: It is crucial to assess whether the reconstruction site is satisfactory by checking for any looseness, breakage, displacement, dislocation, or fractures around the implant.
4. Secondary injuries: It is important to determine whether there are any associated injuries, such as nerve damage, vascular injury, deep vein thrombosis, or bone resorption.
5. Pathology: This evaluation involves detecting infections, rejection, tumor recurrence, and metastasis.
6. Functionality assessment.
7. Survival rate (abbreviated).

5.4 Accelerated Rehabilitation Assessment After 3D-Printed customized Prosthesis Implantations

With the rapid advancement of digital technologies in the medical field, the application of 3D-printed customized prostheses during bone defect reconstruction surgeries has become widespread, significantly enhancing the precision and safety of these procedures. Accurate reconstruction provides the essential anatomical foundation for functional recovery, and postoperative rehabilitation training plays a crucial role in achieving the anticipated functional outcomes for patients. 3D-printed prosthetic reconstruction is typically customized, allowing for personalized plans for early rehabilitation treatment that can expedite recovery beyond what is achievable with standard orthopedic surgery. Currently, there is no one-size-fits-all solution. This discussion initiates a conversation on early rehabilitation following patient reconstruction with 3D-printed customized prostheses, proposing a preliminary treatment plan that is centered on rehabilitation training and supported by health education, nutritional support, complication management, and psychological support (Briguglio et al. 2023; Parikh and Crawford 2003; Vincent et al. 2015; Zheng and Yan 2023).

5.4.1 Rehabilitation Training

Rehabilitation training primarily includes physical rehabilitation and therapeutic rehabilitation. The orthopedic applications of customized 3D-printed prostheses predominantly focus on spinal surgery, joint surgery, and bone trauma surgery. The specific rehabilitation training that is required varies according to the site of surgery. For instance, postoperative physical rehabilitation following the implantation of a customized 3D-printed vertebral body primarily focuses on restoring lower limb strength within the first 10 days to prevent venous thrombosis and enhance leg strength. After this period, exercises to strengthen the lumbar and back muscles, such as strengthening the oblique muscles through McKenzie strengthening exercises, abdominal muscle strengthening exercises, and spinal flexion exercises, can be introduced. The rehabilitation protocols for hip and knee replacements are detailed in Tables 5.9 and 5.10, respectively. Physical therapy modalities include

Table 5.9 Rehabilitation of movement after customized hip joint prosthesis replacement surgery via 3D printing

Timepoint	Training content	Duration and frequency
3 days before surgery	1. Exercises for lifting the buttocks, equal lengthening of the quadriceps, and activation of both the glutes and quadriceps	Depending on the patient's specific conditions
1–3 days after surgery	1. Quadriceps strengthening exercises 2. Gluteal contraction exercises 3. Straight leg raises 4. Patella mobilization exercises	1. 30 reps/set, 4 sets/day 2. 20 reps/set, 3 sets/day 3. 50 reps/set, 5 sets/day 4. 20 reps/set, 3 sets/day
1 week after surgery	1. Leg lifts while keeping the leg straight 2. Exercises for lateral movement on the affected side 3. Hip and knee flexion exercises 4. Transitioning from lying to a semi-reclined position exercises	1. 10 reps/set, 3 sets/day 2. 20 reps/set, 3 sets/day 3. 10 reps/set, 3 sets/day 4. 30 reps/set, 3 sets/day
2–3 weeks after surgery	1. Abduction exercises while lying on the back 2. Transitioning from lying to sitting position exercises 3. Toe-tapping exercises	1. 30 reps/set, 3 sets/day 2. 30 reps/set, 3 sets/day 3. 30 reps/set, 3 sets/day
4 weeks after surgery	1. Squatting practice 2. Up and down stairs practice	1. 30 reps/set, 3 sets/day 2. 20 reps/set, 3 sets/day

Table 5.10 Postoperative rehabilitation after customized 3D-printed prosthetic knee joint replacement

Timepoint	Training content	Duration and frequency
Preoperative training	1. Before surgery, patients should lift their ankles with a weight of 1–2.5 kg and perform leg-lifting exercises 2. Patients should also engage in passive exercises for the knee joint, including isometric exercises for the quadriceps and straight leg raises	1. Perform the exercise for 20 s/repetition, completing 15 repetitions/set, and do 4 sets/day 2. Complete 15 repetitions/set for 4 sets each day
1–2 days postsurgery	1. Quadriceps isometric contraction exercises 2. Straight leg raises	1. 150 repetitions/set, with 4 sets daily 2. Aim for 10 repetitions/set, across 3 sets each day
2–5 days postsurgery	1. Passive training for joint flexion 2. Active training for joint flexion 3. Joint extension exercises	1. Execute 10 repetitions/set for 3 sets daily 2. Accomplish 15 repetitions/set, doing 5 sets/day 3. Spend 15 min/set, completing 3 sets each day
More than 5 days postsurgery	Walk with the aid of a walker	Start with 3–5 min/repetition, gradually increasing to 2–3 times/set

low-frequency pulsed ultrasound stimulation, the application of electromagnetic fields, and infrared therapy, and the appropriate modalities are selected based on the patient's primary condition and characteristics. The use of these treatments should be avoided in patients with specific contraindications, such as those who have undergone surgery for malignant tumors.

5.4.2 Health Education

Health education is currently considered to be an indispensable component of surgical treatment. Educating patients and their families allows them to understand the necessity and significance of surgery as well as the potential complications that may arise. Additionally, education aids in accurately informing patients and their families about the advantages and disadvantages of using 3D-printed prostheses for the repair of bone defects. This knowledge significantly contributes to more effective collaboration between patients and medical staff, thereby reducing patient recovery time.

5.4.3 Nutritional Support

Nutritional support plays a vital role in the comprehensive management of patients undergoing surgical procedures. Before surgery, it is essential to conduct nutritional risk screening and intervention, minimizing the fasting period. Then, after surgery, it is essential to actively provide nutritional support to facilitate the early resumption of oral intake. For orthopedic surgery patients, especially elderly patients or those with osteoporosis, postoperative recovery of bone defect areas is often impaired, necessitating extensive nutritional support to aid in functional restoration.

5.4.4 Complication Assessment and Management

Patients frequently experience complications, such as lower extremity deep vein thrombosis and surgical site infections, postoperatively. Prolonged bed rest can also lead to the development of pressure ulcers or pulmonary infections, which can adversely affect bone defect repair. Therefore, it is essential to manage complications perioperatively, assess the risk of related complications, and provide close observation or prophylactic treatment for patients who are at high risk of complications.

5.4.5 Psychological Support

Psychological support plays a critical role in the surgical process, as surgery can be a significant psychological stressor for patients, leading to issues such as tension and anxiety. These psychological states can adversely affect patient recovery. The use of 3D-printed custom prostheses to repair bone defects represents a novel surgical treatment method. Patients may have overly high expectations regarding the function of these prostheses, or they may have doubts about this new technology. Both psychological states can be detrimental to normal postoperative recovery. Conducting a psychological assessment of a patient before surgery and providing necessary psychological support based on the assessment results can help alleviate tension and anxiety, effectively accelerating patient recovery.

5.5 Conclusion

The evaluation of 3D-printed prosthetic applications includes three critical phases: preoperative, intraoperative, and postoperative assessments. The preoperative evaluation is foundational, ensuring the safe and accurate implantation of a prosthesis and playing a pivotal role throughout its application. Intraoperative evaluation, which assesses a surgeon's skills during the implantation process, is considered the "key" phase. Postoperative evaluation and rehabilitation, which significantly influence the ultimate recovery of limb function, constitute the "support" phase. These three assessments complement each other and collectively determine the success or failure of 3D-printed prosthetic applications.

Despite the widespread application of 3D-printing technology in orthopedic surgery, the accompanying standards and systematic protocols are still evolving toward maturity. For instance, there is no dedicated system for evaluating the osseointegration of 3D-printed prostheses; assessments primarily rely on existing osseointegration imaging systems to evaluate osseointegration in different body parts. Moreover, there is a lack of specialized follow-up and functional scoring systems that can be used after reconstruction with 3D-printed customized prostheses, and most evaluations refer to conventional timelines and scoring systems that are used for different body parts. Furthermore, early rehabilitation treatment after prosthetic reconstruction remains relatively unexplored. The emergence of Enhanced Recovery After Surgery (ERAS) protocols offers new insights into early rehabilitation for patients who undergo 3D-printed prosthetic reconstruction. Effective early rehabilitation requires the active participation of orthopedic surgeons supported by nursing, nutrition, anesthesia, psychology, and other disciplines. A dedicated case manager is essential for managing a patient's journey, including preadmission registration, scheduling, intrahospital case management, and postdischarge follow-up, ensuring that patients receive professional, personalized guidance and support throughout their rehabilitation.

References

Brantigan JW, Steffee AD. A carbon fiber implant to aid interbody lumbar fusion. Two-year clinical results in the first 26 patients. Spine (Phila Pa 1976). 1993;18(14):2106–7.

Briguglio M, Wainwright TW, Southern K, et al. Healthy eating for elective major orthopedic surgery: quality, quantity, and timing. J Multidiscip Healthc. 2023;16:2081–90.

Enneking WF, Dunham W, Gebhardt MC, et al. A system for the functional evaluation of reconstructive procedures after surgical treatment of tumors of the musculoskeletal system. Clin Orthop Relat Res. 1993;(286):241–6.

Jeys L, Matharu GS, Nandra RS, Grimer RJ. Can computer navigation-assisted surgery reduce the risk of an intralesional margin and reduce the rate of local recurrence in patients with a tumour of the pelvis or sacrum? Bone Joint J. 2013;95-B(10):1417–24.

Parikh SN, Crawford AH. Orthopaedic implications in the management of pediatric vertebral and spinal cord tumors: a retrospective review. Spine (Phila Pa 1976). 2003;28(20):2390–6.

Ryd L, Albrektsson BE, Carlsson L, et al. Roentgen stereophotogrammetric analysis as a predictor of mechanical loosening of knee prostheses. J Bone Joint Surg Br. 1995;77(3):377–83.

Sandberg OH, Kärrholm J, Olivecrona H, et al. Computed tomography-based radiostereometric analysis in orthopedic research: practical guidelines. Acta Orthop. 2023;94:373–8.

Siepe CJ, Stosch-Wiechert K, Heider F, et al. Anterior stand-alone fusion revisited: a prospective clinical, X-ray and CT investigation. Eur Spine J. 2015;24(4):838–51.

Vincent HK, Horodyski M, Vincent KR, et al. Psychological distress after orthopedic trauma: prevalence in patients and implications for rehabilitation. PM R. 2015;7(9):978–89.

Zheng Y, Yan Q. Effect of application of short-form video health education on the health knowledge and satisfaction with nursing care of patients with lower extremity fractures. BMC Nurs. 2023;22(1):395.

Clinical Problems of 3D-Printed Customized Prostheses and the Associated Countermeasures

6

Yongquan Zhang and Zheng Guo

6.1 The Concept Clinical Doctors Should Endorse

6.1.1 Customized Prostheses and 3D Printing Technology: Natural Allies

Customized prostheses are not a novel concept. As early as the era of machining, physicians began to think beyond the constraints of the currently available processing techniques, proposing the idea of customized prostheses and suggesting their necessity. The prostheses these doctors envisioned typically have irregular shapes and accessory structures, making it very challenging to produce them using conventional subtractive manufacturing processes. Moreover, since machined customized prostheses are mostly solid structures, achieving good osseointegration at the bone-prosthesis interface is difficult. For enterprises, the design and manufacturing costs of small-batch or single-piece customized products are high, the production speed is slow, and both clinical doctors and patients face long wait times. The difficulties in processing, high costs, long wait times, and poor osseointegration at the bone-prothesis interface greatly limit the widespread application of customized prostheses.

However, with the development of 3D printing technology, especially metal 3D printing technology, the previous challenges have been addressed, comprehensively transforming this situation. 3D printing technology has propelled customized prostheses into a new stage of clinical practicality. Utilizing 3D printing technology to produce customized prostheses results in shorter design and processing cycles,

Y. Zhang
Wedo (Xian) Bio-Medical Technology Co., Ltd, Xi'an, China

Z. Guo (✉)
Department of Orthopedics, Tangdu Hospital, Xi'an, China
e-mail: guozheng@fmmu.edu.cn

Z. Guo et al. (eds.), *3D-Printed Prosthesis in Orthopedic Oncology*,
https://doi.org/10.1007/978-981-95-1454-0_6

lower production costs, the integration of more functional modules into the prostheses, the ability to meet the personalized requirements of patients, and the achievement of favorable biological effects (Li et al. 2018). The technical advantages of 3D-printed customized prostheses are outlined below.

1. Personalization: Customized prostheses are better suited to each patient's bone structure and mechanical requirements. The optimal fit reduces the difficulty of surgical procedures, alleviates the pressure on surgeons, and can shorten the period of patient adaptation, which can be painful and stressful.
2. Complex geometric shapes: Most customized prostheses have complex surface features, and some complex structures based on biomimetic principles cannot be manufactured through traditional methods, such as milling, turning, or casting. These complex geometric shapes and biomimetic structures can only be achieved through 3D printing.
3. Functional integration: Personalized 3D-printed implants can meet the manufacturing needs of various functional implants, can be manufactured in fewer steps, feature porous structures and rough surfaces to improve osseointegration at the bone-prothesis interface, and reduce weight in non-load-bearing areas.
4. Reduced economic burden on patients: Personalized 3D-printed implants can be produced at faster speeds, are characterized by better size fit, which accelerates surgery and recovery, and have improved biocompatibility, which reduces the need for subsequent treatments. Thus, these implants benefit patients by lowering hospitalization and follow-up treatment costs.
5. Reduced technological challenges and economic burden of medical device manufacturers: 3D printing enables the rapid manufacturing of small-batch or single-piece products.

6.1.2 Doctors Lead the Customized Prosthesis Process

Clinical doctors must clearly realize that the design and clinical application of customized prostheses are predominantly led by surgeons. This process completely tests the surgical team's comprehensive application of 3D printing technology and overall process control. Clinical doctors play a crucial role in the various stages of designing, preparing, and applying 3D-printed customized prostheses. They are the leaders in design, supervisors in production, and executors in application. It can be said that the use of 3D-printed customized prostheses revolves around the needs of doctors. Only when surgeons have a thorough understanding of 3D printing technology can they utilize this technology to effectively design and apply customized prostheses and minimize the risk of failure. To guide the design and application of 3D-printed customized prostheses, surgeons need to possess the following qualities:

1. Understanding of clinical indications: Qualified clinical doctors need to have a thorough understanding of the diseases in their field. Precise understanding of disease treatment, especially the accurate diagnosis of surgical indications, and

abundant experience in selecting surgical methods are necessary. Particularly for the clinical application of 3D-printed, personalized, customized prostheses, a good understanding of the relevant elements is essential. Understanding the necessity of 3D printing technology in the process of disease treatment is crucial.
2. In-depth understanding of the overall process of 3D-printed customized prosthesis application: To apply 3D-printed customized prostheses in clinical practice, a thorough understanding of the overall application process is needed. This process begins with a doctor's demand, and then, the engineering personnel propose prosthesis design solutions. Next, the prosthesis is prepared, and finally, the clinical doctor implants the prosthesis and evaluates the outcome. Clinical doctors need to understand this entire process and know the roles they play in it.
3. Proficiency in surgical procedures: As the formulators of surgical plans and designers of prostheses, doctors themselves should be able to perform surgical procedures. The effective implementation of preoperative planning greatly improves the clinical application of the prosthesis. This requires clinical doctors to have profound expertise in the surgeries they perform, as well as rich clinical experience in relevant prosthesis applications, to successfully complete surgeries and maximize the advantages of prostheses.
4. Risk control: Doctors need to have a clear understanding of the risks associated with customized prostheses, such as the inability to adjust or trim the prosthesis during surgery or the fact that changes in the extent of surgical resection affect the normal use of 3D-printed customized prostheses. In such situations, doctors can rely on their extensive clinical experience to adopt alternative plans to complete the surgical procedure without causing harm to the patient.

6.1.3 Elements of Customized Prosthesis Design

Doctors pay more attention to preoperative planning and prosthesis design when using customized prostheses than when using conventional prostheses. Excellent doctors can develop nearly perfect surgical plans before the operation and include some key points in the design of customized prostheses. Thus, surgery is only the real-world implementation of the preoperative plan. The quality of prosthesis design, which is guided by clinical practice, determines the therapeutic effect and lifespan of the prosthesis. When designing customized prostheses, one should not be overly idealistic, avoid pursuing a complete replica of anatomical structures, or integrate too many functions. Instead, focus should be placed on the main contradictions and the primary issues that need to be addressed with the prosthesis.

The design of personalized, customized prostheses using 3D printing first considers clinical needs and practicality while also considering the safety of the prosthesis design and the feasibility of printing (Kranz et al. 2014). From the perspective of the clinician, prosthesis design typically needs to consider the following elements, known as the 7S elements (Table 6.1).

Table 6.1 Seven elements of the design of 3D-printed, personalized, customized prostheses

Design elements	Requirements
Shape	Prosthetic shapes should be designed according to their intended use, considering both appearance and function, and meeting the requirements of complex local anatomical reconstruction, without necessarily requiring a complete anatomical replica.
Structure	The physical structure and internal porous distribution should be reasonable, with pore sizes that are suitable for bone ingrowth and soft tissue attachment requirements. The design of the fixation nail channel should consider both the overall structure of the prosthesis and the local bone condition.
Strength	To meet the support requirements of local mechanics, finite element analysis is beneficial for optimizing prosthesis design.
Surface	The interface between the prosthesis and the bone should have a good fit, and the porous structure of the interface should be designed to promote osseointegration, thereby enhancing the long-term biological stability of the prosthesis.
Survival	It is necessary to overcome the traditional problem of loosening at the interface between metal implants and bones, transforming mechanical reconstruction of implants into implant-bone composite biological reconstruction to ensure long-term biological stability of the implants.
Surgery	When designing implants, it is important to consider ease of operation for the surgeon. If the implant's anatomical structure is too complex, it may require a higher level of precision at the bone interface or exposure. Designing the surface of the implant with grasping and positioning structures can facilitate proper placement.
Setting	When designing prostheses, initial stability requirements must be considered. This can be achieved through the use of self-locking prostheses and auxiliary fixation devices. Customized prostheses are often needed to connect with traditional standardized instruments.

Experience from clinical practice has shown that designing prostheses based on the seven elements can fully leverage the advantages of 3D printing technology, maximizing the functional reconstruction effects while minimizing risks. Figure 6.1 shows an example of a 3D-printed, personalized, customized acetabular prosthesis that was designed with full consideration of the seven elements. In addition to the factors described above, doctors also considered factors such as the patient's life expectancy, bone quality, and compatibility with conventional products.

6.1.4 Customized Prosthetic Mechanical Performance Considerations

Orthopedic implants in the human body must have certain mechanical properties to maintain the integrity of their shape and perform functions such as bearing weight and movement. The same principle applies to 3D-printed orthopedic implants. Currently, the most commonly used 3D-printed metal material is titanium alloy, which is processed using techniques such as electron beam melting

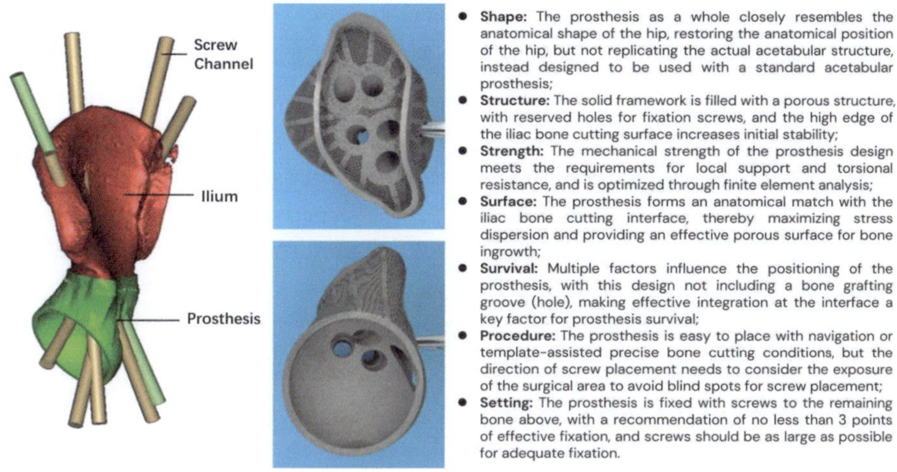

Fig. 6.1 Elements of the design of a customized prosthesis for reconstruction after pelvic acetabular tumor resection using 3D printing

(EBM) and selective laser melting (SLM). Therefore, the mechanical properties of 3D-printed parts made of titanium alloy are discussed using these two methods as examples.

The medical industry standard "Surgical Implants—Forged, Cast, and Ti-6Al-4V. Titanium Alloy Forged Joint Prostheses" (YY0117.1-2005) specifies the mechanical properties of forged titanium alloy parts (Table 6.2). The national standard "Powder Bed Electron Beam Additive Manufacturing of TC4 Alloy Materials" (GB/T 34508-2017) stipulates the mechanical properties at room temperature of TC4 alloy dense materials that are manufactured using powder bed electron beam additive manufacturing technology (Table 6.3). Tests have shown that whether EBM or SLM is used, the mechanical properties of 3D-printed titanium alloy orthopedic implants meet the additive manufacturing standards and exceed the standards of traditionally forged titanium alloy surgical implants; thus, they meet the requirements for use in humans. However, for solid components that are printed using 3D technology, their fatigue performance still cannot match that of traditionally forged titanium alloys. Therefore, in regions where the prosthetic conditions are severe, the use of traditionally forged titanium alloy, such as marrow needles, in conjunction with customized 3D-printed prosthetic components for mechanical processing is still recommended.

3D printing materials are primarily categorized into three main types based on their composition: metal materials, nonmetal materials, and biomaterials. Currently, customized prostheses are predominantly made from metal, but there is also a growing trend toward using nonmetal materials such as polyether ether ketone (PEEK). Regardless of the material that is chosen to manufacture customized prostheses, doctors and designers need to consider the mechanical requirements of the prosthetic's intended use.

Table 6.2 Mechanical properties of forged titanium alloy parts

Item	Tensile strength Rm	Proportional limit yield strength Rp0.2	Elongation A
Value	≥860 MPa	≥780 MPa	≥10%

Table 6.3 Mechanical performance requirements for additively manufactured TC4 alloy materials

Grade	Tensile strength Rm/MPa	Yield strength Rp0.2/MPa	Elongation at break A/%	Reduction of area Z/%
TC4	≥895	≥825	≥10	≥15
TC4ELI	≥855	≥785	≥10	≥15

6.1.5 Methods to Increase the Survival Rate of Customized Prostheses

Doctors aim to increase the survival rate of customized prostheses and reduce the risk of failure by considering both immediate postoperative stability and long-term stability. Immediate postoperative stability is typically achieved through physical methods, such as screw fixation, wing plates, intramedullary nails, and auxiliary steel plate fixation. Long-term stability relies on osseointegration between the customized prosthesis and the host bone interface, as well as the optimization of the prosthesis design to avoid stress concentration and shielding.

In areas that form the interface between the customized prosthesis and the host bone, local configuration design should consider osseointegration at the interface. Osseointegration refers to a bone-to-bone connection that forms between the implant and surrounding bone tissue without fibrous connective tissue. A well-matched interface and a porous structural design facilitate osseointegration, enabling 3D-printed metal prostheses to achieve long-term stability in the body and preventing loosening and sinking that could lead to revision or surgical failure. The importance of porous structures in 3D-printed metal materials is widely recognized (Zhao et al. 2018; Taniguchi et al. 2016). The key parameters that should be considered when designing 3D-printed metal porous structures include their porosity, pore size, and pore connectivity; these parameters significantly impact the mechanical and biological performance of metal scaffolds.

6.1.6 3D-Printed Customized Prostheses to Avoid Joint Surface Design

Due to limitations in prosthesis materials and printing technology, it is currently challenging to generate smooth joint surfaces directly via 3D printing technology. The smoothness of joint surfaces is crucial for the quality and clinical lifespan of implanted joints, and it plays a key role in the success of artificial joints. There are several disadvantages of the use of 3D printing technology to manufacture joint surfaces, and they are related mainly to joint surface design, material selection, and manufacturing technology challenges.

The primary issue with personalized prostheses that include joint surfaces is not related to 3D printing technology but rather to joint surface design. The morphological design of joint surface friction pairs largely determines the wear rate during joint movement. Designing joint surfaces for traditional prostheses requires validation through numerical simulation and wear tests; this requirement results in a lengthy process and increased cost. However, personalized prostheses with joint surfaces are manufactured to match a particular individual, making it challenging to follow the traditional joint surface design and testing process because time constraints do not allow the use of the traditional process. Therefore, achieving personalized joint surface design remains difficult with the currently available design technology.

In terms of materials, the joint surfaces of prostheses are typical friction pairs, and the selection of complementary materials needs to adhere to the principles of tribology. Materials that are commonly used for artificial joints include metal-ultrahigh molecular weight polyethylene (UHMWPE), ceramic-UHMWPE, and ceramic-ceramic materials. Metals that are suitable for manufacturing artificial joints include cobalt-based alloys, titanium-based alloys, and iron-based alloys; cobalt-chromium-molybdenum alloy is the metal material that is most widely used to manufacture joint surfaces due to its high hardness and wear resistance. For a material to serve as a joint surface, it must have extremely high hardness, which typically results in a high elastic modulus. However, a high elastic modulus in a prosthesis can lead to stress shielding effects, causing long-term loosening. Thus, in terms of materials, the conflicting material requirements for the friction pair and other parts of the prosthesis pose a challenge for the production of customized prostheses that include joint surfaces.

Artificial joint friction pairs demand extremely high surface quality, with the surface roughness (Ra) value of metal materials in the joints not exceeding 0.05 μm, typically approximately 0.02 μm, characterized by a misty mirror-like appearance (Fig. 6.2a). This requires methods such as precision grinding, polishing, and superfinishing. In current additive manufacturing processes, parts that

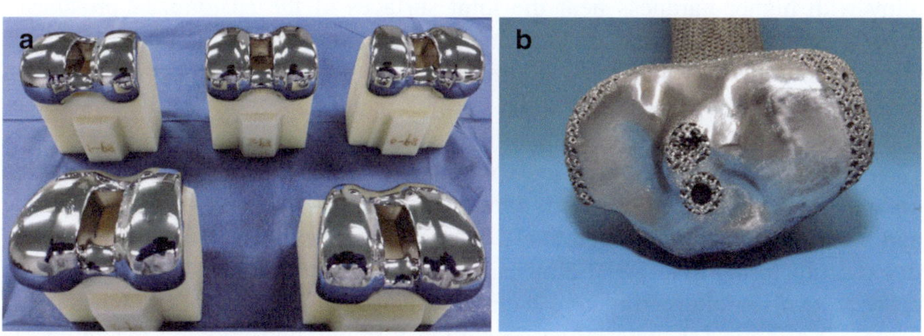

Fig. 6.2 Comparison of conventional human joint surfaces (**a**) and 3D-printed joint surfaces (**b**)

are produced using powder bed fusion technology have relatively low surface roughness, but untreated products can have Ra values below 5 μm, which is still a difference of two orders of magnitude from the roughness of joint surfaces. Although the roughness of joint surfaces of 3D-printed prostheses can be reduced by polishing (Fig. 6.2b), due to the specificity of customized products, the equipment and fixtures that are required for polishing may also need to be customized. Therefore, in terms of manufacturing, the limitations of 3D printing technology in terms of surface quality limit its application in the production of customized prostheses that include joint surfaces.

Currently, for 3D-printed customized prosthetic reconstruction involving joint surfaces, one feasible solution considering the current technological conditions is to use traditional prosthetic joint friction components in conjunction with customized prostheses. The drawback of this assembly-based approach lies in potential fatigue failure and micromotion wear at the interfaces. Another viable solution, considering the current technology, is primarily used to treat cases in which one side of the joint cartilage is preserved. This approach involves utilizing 3D printing technology to manufacture customized prostheses and achieve the required joint surfaces through precise milling, grinding, polishing, and other finishing processes. However, this solution requires a long manufacturing lead time, complex procedures, high costs, and a lack of timeliness.

To address the challenges related to materials and manufacturing technology that were mentioned above in the long term, with advances in additive manufacturing technology, multi-material integrated manufacturing, and composite manufacturing with material addition and subtraction capabilities may provide robust methods for manufacturing personalized custom joint prostheses. Issues, such as prosthetic material limitations and insufficient surface quality, are expected to be overcome, thereby enabling the production of personalized customized joint prostheses that are produced with multiple materials and with high precision. Multi-material controllable shaping and composite manufacturing with material addition and subtraction capabilities will be a powerful approach for the manufacturing of personalized customized prostheses in the future (Bandyopadhyay and Heer 2018). Multi-material composite 3D printing can produce customized prostheses with continuously variable material compositions, for example, using cobalt-chromium-molybdenum alloy with higher hardness near the joint surfaces of the customized prosthesis, using titanium alloy in the main load-bearing areas, and designing a porous configuration at the interface that contacts the bone. This approach balances the hardness requirements of the joint surfaces, the strength requirements of load-bearing areas, and the osseointegration requirements at the bone interface.

Another promising direction to explore is the material addition and subtraction composite manufacturing method, which combines the advantages of 3D printing and traditional machining, effectively compensating for the shortcomings of additive manufacturing in terms of dimensional accuracy and surface quality. The basic process involves alternating or synchronously adding and subtracting materials, using 3D printing for material accumulation forming, and utilizing machining to enhance part accuracy and surface quality. The combination of multi-material 3D printing and material addition and subtraction composite manufacturing methods will provide a robust method for manufacturing personalized custom prostheses with joint surfaces.

6.2 Customized Prostheses and Their Combination with Conventional Products and Prostheses

6.2.1 Limitations of 3D-Printed Customized Prostheses

The emergence and development of 3D printing technology have greatly promoted the development of personalized customized prostheses, expanding the range of customized prosthesis design (Liu 2017). Engineers can incorporate multiple functional modules into the same prosthesis and manufacture them integrally, and this represents a revolutionary change. However, will the 3D-printed customized prostheses completely replace traditional machined prostheses? The answer is definitely no.

Due to the influence of processing technology, the design concepts of 3D-printed customized prostheses and traditional standard prostheses are not entirely the same. Therefore, the physical properties, mechanical properties, and biological properties of these types of prostheses are different, and each type of prosthesis has advantages and disadvantages. Traditional standard prostheses are usually solid in structure and exhibit excellent mechanical performance; this represents an advantage of this type of prosthesis. However, this solid structure leads to poor biocompatibility at the bone-prosthesis interface, making osseointegration difficult. On the other hand, 3D printing technology allows for the design of locally porous interfaces, improving the biological fusion between the prosthesis and surrounding bone tissue. The excellent mechanical performance of traditional standard prostheses can be used to strengthen some weak points in the load-bearing components of 3D-printed customized prostheses. Currently, in scenarios involving joint friction interfaces, 3D-printed customized prostheses still cannot fully meet the safety requirements for prosthesis use and often need to be combined with traditional prostheses or implants.

6.2.2 Clinical Scenarios of Using Conventional Products or Traditional Prostheses in Combination

It must be clearly understood by clinical doctors and design engineers that promoting the use of 3D-printed customized prostheses alone or traditional standard prostheses alone is not the correct approach. One-piece 3D-printed customized prostheses are rarely used alone and often need to be combined with traditional prostheses or implants to leverage the strengths of both types of prostheses.

The short-term stability and long-term stability of 3D-printed, personalized, customized prostheses determine the effectiveness and lifespan of the prostheses. Although the long-term stability of 3D-printed, personalized, customized prostheses can be achieved through osteointegration at porous interfaces, immediate postoperative stability still relies on mechanical fixation. Common prosthesis fixation methods include self-locking fixation and auxiliary fixation; the former uses fixation holes in the prosthesis for fixation, and the latter uses auxiliary steel plates or rods for fixation. Between these approaches, the use of mechanically machined standard screws for fixation is one of the most common approaches for the combined application of 3D-printed customized prostheses and conventional products (Figs. 6.3 and 6.4).

Using machined steel plates for auxiliary fixation is another common approach for the combined application of 3D-printed customized prostheses and conventional products. Due to the unique manufacturing process that is used to produce 3D-printed customized prostheses, the longer the prosthesis is, the poorer its mechanical performance. Therefore, in this usage scenario, standard steel plates are usually used for auxiliary fixation, as shown in Fig. 6.5.

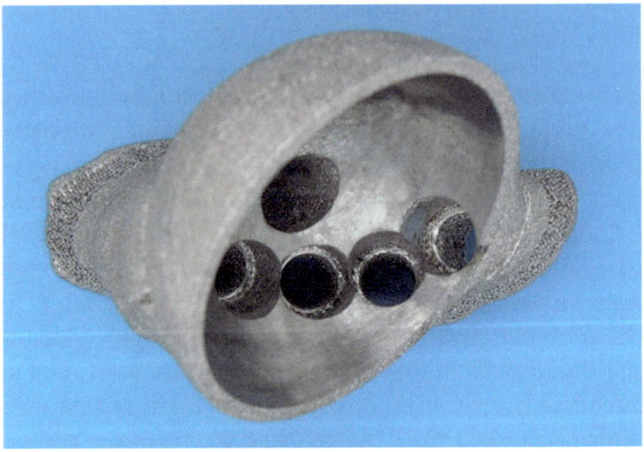

Fig. 6.3 3D-printed customized acetabular prosthesis in one-piece (bottom view) with clearly visible predrilled holes

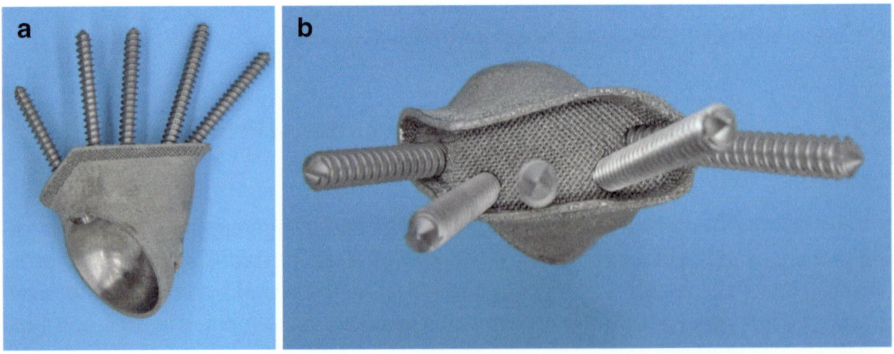

Fig. 6.4 A customized acetabular prosthesis generated by 3D printing for use in conjunction with screws. The prosthesis and screws were made using different manufacturing processes, but both were made of TC4 material. (**a**) Side view. (**b**) Top view

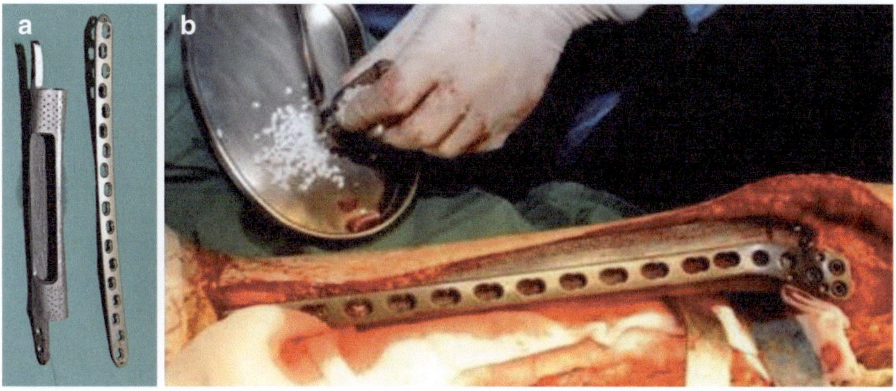

Fig. 6.5 In some anatomical sites with high stress demands, 3D-printed customized prostheses require early clinical mechanical support. This necessitates their combination with traditional standard prostheses. (**a**) Standard femoral anatomical plates are used in conjunction with 3D-printed customized femoral shaft defect prostheses. (**b**) Image of a surgical operation in which the 3D-printed customized tibial shaft defect prosthesis was used with a standard bone plate and screws (Yu et al. 2022)

In the treatment of segmental bone defects in long bones, especially large segmental bone defects in long bones, custom-made implants that are made via 3D printing are often used for reconstruction. However, due to concerns about the fatigue performance of solid components that are generated by 3D printing, these implants are often designed in a modular fashion. This means that the main body of the implant is 3D printed, while the intramedullary fixation components are machined standard intramedullary nails. The two parts are securely combined through a well-designed interface, exploiting the technical advantages of both types of implants (Fig. 6.6).

The common approach for combining custom-made artificial vertebral bodies with conventional products involves the use of conventional spinal pedicle screw-rod systems for additional fixation. Custom-made artificial vertebral bodies that are printed in 3D for fusion purposes are increasingly replacing traditional titanium mesh and are increasingly being used in clinical practice. Short segment or simple custom-made artificial vertebral bodies usually do not have additional fixation structures, requiring the use of posterior spinal pedicle screw-rod systems for stability.

The common approach for combining standard modular joint components with custom-made 3D-printed implants involves the reconstruction of tumor joints with custom and conventional implants. Due to differences among individuals in terms of the extent of tumor resection around the joint, the use of standard modular implants alone may not always meet the requirements. In such cases, custom-made implants play a significant role. Customized implants are typically implanted on one side of the joint, while standard modular components of artificial joints can be use on the articulating surface of the artificial joint and the opposite side (Fig. 6.7).

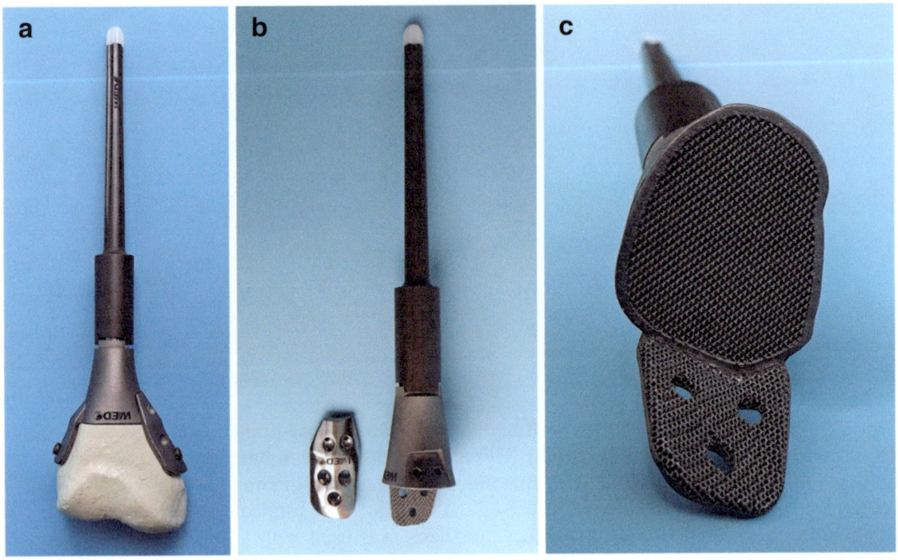

Fig. 6.6 Customized prostheses that combine 3D printing and machining: The main body of the prosthesis was manufactured using 3D printing technology, with a porous structure at the interface to promote integration with the host bone, while the core pins were produced using machining processes. (**a**) Front view of the assembling prostheses. (**b**) Side view. (**c**) Bottom view

The combination of a 3D-printed acetabular cup with a conventional UHMWPE liner is a typical example of this method, along with the use of standard femoral head and stem implants. This method leverages the advantages of 3D printing to provide tailored fitting while avoiding issues with joint surface printing, effectively exploiting the strengths of custom-made 3D-printed implants and traditional standard implants.

It is worth noting that the methods for the production of standard prostheses differ from those for the production of 3D-printed customized prostheses, and sometimes even the manufacturers may vary. Therefore, before proceeding with the production of 3D-printed customized prostheses, it is essential to understand the specifications of standard prostheses to facilitate compatibility. Additionally, it is necessary to understand the materials of metal prostheses further and preferably select materials of the same metal for 3D printing to avoid electrolytic reactions inside the body when the two types of prostheses are combined.

In conclusion, 3D-printed customized prostheses and conventional or traditional products have their own advantages and disadvantages. Doctors must have a thorough understanding of these advantages and disadvantages, make reasonable choices, and combine the two types of prostheses, leveraging their strengths and mitigating their weaknesses, during the surgical planning stage, according to the specific needs of disease treatment.

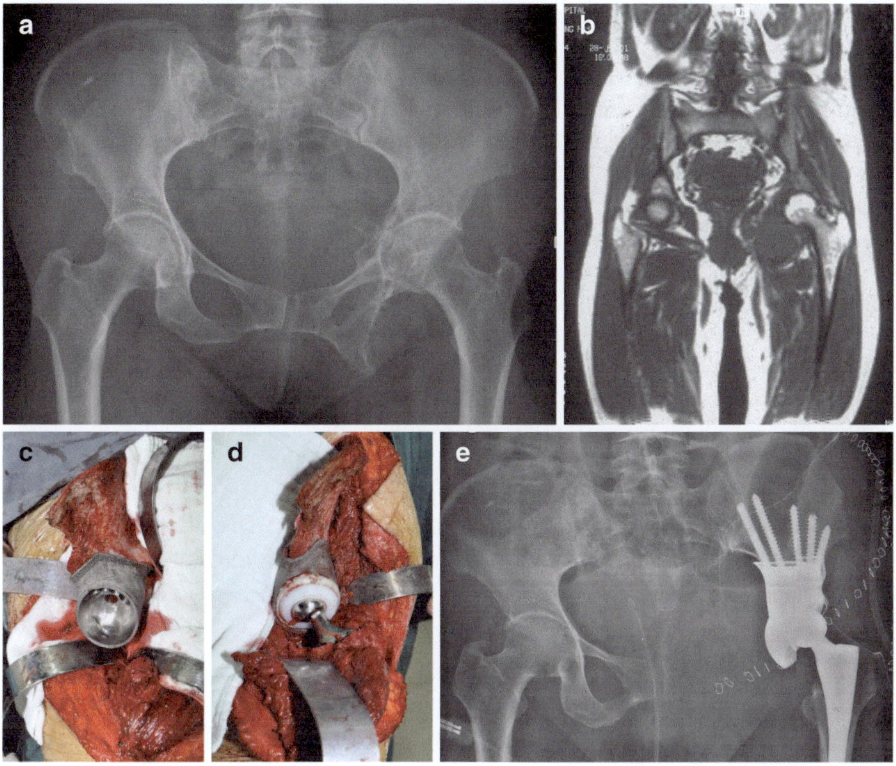

Fig. 6.7 After the resection of a malignant tumor around the acetabulum, a 3D-printed customized acetabular prosthesis was used in conjunction with a standard hip joint prosthesis for repair. (**a**) Preoperative pelvic X-ray (anteroposterior view) of a patient with left acetabular chondrosarcoma. (**b**) Preoperative MR image (coronal section). (**c**) Photo of the 3D-printed customized acetabular prosthesis that was installed during surgery. (**d**) Photo of the combination of the 3D-printed customized acetabular prosthesis and standard hip joint prosthesis during surgery. (**e**) Postoperative pelvic X-ray (anteroposterior view) of the patient

6.3 Precise Installation of Customized Prostheses

6.3.1 Requirements for Customized Prosthesis Installation

The diversity in the design and manufacturing processes of 3D-printed, personalized, customized prostheses sets them apart from traditional prostheses in terms of risk control. Clinical doctors lead the entire process of customized prosthesis design, manufacturing, and application. During the preoperative planning and prosthesis design phase, clinical doctors need to clearly define the requirements for prosthesis design and the methods of installation and fixation. By the time the prosthesis design is completed, the shape of the prosthesis, the installation position, and the fixation method should already be specified. The installation of customized prostheses is essentially the real-world realization of the virtual preoperative planning. The accuracy of prosthesis installation during surgery is based on the actual implementation of the surgical plan. While traditional prostheses also involve preoperative planning, they are usually not detailed, and surgeons often need to further measure and use trial models to select the appropriate size and type of prosthesis. These two types of prostheses are significantly different in terms of installation requirements, with 3D-printed customized prostheses having stricter installation requirements and higher precision requirements.

The consistency between the clinical use of 3D-printed customized prostheses and preoperative design planning determines the therapeutic effect. Undoubtedly, good preoperative planning and prosthesis design play crucial roles. However, precise installation is a critical aspect of the clinical use of prostheses. During the actual installation process, the use of digital technology to assist in prosthesis positioning and installation is essential. For example, preoperative simulation surgery can be performed using 3D-printed models, and during the surgical process, precise installation of the customized prosthesis can be achieved with the help of surgical guides, computer-assisted navigation, or surgical robots. The digital technology-assisted technique for the precise installation of 3D-printed, personalized, customized prostheses (Fig. 6.8).

6.3.2 Auxiliary Installation Tools: 3D-Printed Models

During the preoperative stage, surgical simulation can be conducted using 3D-printed models, which is an important means by which surgeons can familiarize themselves with the surgical plan and increase the accuracy of surgical procedures.

Through nonmetal 3D-printing technology, a skeletal outline of the surgical area can be processed, creating 3D-printed skeletal models. These models do not require

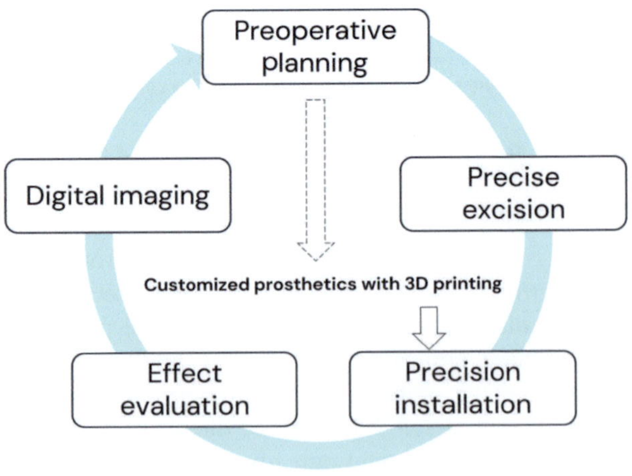

Fig. 6.8 Digital technology assists in the precise installation of 3D-printed, personalized, custom prostheses

separate designs; they serve as preliminary materials for customized prosthesis design alongside individualized prosthesis design. Based on our team's practical experience, the 3D printing of skeletal models of the surgical area, including models before and after tumor resection, is recommended before the clinical application of 3D-printed customized prostheses. The main functions of these models are as follows:

1. Familiarization with the surgical plan

Utilizing 3D-printed physical models before surgery to practice the operation and simulate prosthesis installation can help doctors better familiarize themselves with the surgical plan (Fig. 6.9). Through the combination of 3D-printed customized prostheses and solid models, doctors can understand the potential difficulties in prosthesis installation that may occur during the actual surgical operation; this is especially helpful for doctors with less surgical experience or those with less experience with 3D-printed customized prostheses.

2. Surgical guidance

During surgery, 3D-printed solid models can play a crucial role in assisting surgical teams. While design software can completely cover soft tissues to expose the skeleton during the surgical planning stage, during the operation, it is essential to minimize damage due to limitations, such as incision limitations, soft tissue exposure limitations, and crucial neurovascular limitations, resulting in a limited range of exposed bone surfaces. At this point, the surgeon can rely on the 3D-printed solid model, which can provide valuable guidance related to anatomical positioning (Fig. 6.10a). Furthermore, after tumor resection and before prosthesis installation, the 3D-printed solid model can be compared with the actual surgical situation to verify the accuracy of bone resection (Fig. 6.10b), and the prosthesis can be adjusted to the correct installation position according to the model's guidance.

Although 3D-printed three-dimensional models serve as byproducts in the process of 3D-printed prosthesis design, their value in clinical application should not be underestimated. Proper utilization of 3D-printed solid models can provide significant assistance for the precise installation of 3D-printed customized prostheses.

6.3.3 Auxiliary Installation Tools: 3D-Printed Customized Surgical Guides

A 3D-printed customized surgical guide is an auxiliary tool that is used in orthopedic surgery. Such guides are customized according to the patient's bone structure and the surgeon's surgical plan, and they help the surgeon to more accurately locate the target site and operate during surgery. Before the adoption of 3D-printed guides, surgeons mainly used positioning blocks that were provided by surgical instrument

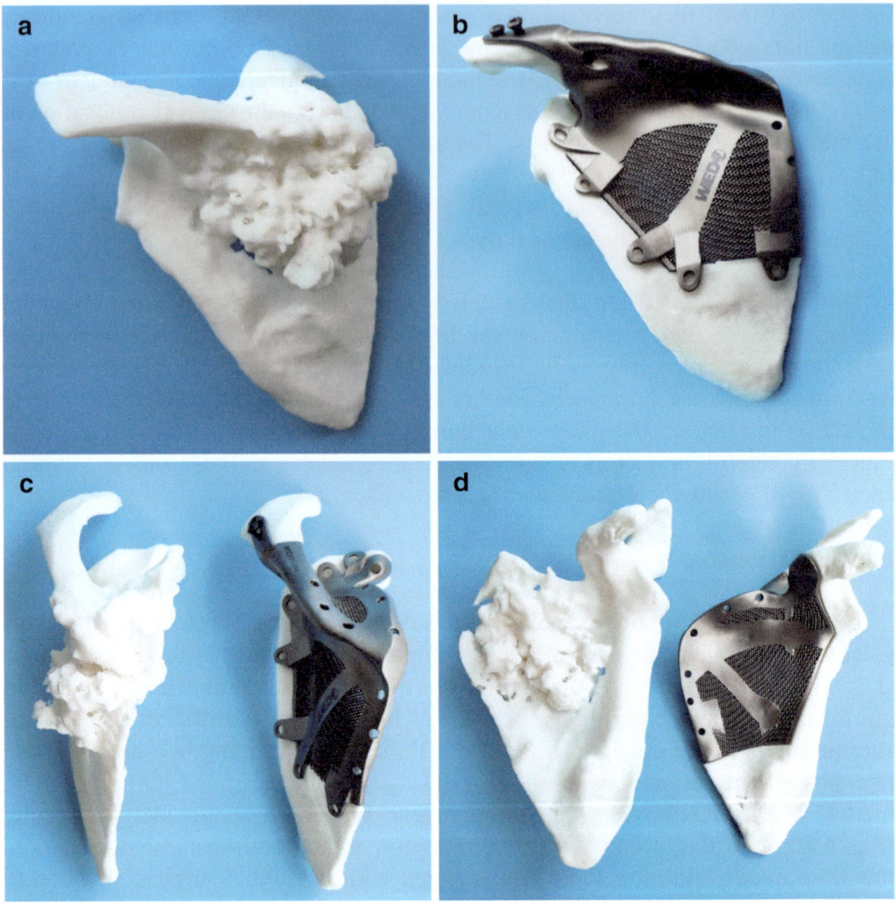

Fig. 6.9 After the completion of the customized titanium alloy scapular prosthesis manufactured through 3D printing, a 3D printed skeletal model is used in conjunction before surgery for simulated installation. This allows for the assessment of the prosthetic installation effect. (**a**) Rear view of the 3D printed scapula model. (**b**) Rear view of the installation model for the 3D printed scapular prosthesis. (**c**) Side view. (**d**) Frontal view

manufacturers; these positioning blocks typically had conventional shapes, such as rectangles or circles, and relied more on the surgeon's own experience with implant placement during surgery. In contrast, 3D-printed customized guides are personalized according to the patient's specific condition; CT or MR images are used in combination with the surgeon's plan to generate guide models, ensuring a complete match between the surgical guide and the patient's bone structure. Therefore, 3D-printed surgical guides can assist surgeons in performing precise surgeries, especially complex tissue structure nailing and excision, as well as customized implant installations. These 3D-printed customized guides assist surgeons during

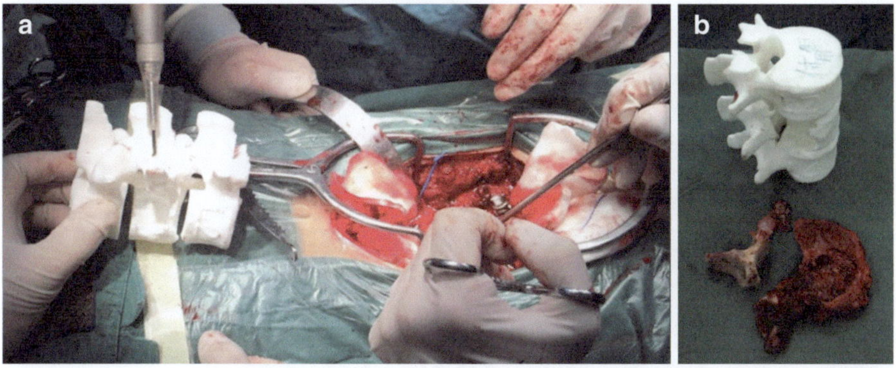

Fig. 6.10 3D-printed skeletal models play a crucial role in guiding tumor resection procedures. (**a**) Prior to tumor removal, these models assist in locating the tumor and defining the resection boundaries. (**b**) They enable a comparison with the actual tumor during surgery to ensure the completeness of the resection

surgery by providing three-dimensional spatial guidance, such as guidance related to direction, cross-section, and depth, making surgeries more accurate and safer.

In cases where surgeons do not have access to computer-assisted navigation or surgical robots, 3D-printed customized surgical guides remain an easily accessible auxiliary tool for surgeons, making them a favorable choice.

6.3.4 Auxiliary Installation Tools: Computer-Assisted Navigation

Computer-assisted navigation, a digital technology, is a powerful auxiliary tool for the precise installation of 3D-printed customized implants (Guo 2019). For patients undergoing bone tumor resection and reconstruction using 3D-printed personalized implants, computer-assisted navigation offers the following advantages: (1) Intraoperative visualization of the tumor location, determination of safe tumor margins, and bone cutting according to preoperative planning; (2) Preoperative simulation of personalized implant installation and evaluation of the safety and effectiveness of implant design; (3) Intraoperative visualization of screw placement for implant fixation, reducing the risk of damage to vital structures; (4) Accurate measurement of screw direction and size to maximize implant stability; (5) Assurance of anatomical compatibility between bone cutting surfaces and custom implants to facilitate bone-implant integration; and (6) Postimplantation verification that the anatomical implant position and preoperative design matched and that precise installation of the personalized customized implants are achieved. Figure 6.11 illustrates the precise resection of a periacetabular tumor and accurate reconstruction with a customized acetabular implant utilizing computer-assisted navigation technology for intraoperative spatial positioning.

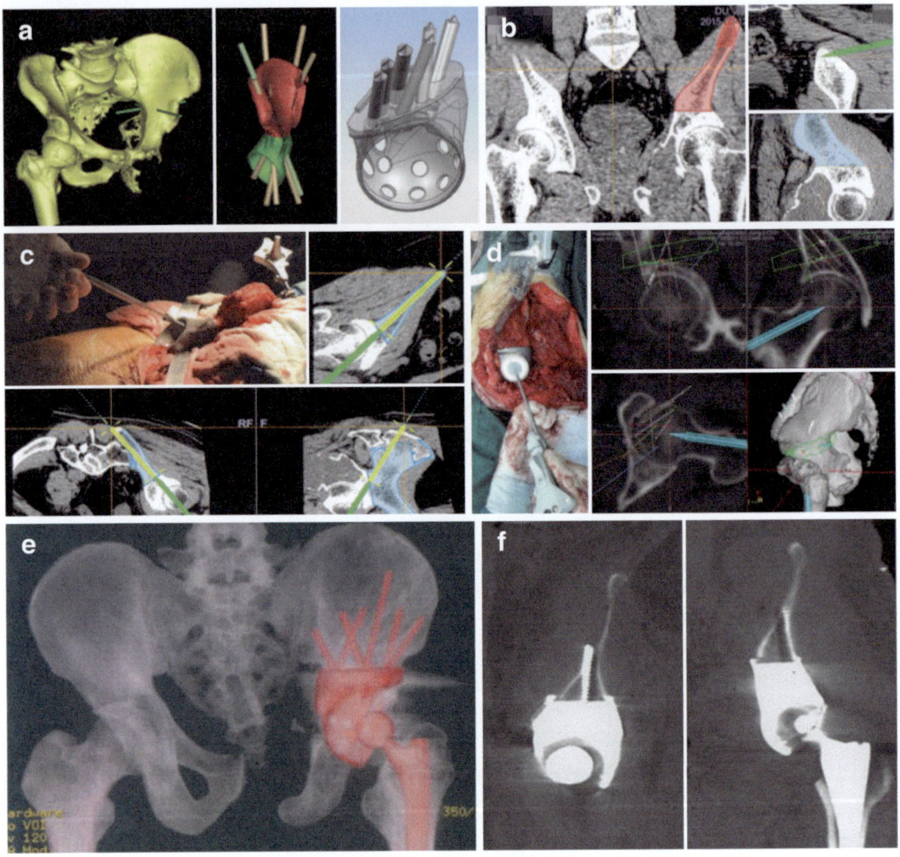

Fig. 6.11 Navigation-assisted precise resection of a periacetabular tumor and accurate reconstruction with an individualized, customized acetabular prosthetic. (**a**) Preoperative osteotomy and prosthesis design for acetabular tumors. (**b**) Intraoperative navigation-guided osteotomy of the acetabular margin. (**c**) Installation of custom-made prostheses and navigation-guided screw fixation. (**d**) Intraoperative navigation verification of the central position of the acetabular prosthesis. (**e**) Postoperative CT three-dimensional reconstruction showing the precise anatomical position of the individualized customized acetabular prosthesis. (**f**) Postoperative CT sectional images showing the intact anatomical match of the prosthesis-bone interface (Li et al. 2018)

6.3.5 Auxiliary Installation Tools: Surgical Robots

With continuous advances in science and technology, the development of surgical robots is becoming increasingly mature. Robot-assisted surgery does not involve the replacement of doctors by robots for performing surgeries; rather, robot-assisted surgery is an advanced technology by which robots assist doctors during surgeries. Similar to computer-assisted navigation, surgical robots can provide precise spatial positioning for surgeons and enable direct control of surgical instruments through a robotic arm system.

In traditional surgical methods, surgeons directly control surgical instruments, and the proficiency and fatigue of the surgeon directly affect the precision and stability of the operation. Robot-assisted surgery can significantly reduce the amount of physical exertion of doctors. Additionally, the stability of instrument manipulation by robots is notably superior to that of humans, and stability is often crucial for surgeons who are working with complex anatomical structures or performing high-risk surgeries. Therefore, robot-assisted surgery can provide greater precision during surgical procedures, reducing errors and risks during surgeries.

However, surgical robots have some disadvantages; for instance, they are expensive, must be operated by experienced and extensively trained surgical teams to ensure the success and safety of surgeries, and are associated with risks, such as system failures and program errors, that are inherent to robotic systems.

6.4 Intraoperative Failure to Execute the Surgical Plan

The precise installation of 3D-printed, personalized, customized prostheses is crucial, and it requires not only the rationality from design to implantation but also the user's clinical experience and overall control of the technology. Adhering strictly to the procedures for the precise installation of 3D-printed, personalized, customized prostheses typically ensures the execution of the installation plan. However, certain factors may hinder smooth prosthesis placement, necessitating timely adjustments to the surgical plan and reconstruction strategy.

1. Inadequate consideration of the exposure range and obstruction of important tissue structures during the design of customized prostheses may result in oversized prostheses or mismatched local shapes, making implantation difficult (Fig. 6.12).
2. Temporary changes to the surgical plan during surgery may lead to an increase or decrease in the extent of bone resection, causing the customized prostheses, which were designed preoperatively, to not completely match the bone defect area, thus requiring the formulation of alternative plans. In such cases, traditional reconstruction methods or conventional prostheses from alternative plans should be used for reconstruction.
3. If no alternative reconstruction materials are available during surgery, the procedure should be terminated. A personalized prosthesis should be redesigned and prepared based on the range of bone and joint defects, and a two-stage implantation should be performed.
4. If residual defects or gaps are found around the customized prosthesis after placement, bone grafting should be performed to increase the attachment of the prosthesis to the bone and enhance its stability.
5. If the customized prosthesis cannot be smoothly implanted according to the original surgical plan due to reasons related to its shape or size, appropriate adjustments to the defect area or expansion of exposure should be made to facili-

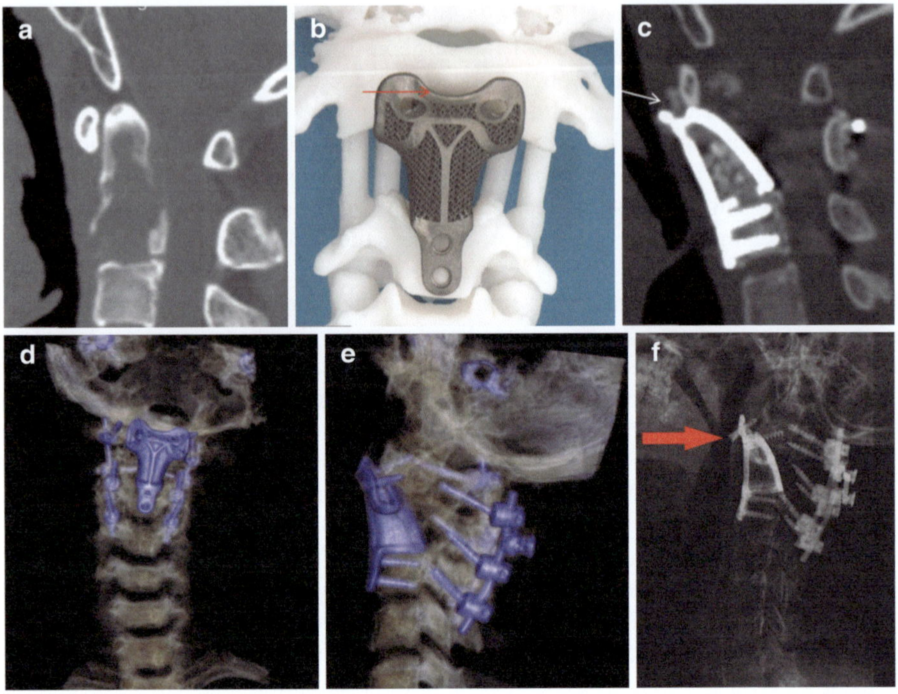

Fig. 6.12 Surgical removal of a thoracic spinal tumor with 3D-printed, customized artificial vertebral body reconstruction. (**a**) CT scan of the thoracic spine tumor showing bone destruction. (**b**) Preoperative installation of a customized thoracic artificial vertebral body on a physical model, with a red arrow indicating perfect anatomical alignment with the anterior arch of the atlas vertebra. Due to the overly anatomically consistent design of the upper edge groove, it was challenging to fully expose the area and place the artificial vertebral body during surgery. However, the intraoperative assessment of the position was acceptable, and the surgical plan was not altered. (**c**) Immediate postoperative CT revealed that the upper edge of the artificial vertebral body did not lock with the anterior arch of the atlas vertebra (indicated by a white arrow), indicating an unsatisfactory placement position. (**d**, **e**) Immediate postoperative CT three-dimensional reconstruction image. (**f**) Thirty months after surgery, there was no significant change in the position of the implant, but there was a complication of screw loosening (indicated by a red arrow)

tate prosthesis installation, or the surgical approach should be altered to allow easier installation. For example, when reconstructing the fifth lumbar vertebra after pathological collapse and vertebral body reconstruction, if the personalized custom artificial vertebral body is too large to be placed from the posterior due to nerve root obstruction on both sides, the artificial vertebral body often needs to be inserted through an anterior approach.

6. If positional effects or surgical operations cause deformation of the defect area, thus preventing the customized prosthesis from matching the original defect area well, auxiliary instruments should be used to restore the original defect morphology to promote prosthesis alignment. For instance, during the placement of personalized artificial vertebral bodies, auxiliary fixation rods are often used to

open, compress, or bend to ensure tight attachment of the artificial vertebral body to the upper and lower endplates while restoring the physiological curvature of the spine.

The successful and accurate installation of 3D-printed, personalized, customized prostheses determines the outcome of the reconstruction. Surgeons should specify the requirements for the design of customized prostheses based on surgical procedures and potential changes that could occur in the defect area during surgery, adequately prepare alternative reconstruction plans preoperatively, and be capable of adjusting prosthesis installation during surgery.

6.5 Customized Prosthesis Failure After Surgery

6.5.1 Analysis of the Current Situation

Due to their personalized nature, 3D-printed customized prostheses face challenges in standardization from design and preparation to clinical application, potentially posing a greater risk of failure than traditional standardized prostheses. Currently, several domestic hospitals have conducted clinical trials on 3D-printed, personalized, customized prostheses, and a few cases of prosthesis failure have been reported. The reasons for this phenomenon may include the following factors that are related to the surgeons and the advantages of 3D-printed prostheses themselves:

1. The short duration of clinical trials and the limited number of cases make it difficult to evaluate some complications (such as aseptic loosening, prosthesis fatigue fracture, and joint wear).
2. Clinical doctors who apply this novel treatment model generally have extensive clinical experience, and users are more cautious in the initial stages.
3. Surgical planning is more precise, reducing the exposure time of surgical wounds.
4. Current prostheses mainly focus on fusion, with additional internal fixation support or a combination with other standardized products in weight-bearing areas.
5. The individualized matching of prostheses is more accurate, and the design of prosthesis fixation nails is more reasonable, leading to better stability immediately after surgery.
6. The porous structure of prostheses not only promotes osseointegration but also facilitates the attachment of soft tissues around the prosthesis, reducing dead space.

6.5.2 Reasons for Failure

3D-printed, personalized, customized prostheses, similar to traditional standardized prostheses, face postimplantation failure issues, but there are differences between the two types of prostheses. Risk factors for postoperative prosthesis failure include patient factors, surgical factors, and prosthesis factors. The main reasons for failure are aseptic prosthesis loosening, infection, periprosthetic bone fractures, prosthesis fractures, and prosthesis dislocation. For large bone tumor segmental prostheses, failure occurs due to two main causes: mechanical causes and nonmechanical causes (Table 6.4).

Traditional standardized prostheses are subjected to effective systematic validation before use, and their biological, mechanical, and frictional performance are all tested via standard procedures. Therefore, the failure of traditional prostheses after surgery mostly occurs due to the improper selection of prosthesis type or model, inadequate understanding of surgical indications, and nonstandard surgical procedures, and fewer cases of failure are attributed to prosthesis design defects. However, the most common mechanical reasons for the early failure of 3D-printed, personalized, customized prostheses are fracture of the load-bearing components of the prosthesis and improper placement; these causes are related to the design, preparation, and utilization of the prosthesis (Du et al. 2016).

Figure 6.13 illustrates reconstruction after the segmental resection of a malignant bone tumor in the lower segment of a child's femur (retaining the epiphysis) using

Table 6.4 Types of prosthesis failure

Type	Reason	Explanation
Mechanical	Soft tissue issues	Ligament tear, wound split
	Aseptic loosening	Displacement of the prosthesis, unstable support, localized pain
	Structural failure	Implant rupture, surrounding bone fractures, loss of bony support
Nonmechanical	Deep infection	Inability to retain prosthetic infections
	Tumor progression	Tumor recurrence or progression involving prostheses

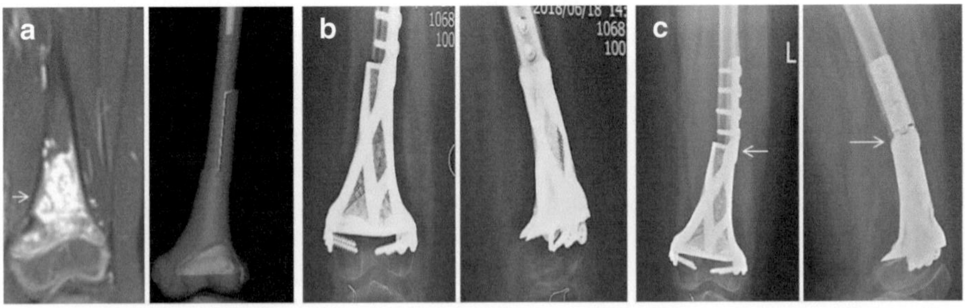

Fig. 6.13 Pediatric malignant bone tumor segment resection (retaining the epiphysis) with 3D-printed customized prosthesis reconstruction. (**a**) Preoperative MR images showing the extent of the tumor (indicated by white arrows) and simulating reconstruction with a personalized customized prosthesis after tumor resection. (**b**) Postoperative X-ray at 1 month showing good prosthesis fitting and satisfactory positioning. (**c**) At 10 months postsurgery, the child experienced a fracture at the base of the prosthesis support plate (indicated by white arrows) and tilting of the prosthesis after weight-bearing walking

a 3D-printed, personalized, customized prosthesis. A base plate fracture occurred in this prosthesis after weight-bearing walking 10 months postsurgery. Figure 6.14 provides an analysis of the reasons for the failure of this prosthesis.

Figure 6.15 shows a case of personalized artificial vertebral body reconstruction using 3D-printed customized implants after total vertebral body resection due to a malignant tumor in a single lumbar segment. The artificial implant showed no obvious abnormalities immediately after surgery or at the 2-year follow-up. The patient did not follow the annual follow-up schedule and presented

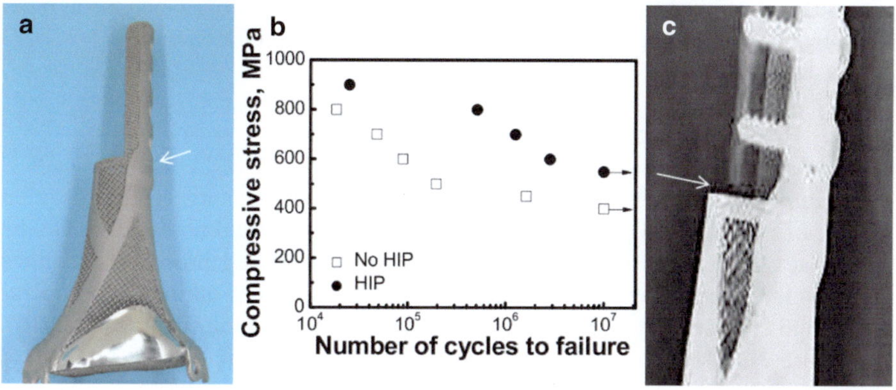

Fig. 6.14 The impact of personalized customized prosthesis design, preparation, and application defects on prosthesis fracture. (**a**) The side support wing base of the personalized customized femoral end prosthesis is a point of stress concentration (indicated by white arrows), and the design lacked local reinforcement. (**b**) The influence of post-printing hot isostatic pressing (HIP) treatment on material fatigue performance. (**c**) The mismatch at the prosthesis placement interface created gaps, affecting bone healing and further concentrating stress at the support wing base (indicated by white arrows)

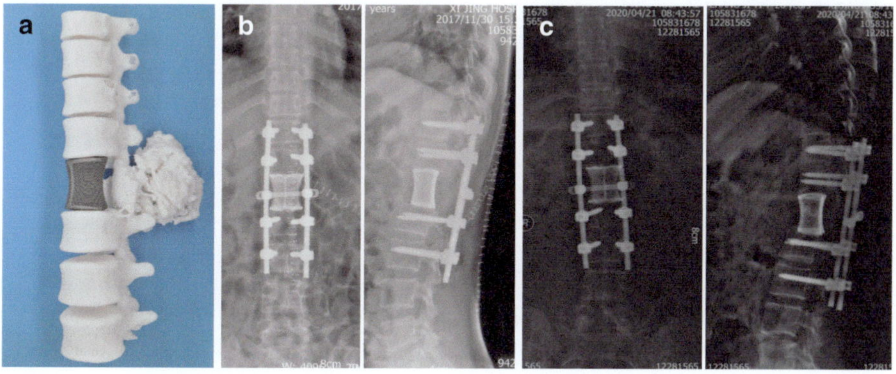

Fig. 6.15 Customized artificial vertebral body reconstruction using 3D printing after total resection of a malignant tumor in a single segment of the lumbar spine. (**a**) Preoperative installation simulation. (**b**) Immediate postoperative assessment. (**c**) A 2-year follow-up revealed excellent positioning of the prosthesis with no abnormalities detected

with implant failure and rod breakage at the 6-year follow-up, leading to a secondary revision surgery. Figure 6.16 shows the imaging results at the time of implant failure and after the removal of the fractured artificial vertebral body during surgery.

The primary cause of nonmechanical failure is infection. Periprosthetic infection can be catastrophic. Our surgical team encountered a patient who underwent 3D-printed personalized heel bone reconstruction, and 6 months after surgery, the patient had to undergo a second surgery to remove the heel bone prosthesis due to periprosthetic infection. This case highlights the risk of infection and other soft tissue issues in weight-bearing areas with poor soft tissue conditions when metal prosthetic reconstructions are performed, emphasizing the need for caution.

6.5.3 Prevention of Failure

To avoid or reduce the probability of failure after prosthetic surgery, the selection and use of conventional prostheses need to be standardized and normalized. On the other hand, the use of 3D-printed, personalized, customized prostheses requires thorough interactions between medical and engineering teams during the preoperative design and preparation stages, along with surgical planning (Pang et al. 2016). This approach ensures that the ideal prosthesis is designed and prepared, and proper preoperative planning is conducted to mitigate potential risks of postoperative failure. Key areas of focus include (1) Optimizing prosthesis design to reduce the risk of fracture (Figs. 6.17 and 6.18); (2) Preventing mechanical defects in 3D printing materials and enhancing fatigue resistance through necessary postprocessing techniques such as hot isostatic pressing; (3) Avoiding the design of overly complex

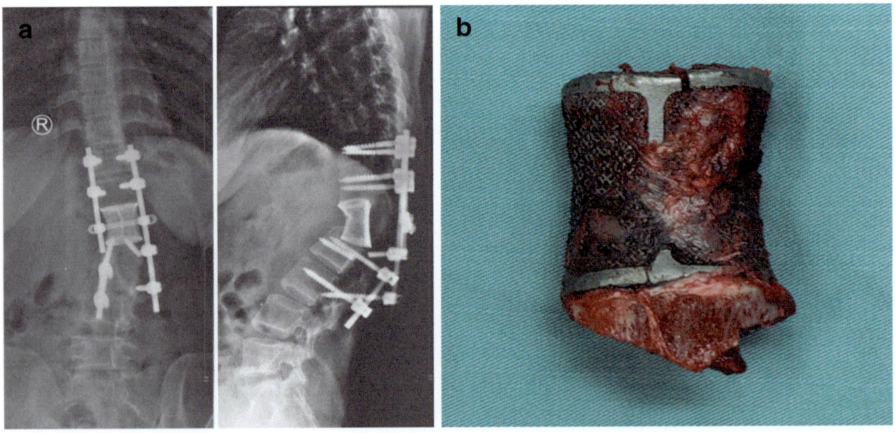

Fig. 6.16 (**a**) A personalized 3D-printed artificial vertebral body failed 6 years after surgery, showing fractures, anterior compression, and fractures in the posterior pedicle screw-rod system. (**b**) The image shows the artificial vertebral body after its removal, revealing a fracture in its anterior solid framework and anterior compression of the vertebral body

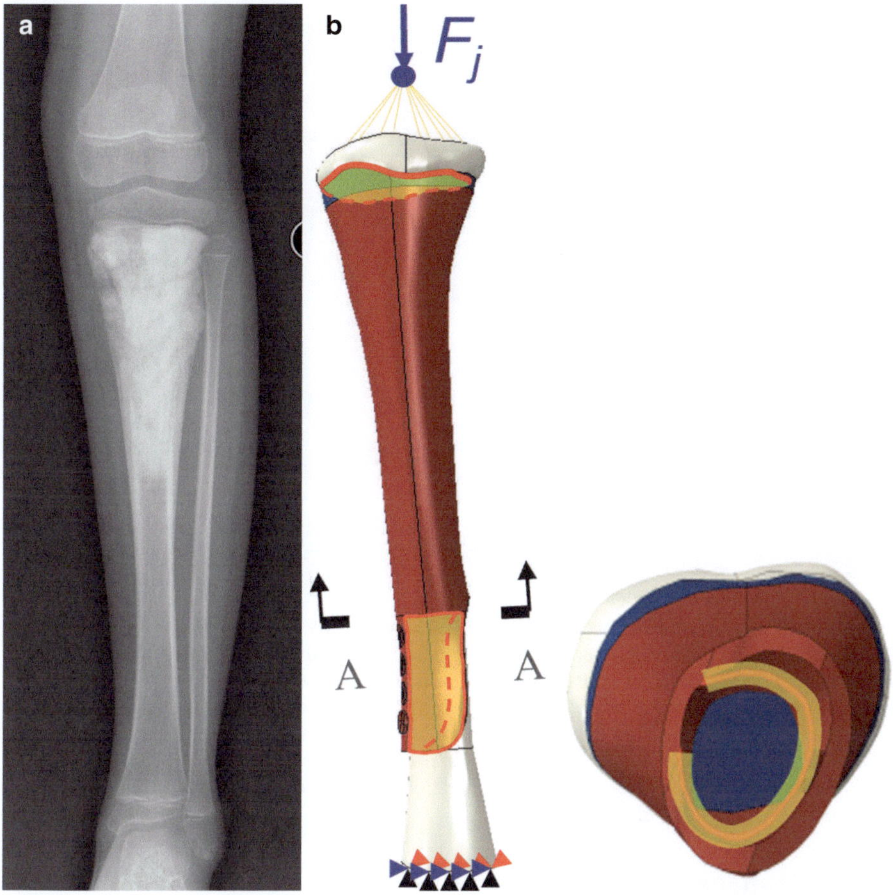

Fig. 6.17 Initial design for the resection of a malignant bone tumor segment in the middle and upper part of the tibia of a 7-year-old child (retaining the growth plate), with a plan to proceed with 3D-printed, personalized, customized prosthesis reconstruction. (**a**) Front view. (**b**) Bottom view (Pei et al. 2020)

prosthesis structures to facilitate easier placement and fully evaluating the feasibility of prosthesis design during surgical procedures; and (4) Designing specific prosthesis regions to have porous structures to promote osseointegration and soft tissue attachment around the prosthesis, reducing dead spaces.

Furthermore, surgical factors require increased attention, such as (1) The use of digital technology to assist in precise lesion resection and precise matching of personalized custom prostheses to reduce local stress and (2) The use of composite reconstruction techniques, such as combined bone grafting, to accelerate interface bone healing.

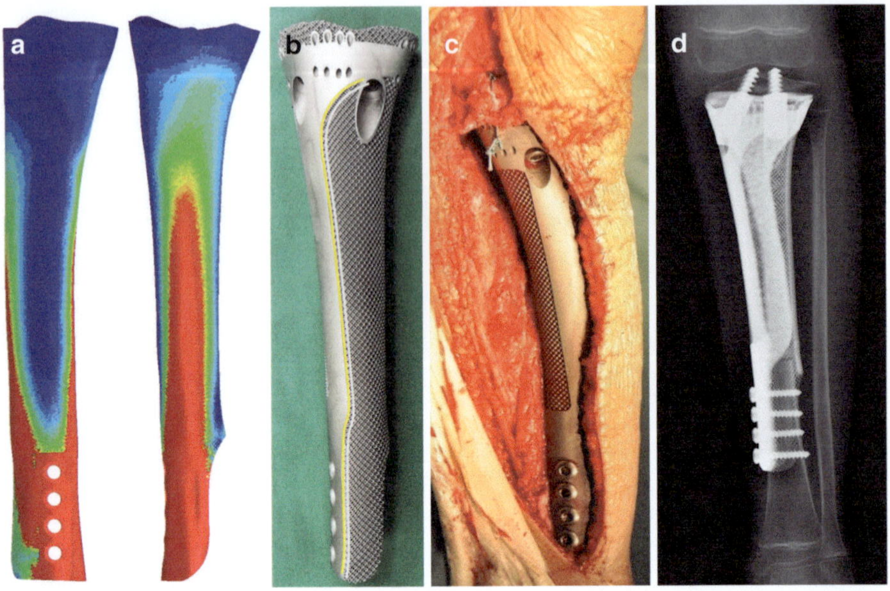

Fig. 6.18 (**a**, **b**) Based on the initial design, finite element analysis was conducted to optimize the design: (1) Enhanced body contour: the solid wing extended to the top of the prosthesis, forming a reinforced body. (2) Gradient transition: In the initial design, there was no transition between the solid part and the porous part of the prosthesis, which could lead to stress concentration and potential failure, such as separation between the solid and porous parts. The optimization included a gradual transition where the modulus of the porous/solid parts decreased gradually, avoiding potential failures that could be caused by sudden changes in porosity. (**c**, **d**) Intraoperative and postoperative images (Pei et al. 2020)

6.5.4 Management of Failure

The principles for managing the failure of personalized 3D-printed implants are similar to those for managing the failure of conventional implants. Revision surgery is usually the clinical remedy that is used to address the failure of personalized 3D-printed implants. Revision procedures need to address the specific reasons for failure.

For aseptic loosening, implant fracture, dislocation, and other noninfectious situations, clinicians may choose to prioritize revising the implant by producing a new customized implant. Manufacturers of customized implants retain the original design drawings. Therefore, when an implant needs to be redesigned, a thorough analysis of the reasons for the initial implant failure can be conducted, facilitating improvements and optimizations in the design based on the original implant drawings. Once the patient is satisfied with the new implant, a second revision surgery can be performed. This is one advantage of personalized 3D-printed implants that is not shared by traditional implants.

The most challenging aspect of implant failure is infection. Periprosthetic infections can have catastrophic consequences. When periprosthetic infection is diagnosed, for some patients with early-stage infections, it may be possible to perform thorough debridement while retaining the implant, followed by antibiotic therapy. However, for the majority of patients, revision surgery, which is typically conducted in two stages, is necessary. The first stage involves complete removal of the implant, thorough debridement, and insertion of a spacer, followed by antibiotic therapy to combat the infection. After a successful bacterial culture test 3 months after surgery, the spacer is removed, and a new implant is inserted. The duration of antibiotic therapy varies among different clinical centers, but the final determination requires confirmation of the absence of bacteria.

The most challenging aspect of such revision surgeries is dealing with soft tissues. Thorough debridement may lead to significant soft tissue damage. During the process of inserting a spacer to control infection, the surrounding soft tissues often exhibit increased adhesions and contractures, as well as poor blood supply. In the past, when using traditional implants for revision surgeries with poor soft tissue conditions, the surgical risks were high, and there was a high probability of poor wound healing after surgery or secondary infections around the implant. However, utilizing 3D-printed personalized implants for revision and reconstruction allows specific areas of the implant to be designed with a porous structure, facilitating soft tissue adhesion and reducing dead space, thereby reducing these risks.

In conclusion, the clinical application (clinical trials) of personalized 3D-printed implants in orthopedics has not been extensive. The initial outcomes have been generally positive; this is particularly true in cases of failed metal implants, where porous 3D-printed implants are significantly superior to traditional customized implants. However, the issue of 3D-printed implant fatigue fracture requires close attention, and strict control measures in design, preparation, and surgical procedures must be emphasized to minimize failure rates.

6.6 Summary

The emergence of new technologies often drives the evolution of treatment concepts. The maturity of 3D printing technology has profoundly changed the clinical application of personalized customized prostheses, and an increasing number of doctors have accepted 3D-printed personalized prostheses and recognized their value. Due to the wide range and diverse products among 3D-printed personalized customized prostheses, different from traditional processing methods for medical devices, as the clinical use of 3D-printed personalized prostheses increases, more clinical issues are being revealed, prompting doctors and related personnel to consider, explore, and optimize improvements to these processing methods. Surgeons play crucial roles in the design and clinical application of customized prostheses, conducting in-depth research based on patients' individual characteristics and incorporating the unique features of the prosthesis into a rational design to prevent and minimize potential failure risks.

References

Bandyopadhyay A, Heer B. Additive manufacturing of multi-material structures. Mater Sci Eng R Rep. 2018;129:1–16.

Du W, Bai Q, Zhang B. A novel method for additive/subtractive hybrid manufacturing of metallic parts. Procedia Manuf. 2016;5:1018–30.

Guo Z. Digital orthopedic technology assisted precise surgical treatment of pelvic tumors. Natl Med J China. 2019;99(37):2885–8.

Kranz J, Herzog D, Emmelmann C. Design guidelines for laser additive manufacturing of lightweight structures in TiAl6V4. J Laser Appl. 2014;27(S1):16.

Li S, Li X, Hou W, et al. Fabrication of open-cellular (porous) titanium alloy implants: osseointegration, vascularization and preliminary human trials. Sci China Mater. 2018;61(4):525–36.

Liu Z. Analysis of the application status and development trend of metal 3D printing orthopedic implants. J Orthop Clin Res. 2017;2(2):65–7.

Pang X, Wang L, Wang Z, et al. Finite element analysis of total knee replacement with various misalignment angles in the sagittal plane. J Mech Med Biol. 2016;16(7):1650096.

Pei Y, Fu J, Li J, et al. Biomechanical analysis and clinical application of 3D printed bone tumor prosthesis of lower limb. Chin J Orthop. 2020;40(12):760–8.

Taniguchi N, Fujibayashi S, Takemoto M, et al. Effect of pore size on bone ingrowth into porous titanium implants fabricated by additive manufacturing: an in vivo experiment. Mater Sci Eng C Mater Biol Appl. 2016;59:690–701.

Yu D, Wu S, Zhao J, et al. Exploration and clinical application of 3D printed personalized titanium alloy for bone repair prosthesis. Metal World. 2022;4:55–67.

Zhao D, Huang Y, Ao Y, et al. Effect of pore geometry on the fatigue properties and cell affinity of porous titanium scaffolds fabricated by selective laser melting. J Mech Behav Biomed Mater. 2018;88:478–87.

Part III

Regulations and standards for 3D-printed custom-made prostheses Overview

1.1 Regulations and Standards for 3D-Printed Custom-Made Prostheses Overview

Custom-made medical devices can be designed and manufactured according to the different individual needs of patients, facilitating the personalized matching of these products. A custom-made medical device is designed based on the needs of a specific patient, and it is characterized by strong anisotropy and the generation of few products. 3D printing is an emerging manufacturing technology by which physical objects are manufactured via the layer-by-layer accumulation of materials via a digital model. This approach has had a profound impact on traditional manufacturing processes, production lines, factory models, and industrial chain combinations, and it is a representative technology that is disrupting the manufacturing industry. Because of its innovative processing methods, 3D printing has greatly expanded the innovative design of products, shortened development cycles, and reduced material consumption, thus playing a major role in promoting the development of medical products and allowing their full use in the manufacture of custom-made medical devices. We fully exploit the ability of this approach to achieve efficient, accurate, and complex manufacturing as well as meet the goals of personalized medicine.

Preclinical studies and clinical trials typically cannot be conducted on custom-made medical devices because of the sample size requirements of studies and trials that are conducted on standardized medical devices. The supervision, laws, and registration systems that are applicable to standardized medical devices are not fully applicable to custom-made medical devices. Therefore, although custom-made medical devices are advantageous to the development of medicine, such products also challenge the model of supervision that is used for generally standardized products. Thus, regulatory authorities and scholars in various countries have conducted active investigations and research. Many countries have passed regulatory laws and produced guidance documents for 3D-printed custom-made medical devices. The first authority to do so was the U.S. Food and Drug Administration (FDA). In the Medical Device Amendments to Federal Food, Drug, and Cosmetic Act, which was published in 1976, the FDA proposed a custom-made device for the first time. Then, the Food and Drug Administration Safety and Innovation Act, which was published on July 9, 2012, announced the clinical use of these devices as well as restrictions on postmarketing management. In September 2014, the FDA released the Custom Device Exemption, which explained in detail the regulatory provisions and relevant requirements for custom-made devices (Min and Liu 2017; Wu and Liu 2020). The European Union, which also began to regulate medical devices relatively early, defined custom-made medical devices according to the Regulations on Medical Devices of the European Parliament and the Council, which was released in May 2017. The Personalized Medical Devices Working Group, which is part of the International Medical Device Regulators Forum and the main research group focusing on personalized medical device terminology and regulatory requirements, released the Definitions for Personalized Medical Devices in November 2018. This guidance also represents the preliminary international unification of the understanding of personalized medical devices; according to the degree of personalization (from high to low), personalized medical devices are divided into custom-made medical devices, patient-matched medical devices, and adaptable medical devices. The Personalized Medical Devices-Regularity Pathways, which were released in March 2020, described the regulatory pathways and requirements for these three types of personalized medical devices. In China, the National Medical Products Administration (NMPA) and the National Health Commission released the "Regulations on the Supervision and Administration of Customized Medical Devices (Trial)," defined custom-made medical devices and patient-matched medical devices, and clarified the regulatory pathways and specific requirements for custom-made medical devices. The regulation of custom-made medical devices in China began relatively late, but it developed quickly.

3D-printed custom-made medical devices are an important area of development. Moreover, the safety and effectiveness of medical devices that are manufactured by 3D printing technology are influenced by increasingly complex factors; this has resulted in the generation of corresponding standards and guidance documents for 3D-printed medical devices, which regulate and guide the development of the industry. This section will introduce and comparatively analyze the regulatory laws and regulations of the USA, the European Union, and China as well as the standards and guidance documents related to the supervision of 3D-printed medical devices.

References

Min Y, Liu B. Study of regulatory requirements of customized device in the U.S. Chin J Med Instrum. 2017;41(01):43–7.

Wu J, Liu B. Overview of domestic and foreign regulatory regulations about customized additive manufacturing medical devices and considerations of the industry development. Orthopaed Biomech Mater Clin Study. 2020;17(05):65–70.

US Regulations and Standards

7

Jintao Gao, Dan Han, Hainan Shen, Niya Li, Chang Yang, and Bin Liu

7.1 Introduction

The United States began supervising medical devices early; medical devices were mentioned in the Food and Drug Act of 1906, and the management of medical devices was added to the Federal Food, Drug, and Cosmetic Act of 1938. In 1976, the Medical Device Amendment was released, and it confirmed the classification system of medical devices, enhanced supervision, and proposed custom-made medical devices for the first time. In 1990, the US Congress passed the Safe Medical Devices Act, which authorized the FDA to conduct postmarket safety supervision of companies that produce permanently implanted devices and gave the FDA the power to require the recall of noncompliant devices. In July 2012, the FDA Safety and Innovation Act officially went into effect, adding restrictions on the clinical use and postmarket management of custom-made medical devices. In September 2014, the FDA officially released guidance on "Custom Device Exemption," which clarified the regulatory model for custom-made medical devices. From 2012 to 2021, the FDA strengthened its work on international standards related to medical devices, including the announcement of international standards recognized by the FDA and the development of compliance guidelines. In December 2017, the FDA officially released the Guidance Document Technical Considerations for Additive Manufactured Medical Devices to regulate the manufacturing of 3D-printed medical devices.

J. Gao · D. Han · H. Shen · N. Li · C. Yang · B. Liu (✉)
Shenzhen, China
e-mail: gaojt@mdei.org.cn; handan@mdei.org.cn; shenhn@mdei.org.cn; liny@mdei.org.cn; yangchang@mdei.org.cn; liubin@mdei.org.cn

Z. Guo et al. (eds.), *3D-Printed Prosthesis in Orthopedic Oncology*,
https://doi.org/10.1007/978-981-95-1454-0_7

7.2 Regulations and Guidance for Custom-Made Medical Devices

7.2.1 Regulatory Laws and Regulatory Pathways of Medical Devices

7.2.1.1 Product Classification

The FDA implements classification management of medical devices, which can be divided into three main classes: Class I products, Class II products, and Class III products. Class I products have relatively low risk, and premarket notification is not required; premarket notification (510(k)) is required for Class II products (US Food and Drug Administration 2023), and premarket approval (PMA) is required for Class III products (US Food and Drug Administration 2019).

Class I products (commonly managed products) include medical gloves, tongue depressors, manual surgical instruments, etc., and they do not require premarket notification as long as they meet GMP requirements and are registered.

For Class II products (common and specially managed products), a 510(k) application is required, and they can be marketed for sale after FDA review.

Class III products (premarketing approval-managed products), such as artificial heart valves and cardiac pacemakers, have relatively high risks or hazards, and the submission of a PMA application and approval from the FDA are required before they can be marketed.

Most medical devices can be classified by searching for a matching description for medical devices in Chapter 21 of the Federal Regulations (CFR) Parts 862–892. The FDA has classified and described more than 1700 different types of medical devices, such as cardiovascular medical devices or ENT medical devices, and organized them into 16 medical specialty "groups" in the CFR. These panels can be found in CFR Parts 862 through 892. For each medical device that has been classified by the FDA, the CFR provides a general description, including the intended use, the class to which the device belongs (i.e., Class I, II, or III), and information on marketing requirements. A medical device should meet the definition in the 21 CFR 862–892 classification regulation. The FDA has clarified how to search for classification rules (US Food and Drug Administration 2018).

7.2.1.2 Registration Forms and Approval Process

In the United States, the supervision of medical devices is a complex and important part of medical supervision, and it is the responsibility of the Center for Devices and Radiological Products Health (CDRH) under the FDA. The CDRH plays a key role in protecting the health and well-being of Americans, ensuring that medical devices and radiating electronic products meet strict safety and effectiveness standards. This regulatory framework is critical for enhancing the confidence of the public and health care professionals in the devices that are used in patient care. The CDRH is responsible for the protection and promotion of public health. Patients and medical service providers must have timely and continuous access to safe, effective, and high-quality medical devices. The CDRH provides consumers, patients, patient caregivers, and health care providers with understandable and accessible scientific information about the products that are regulated. The CDRH promotes medical device innovation by advancing regulatory science, providing predictable, consistent, transparent, and efficient regulatory pathways for the industry, and ensuring that patients have confidence in the devices that are sold in the United States.

The CDRH is mainly responsible for:

(a) Conducting reviews of medical device applications for scientific research or clinical use.
(b) Collecting, analyzing, and processing information related to injuries and other experiences in the use of medical devices and radioactive electronic products.
(c) Establishing and organizing the implementation of GMPs and performance standards for radioactive electronic products and medical devices.
(d) Supervising the conformity of medical devices and radioactive electronic products.
(e) Providing technical and other noneconomic assistance to small-scale medical device manufacturers.

In the United States, the premarket approval of medical devices falls under the unified management of the FDA headquarters. Although some products can be reviewed by a third-party organization, the final approval rights remain at the FDA headquarters. Local institutions have no power in premarket approval and mainly play a role in daily supervision and assistance of the FDA headquarters in completing other tasks.

This section provides a brief overview of the basic requirements of medical device supervision in the United States (Table 7.1), including institutional registration, premarket notification (510(k)), premarket approval (PMA), investigational device exemption (IDE), quality system supervision and medical regulatory models such as device reporting (MDR), highlighting the essentials of each regulatory model.

Medical devices that are exempt from premarket notification: For most Class I medical devices and a small number of Class II medical devices, premarket notification is not required, and they can be marketed as long as they comply with relevant regulations and GMP requirements.

Medical devices that require premarket notification (510(k)): For most Class II medical devices, a 510(k) application must be submitted, and they can be marketed after an FDA review. The review process includes the issuance of the confirmation letter, the amendment, and the determination of substantive equivalence.

Medical devices that require premarket approval (PMA): For all Class III medical devices and innovative medical devices, a PMA application must be submitted, and they can be marketed after being reviewed by the FDA. The review process included filing reviews, scientific reviews, regulatory reviews, advisory committee reviews, PMA amendments, and final decisions.

Table 7.1 Requirements of the US medical device regulatory model

Supervision model	Requirement
Institutional registration and listing	Manufacturers and initial distributors must register their establishments with the FDA Registration information must be verified annually Foreign manufacturers must appoint a US agent for communication Institutional registration fees were introduced in October 2007
Premarket notification 510(k)	There are requirements for equipment that has been proven to be basically equivalent to existing equipment Most class I and some class II devices are exempt The device must be thoroughly evaluated before entering the market
Premarket approval (PMA)	Class III and some class II devices require strict evaluation and the submission of clinical data
Investigational device exemption (IDE)	The use of investigative equipment in clinical research is permitted Devices with significant risk require approval from the FDA and the institutional review board Safety and efficacy testing must be conducted before market access
Quality system regulations	All aspects of device design, manufacturing, and labeling must be managed Factories are inspected by the FDA to ensure compliance Clear and accurate labeling is critical for patient safety
Medical device reporting (MDR)	Timely reporting of device-related deaths, injuries, and failures is needed It is convenient for the Food and Drug Administration and the manufacturer to monitor adverse events Custom-made devices that meet specific criteria are exempt

Medical devices that can be audited by a third party: Several Class II medical devices can be audited by a third-party organization to accelerate the market access process. Audit agencies need to meet the requirements of the FDA, including independence and audit experience.

7.2.1.3 Postmarket Surveillance

The FDA requires manufacturers to ensure that medical devices are produced under conditions that meet GMP requirements. The supervision includes quality system inspection, traceability systems, and adverse event reporting and recall. The FDA may take administrative punishment measures, such as issuing warning letters, seizing products, and compulsory recall.

Quality system inspection: The frequency of risk is determined according to the risk level of the medical device.

Traceability system: This system ensures that medical devices are traceable from production to use by patients.

Adverse event reporting: Manufacturers, importers, and user units are required to report the number of deaths and serious injuries.

Recall: Manufacturers may recall medical devices with quality problems, and the FDA may also issue a recall order.

These measures are designed to ensure the quality and safety of medical devices to protect the health of patients.

7.2.2 Regulatory Pathways for Custom-Made Medical Devices

7.2.2.1 Regulations for Custom-Made Medical Devices

The concept of custom-made medical devices was proposed for the first time in 1976 in the amendment to the Federal Food, Drug, and Cosmetic Act, which laid the foundation for the regulation of these devices. This act provided the FDA with regulatory power to ensure the safety and effectiveness of medical devices. However, with the continuous development of medical technology, more specific and differentiated supervision of different types of medical devices is needed. Therefore, in 2012, the Food and Drug Regulatory Safety and Innovation Act increased the restrictions on custom-made medical devices and strengthened regulatory requirements, paying special attention to clinical use and postmarketing management. Thus, the regulatory requirements for custom-made medical devices have improved in terms of supervision and regulation.

Custom-made medical devices are generally defined as medical devices with the characteristics of "personalized design" and "customized production". In the United States, personalized custom-made medical devices can include custom-made medical devices and patient-matched medical devices, and the FDA adopts different models for the supervision of these different devices. The regulation of patient-matched medical devices follows the model that is used to regulate conventional medical devices, while a simplified model is used to regulate custom-made medical devices according to specific requirements.

Patient-matched medical devices and custom-made medical devices are personalized custom-made medical devices, but there are certain differences between these two kinds of devices. Usually, patient-matched medical devices have a series of different specifications that can be approved for the treatment of patient populations and can be used to conduct clinical studies. On the other hand, custom-made medical devices are used for patients with rare diseases or to meet the unique needs of physicians, and they have unique specifications and sizes, making it difficult to carry out clinical studies. One type of custom-made medical device is patient-centered, while the other is physician-centered, and both patients and physicians cannot be centered at the same time.

An analysis and comparison of seven aspects of custom-made medical devices and patient-matched medical devices, including the applicable population, indications, use restrictions, specifications and sizes, processing technology, approval requirements, and postmarket supervision, is presented (Table 7.2), to help

Table 7.2 Comparison of custom-made medical devices and patient-matched medical devices in the United States

	Personalized, customized medical devices	
	Custom-made medical devices	Patient-matched medical devices
Applicable population for each product	A doctor or a patient	A patient
Applicable situation	The unique physiological condition or pathological anatomy of the patient, or the special operational needs of the doctor	Unlimited
Restriction on use	No alternative device	Unlimited
Production process	Traditional production technology or emerging production technology (such as 3D printing)	
Specifications and sizes	Only the specification size, which is different for each product, is approved	Approved size range
Approval requirements	Custom-made medical device requirements	510(k) or PMA requirements
Postmarket supervision	Annual production volume of each product cannot exceed five pieces, and an annual report must be submitted to the FDA every year	510(k) or PMA requirements

elucidate the similarities and differences between these devices. These comparisons can help medical professionals and manufacturers better understand different types of personalized, custom-made medical devices and provide guidance for their compliance and safety. This helps to ensure that patients receive the medical devices that best suit their needs.

In the United States, custom-made medical devices and patient-matched medical devices are personalized, custom-made medical devices that not only solve the problem of nondevice use, which patients with unique conditions face, but also meet the needs of personalized medicine in treating patients with common conditions. Although these two types of devices both have "custom-made" characteristics, the focus of FDA supervision is different, focusing on postmarketing supervision and premarket approval. The reasons may be as follows (Min and Liu 2017): first, because custom-made medical devices are suitable for patients with unique anatomical structures, the design features of the products are either limited in size or very rare structural shapes. The "substantial equivalence" of marketed devices cannot prove the safety and effectiveness of the declared products. Moreover, the patient population that is treated with custom-made medical devices is too small to verify the safety and effectiveness of the products through clinical trials. Therefore, neither the traditional 510(k) nor PMA approval modes are suitable for custom-made medical devices. Therefore, in the revision of the Medical Devices Regulations in 1976, the FDA separately formulated regulatory requirements for custom-made medical devices, turning the strict premarket approval system that is applicable to conventional devices into strict postmarket regulatory requirements that are more suitable for custom-made medical devices; this reflects the "minimum burden principle" of the FDA. Second, with the application and popularity of 3D-printing technology in the medical device field in recent years, the general patient population is not satisfied with the "cut the foot to fit the shoe" treatment method and has come to prefer "tailor-made" personalized medicine. The FDA has gradually distinguished the product category of patient-matched medical devices from that of conventional medical devices to ensure that the products have certain personalized applications within a range that is suitable for the general patient population. Therefore, patient-matched medical devices can still use the criteria of substantial equivalence comparison or clinical trial validation data to support premarket approval.

7.2.2.2 Premarket Approval Process and Guidance for Custom-Made Medical Devices

The regulatory model that is implemented in many countries involves the use of guidance to evaluate the premarket safety and effectiveness of medical devices. The USA began to regulate medical devices early, and after long-term experience had accumulated, the construction of the FDA's guidance system became relatively mature. The CDRH is responsible for the formulation of medical device guidance in the United States. The FDA released the draft good guidance specification in 1997, which clarified the basic requirements for the development, release, and use of FDA guidance documents. This document affirmed that FDA guidance is not mandatory but also emphasized the binding force on FDA staff. The FDA staff may conduct review work in violation of the guidance document requirements only for legitimate reasons and with regulatory consent.

In terms of custom-made medical device supervision, in September 2014, the FDA officially released the guidance document "Custom Device Exemption" (US Food and Drug Administration 2014), which explained in detail the regulatory provisions and relevant requirements for custom-made medical devices and provided guidance for manufacturers and medical professionals. This guidance helps to regulate and manage custom-made medical devices more clearly and ensures their compliance with relevant laws and regulations.

In this guidance, the FDA specifically emphasized that a custom-made medical device must meet all the requirements of Section 520(b) of the Food and Drug Chemical Law before it can be identified as a custom-made medical device. The guidance also noted that custom-made medical devices do not need to meet premarket approval requirements and do not need to follow mandatory performance standards, but they cannot be exempt from the requirements of quality system specifications. The guidance further noted that the postmarket supervision of custom-made medical devices should be more stringent, stipulating that the annual production number of each type of product should not exceed five and that manufacturers should be required to produce these devices as needed and submit an annual report to the FDA each year. The guidance also indicated that the final custom-made devices should not usually be sold through marketing or advertising.

The FDA does not require a review or approval for the use of custom-made medical devices, but the FDA recommends prudence in taking as many measures to protect patients as possible. Ethics committees (IRBs) should have an in-depth understanding of the regulatory requirements for custom-made medical devices because doctors or medical institutions may consult an IRB for information on the use of medical devices in their medical institutions. IRBs can develop procedures that are applicable to the use of medical devices to ensure that patient protection measures are carefully implemented, thereby safeguarding the rights and safety of patients. This helps to ensure the rational use of custom-made medical devices and provides doctors with a legal framework to meet the unique needs of their patients.

Section 520(b) of the Food and Drug Administration Act specifies the exemption for custom-made medical devices, allowing them to meet specific requirements for 510(k) and PMA approval based on the characteristics of their design, production, and clinical application. Nevertheless, as medical device products, custom-made medical devices still need to meet the basic requirements of the quality management system, including enterprise registration, device listing, design control, and reporting of medical device adverse events. In addition, relevant information on custom-made medical devices should be clearly indicated on their labels.

Compared with general medical devices, the requirements for the premarket approval of custom-made medical devices are looser, but the FDA also has detailed postmarket regulatory requirements, the most important of which is that manufacturers need to submit an annual report for each custom-made medical device. Manufacturers must prepare a corresponding annual report based on the intended user of a custom-made medical device, whether it is a patient or a doctor. These measures aim to ensure the safety and effectiveness of custom-made medical devices that are on the market and provide regulatory agencies with necessary information about these medical devices to continue to ensure the health and safety of patients.

7.3 Standards and Guidance for Medical 3D-Printing Technology

7.3.1 Medical Device Standards

7.3.1.1 US Medical Device Standard Management (Yu et al. 2020)

(a) American National Standards

The American standards system is a highly decentralized, independent, private organization-led, and market-oriented combination of voluntary and mandatory standards. The formulation of American standards is organized mainly by associations, societies, alliances, committees and other private groups, such as the Association for the Advancement of Medical Instrumentation (AAMI), the Institute of Electrical and Electronics Engineers (IEEE), the American Society for Testing and Materials (ASTM), the American Society of Mechanical Engineers (ASME), and Underwriters Laboratories (UL).

The American national standards are implemented by an accreditation system, and the American National Standards Institute (ANSI) is responsible for accrediting standard development organizations. The American national standards are all voluntary consensus standards. If the standards are cited by regulations or appear in contracts, the standards are mandatory.

(b) American National Standards Institute

Founded in 1918, the American National Standards Institute (ANSI) is a private nonprofit organization that has served as the administrator and coordinator of the voluntary standardization system in the private sector in the United States for more than 100 years. The mission of the ANSI is to enhance the global competitiveness of US enterprises and quality of life in the United States by promoting voluntary consensus standards and conformity assessment systems and maintaining their integrity. The ANSI is the official US representative of the International Organization for Standardization (ISO) and the International Electrotechnical Commission (IEC). It represents the United States in international standardization activities around the world and acts as a bridge between private industry and governmental organizations, such as the National Institute of Standards and Technology (NIST) and the US Department of Commerce.

The ANSI is neither a governmental organization nor a standard setter. Its responsibility is mainly to accredit the Standards Developing Organization (SDO) and the US Technical Advisory Groups (TAGs), and the scope of its work is similar to that of the Standardization Administration of China (SAC).

The accreditation process of the ANSI includes the following: stakeholders must reach a consensus; when any public figures post comments, the standards need to be reviewed by the public; and the comments of the consensus agencies and public commentators must be based on the respondent in a sincere manner.

In the United States, only standard developers can submit a standard to be approved as an American national standard. An American national standard is approved by the ANSI in accordance with the requirements stipulated in the American National Standards Procedures, such as ANSI IEEEc63.27-2017 and ANSI AAMI EC53:2013.

(c) US Medical Device Standard Management

Medical device standards in the United States are supervised by the FDA. In the USA, the enactment of the Food and Drug Administration Modernization Act (FDAMA) in 1997 allowed the FDA to formally recognize standards. Currently, conformity assessment of medical device standards is performed by the Center for Devices and Radiological Health (CDRH).

1. Consensus Standard

The American voluntary consensus standards are the standards that were developed or adopted by the SDO according to the strict consensus principle. Consensus standards help improve regulatory quality because consensus-based, standard-setting organizations must abide by the principles of transparency, openness, and fairness to participants and stakeholders.

2. Recognition of the Requirements of the Consensus Standards

The FDAMA stipulates that the Standards Management Staff (SMS) is responsible for promoting the acceptance of national and international consensus standards for medical devices. Section 514(c) was added to the FDAMA, and it stipulates that the FDA shall publish in the Federal Register and recognize all or part of the appropriate standards that were developed by nationally or internationally recognized standard-setting organizations. Individuals may submit the Declaration of Conformity applicable to this standard in accordance with the premarket submission requirements of this act or other requirements. Any interested party can propose accreditation standards. The submission procedures and requirements are specified in the relevant laws and regulations, and the list of accreditation results is published in the Federal Register. The standards on the accreditation list that cannot be used in the declaration of conformity are removed as needed.

The FDA usually approves or disapproves of the consensus standards of national or international standard-setting organizations in whole or in part according to the following procedures. The accreditation of medical device standards is organized and implemented by the SMS designated by the CDRH. Under the organization of the SMS, different Standards Task Groups (STGs) coordinate the assessment of consensus standards and propose candidate standards, collect information on relevant consensus standards, periodically evaluate newly developed or revised standards, propose accreditation and technical suggestions for delayed or disapproval, identify whether the FDA has corresponding guidance, evaluate the issue of consistency or conflict, and identify the devices to which the accreditation standards apply. The SMS summarizes the opinions of each STG and proposes a list of proposed accreditation standards. Then, the opinions of all parties are solicited and coordinated, the list of accreditation standards is revised and improved, the federal notice is drafted, and the results of accreditation standards are released after approval. Moreover, the SMS coordinates the maintenance of the accreditation consensus standards database, notifies the affected departments, and guides relevant personnel to become familiar with the standard requirements in advance and prepare for standard implementation.

7.3.1.2 Relevant Standards of 3D-Printing Technology in the United States

ISO/TC 261 and ASTM F42 are engaged in relevant standardization work and research in the field of additive manufacturing in the machinery industry. ISO/TC

261 is divided into four working groups, namely, term, methods, technique, and test methods, and data and design; ASTM covers test terminology, methods, design, materials, and techniques. As of November 2023, approximately 40 additive manufacturing-related standards were compiled by ASTM F42, covering terminology specifications, data and software, equipment, material, process, and product. More details are provided in Appendix (Tables 7.3, 7.4, 7.5, 7.6, 7.7 and 7.8). However, the standards that have been formulated or published involve only the machinery industry and the aerospace field, not the medical field, and there are no corresponding specific medical device standards.

7.3.2 Relevant Guidance for Medical 3D-Printing Technology

The FDA defines 3D printing as "a process of creating a three-dimensional object by creating a continuous layer on a raw material such as metal or ceramics." 3D printing is a type of additive manufacturing, but the FDA uses the two terms interchangeably. Since the early 2000s, this technology has been used in the medical field to produce products such as implants, surgical instruments, pharmaceuticals, and cells and tissues. 3D printing can create devices with complex internal geometries, such as spinal implants with porous structures, that can promote tissue outgrowth and integration. 3D-printed devices can also be manufactured as monolithic products, eliminating the need for the assembly of many individually created components.

On December 5, 2017, the FDA officially released the "Guidance Document: Technical Considerations for Additive Manufactured Medical Devices" to regulate the manufacturing activities of the medical 3D printing industry (US Food and Drug Administration 2017). This guidance not only provided clear operational suggestions for the additive manufacturing process and the testing of related medical devices but also set specific requirements for the 3D printing method, design, functionality, and quality system of relevant medical devices. To ensure that the regulatory method is suitable for this unique and innovative technology, the guidance is based on the experience of the US FDA in reviewing more than 100 medical products that use 3D printing, including knee joint prostheses and cranial reconstruction.

This guidance was issued to ensure the safety of innovative 3D-printed medical products and promote their marketing. This approach provides suggestions for 3D-printing technology and elaborates on the specific content that must be submitted to the FDA for the marketing of 3D-printed medical devices. This guidance is divided into seven parts, and each part includes detailed considerations on the design, manufacturing, and testing of 3D-printed medical devices. In the section on design and manufacturing process considerations, the importance of patient matching is emphasized, and key factors such as material control and postprocessing are discussed. In the section on equipment testing, mechanical testing, material property testing, and biocompatibility testing are included.

It is worth mentioning that this guidance also highlights the influence of different processes during 3D printing on the performance of the final product. Without completely understanding each process flow, it is very difficult to determine the root cause of product failure. Therefore, it is recommended that manufacturers use production flowcharts during production and establish constructive tips and conclusions in each key process flow to ensure product quality and performance.

In addition, even if the same 3D printer model, same parameters, process flow, or materials are used to manufacture the same medical device, the quality of the products may be different. Therefore, the FDA strongly recommends that manufacturers clearly understand the variability of each input parameter and processing flow and how they affect the quality of the final product or part of the material. If the result of a certain process cannot be verified by subsequent inspection and testing, then strict verification procedures must be implemented, and approval should be obtained according to the prescribed procedures.

Additionally, for 3D-printed, custom-made medical devices, the applicability of the system for scanning and creating 3D structural images also needs to be considered, as this system is critical for the generation of the final products. Various factors, such as image quality, resolution, smoothness, and image processing algorithms, may affect the initial model design of the product. Therefore, it is necessary to customize the anatomical landmarks to establish a clearer model to ensure that the needs of customers are met. The guidance recommends that before submitting a marketing application for a 3D-printed medical device, the manufacturer should prepare documents of device description, mechanical testing, dimensional measurement, material property testing, methods for removing manufacturing material residues, sterilization, and biocompatibility testing, etc., to meet FDA requirements. These documents will be very important to the FDA review process.

In the field of biomedical engineering, 3D-printing technology has enormous potential, and it is widely used in medical hard implant markets, such as dentistry, orthopedics, and neurosurgery. Although many products, such as medical models, surgical guides, surgical molds, vascular stents, and postoperative orthopedic instruments, have appeared on the market, there are still uncertainties in their development in the absence of a clear regulatory framework.

Therefore, this guidance from the FDA provides manufacturers with a clear regulatory framework and helps promote the customization and high-quality development of medical devices. In addition, the FDA plans to further review the regulatory issues related to 3D bioprinting of biological, cell, and tissue products to determine whether regulatory guidance is needed for regenerative medicine products, and additional guidance needs to be provided. This will provide a clearer direction for the development of 3D printing for wound treatment and for soft implantable organs, yielding additional innovations and opening additional possibilities in the medical field in the future.

Different from most guidance documents, the FDA characterizes this guidance as tentative and evolving, acknowledging that 3D-printing technology is still being developed and that any guidance may be changed accordingly. Additionally, while

3D printing may cause additional technical considerations to occur, these aspects are not discussed further.

However, the FDA does not regulate the 3D printing equipment itself but rather the manufacturing process and output of this printing equipment (if the output is a medical device). The CDRH commented on the supervision of 3D-printed medical devices through public forums, formal guidelines, and demonstrations, and it stated that, given the constantly evolving nature of the technology, its guidance on this topic is tentative and subject to change. The FDA has solicited opinions on its future-oriented regulatory framework to ensure the quality of 3D-printed medical devices and improve its upcoming regulation of 3D-printed medical devices as much as possible.

In 2021, the FDA released a discussion paper on 3D printing for point of care (POC). This document not only outlined the regulation of point-of-care 3D printing but also identified the challenges of its end use and provided revised potential rules. The FDA said the recommendations were not meant to be guidance but were designed to "raise questions" that would help inform future regulation. According to the FDA, the use of 3D printing in hospitals and surgeries can rapidly lead to the production of patient-specific medical devices, such as anatomical models and other point-of-care medical devices. The FDA emphasized the role of 3D-printing technology in helping solve supply chain problems, such as the worldwide shortage of medical resources for the treatment and prevention of COVID-19 in the early stage of the pandemic. However, the FDA also admitted that there are challenges in the large-scale promotion of this type of medical device, including the fact that suppliers are unlikely to have the same level of production knowledge as traditional manufacturers. Therefore, to ensure that the devices remain safe and fit for purpose, the FDA is now seeking feedback on the so-called "preliminary outline of a regulatory approach."

In its document, the FDA emphasized the differences in technology and training between manufacturers of 3D printing equipment and those of other medical device equipment and how related mismatches lead to differences in the quality of the final products. These mismatches ranged from the development of internal processes and clinical application guidelines to the availability of reprocessing equipment. In some cases, these mismatches may have a critical impact on product safety. Ultimately, the FDA emphasized that "communication among all stakeholders" is critical to creating an environment that is conducive to the growth and development of technology. 3D printing-technology is developing so rapidly that the current regulatory framework may not be able to keep up with the pace of technological development in the next few years. Therefore, the FDA's goal is to develop a set of revised rules to promote innovation while maintaining regulatory balance.

In addition, to better understand the nature of 3D printing technology, the US FDA has conducted studies and used the most advanced 3D printing equipment to promote and establish a management framework for the quality and safety of 3D-printed products and to promote the development of regulatory science. For example, the Center for Drug Evaluation and Research (CDER) is focused on the effect of 3D printing on the quality control of inactive ingredients and other pharmaceutical ingredients in drugs as well as the manufacturing process, while the CDRH uses 3D printing equipment to study whether changes in the manufacturing method can affect the safety and performance of medical devices and whether each product manufacturer or iteratively updates to the instrument will change the safety and performance of the product, for example, whether the applicability and comfort of prosthetic limbs will be affected.

Appendix: Relevant Standards for 3D Printing in the United States

Table 7.3 Basic US 3D printing standards

Standard number	Standard name
ASTM F2971-13(2021)	Standard practice for reporting data for test specimens prepared by additive manufacturing
ISO ASTM 52900-2021	Additive manufacturing—general principles—fundamentals and vocabulary
ISO ASTM 52901-16	Standard guide for additive manufacturing—general principles—requirements for purchased AM parts
ISO ASTM 52910-2018	Additive manufacturing—design—requirements, guidelines, and recommendations
ISO ASTM 52915-2020	Specification for additive manufacturing file format (AMF) version 1.2
ISO ASTM 52936-1-2023	Additive manufacturing of polymers—qualification principles—part 1:General principles and preparation of test specimens for PBF-LB
ISO ASTM52921-13(2019)	Standard terminology for additive manufacturing—coordinate systems and test methodologies

Table 7.4 US 3D printing data/software standards

Standard number	Standard name
ASTM F3413-19e1	Guide for additive manufacturing—design—directed energy deposition
ISO ASTM 52950-2021	Additive manufacturing—general principles—overview of data processing
ISO ASTM TR 52916-2022	Additive manufacturing for medical—data—optimized medical image data
ISO IEC 3532-1-2023	Information technology—medical image-based modeling for 3D printing —part 1: general requirements

Table 7.5 US 3D printing equipment standards

Standard number	Standard name
ISO ASTM 52903-2-2020	Additive manufacturing—material extrusion-based additive manufacturing of plastic materials—part 2: process equipment
ISO ASTM TS 52930-2021	Additive manufacturing—qualification principles—installation, operation, and performance (IQ/OQ/PQ) of PBF-LB equipment
ISO IEC 23510-2021	Information technology—3D printing and scanning—framework for an additive manufacturing service platform (AMSP)

Table 7.6 US 3D printing material standards

Standard number	Standard name	Standard number	Standard name
ASTM F2924-14(2021)	Standard specification for additive manufacturing Titanium-6 Aluminum-4 vanadium with powder bed fusion	ASTM F3213-17	Standard for additive manufacturing—finished part properties—Standard specification for Cobalt-28 Chromium-6 molybdenum via powder bed fusion
ASTM F3001-14(2021)	Standard specification for additive manufacturing Titanium-6 Aluminum-4 vanadium ELI (extra low interstitial) with powder bed fusion	ASTM F3489-23	Standard guide for additive manufacturing of polymers—Material extrusion—Recommendation for material handling and evaluation of static mechanical properties
ASTM F3049-14(2021)	Standard guide for characterizing properties of metal powders used for additive manufacturing processes	ASTM F3522-22	Standard guide for additive manufacturing of metals—feedstock materials—assessment of powder spreadability
ASTM F3055-14a(2021)	Standard specification for additive manufacturing nickel alloy (UNS N07718) with powder bed fusion	ASTM F3571-22	Standard guide for additive manufacturing—feedstock—particle shape image analysis by optical photography to identify and quantify the agglomerates/satellites in metal powder feedstock
ASTM F3056-14(2021)	Standard specification for additive manufacturing nickel alloy (UNS N06625) with powder bed fusion	ASTM F3606-22	Standard guide for additive manufacturing—feedstock materials—testing moisture content in powder feedstock
ASTM F3091-14(2021)	Standard specification for powder bed fusion of plastic materials	ISO ASTM 52907-2019	Additive manufacturing—feedstock materials—methods to characterize metallic powders
ASTM F31222-14(2022)	Standard guide for evaluating mechanical properties of metal materials made via additive manufacturing processes	ISO ASTM 52925-2022	Additive manufacturing of polymers –feedstock materials—Qualification of materials for laser-based powder bed fusion of parts
ASTM F3184-16	Standard specification for additive manufacturing stainless steel alloy (UNS S31603) with powder bed fusion	ISO ASTM 52903-1-2020	Additive manufacturing—material extrusion-based additive manufacturing of plastic materials—part 1: feedstock materials

Table 7.7 US 3D printing process standards

Standard number	Standard name	Standard number	Standard name
ASTM F3456-22	Standard guide for powder reuse schema in powder bed fusion processes for medical applications for additive manufacturing feedstock materials	ASTM F3626-23	Standard guide for additive manufacturing—test artifacts—accelerated build quality assurance for laser beam powder bed fusion (PBF-LB)
ASTM F3187-16	Standard guide for directed energy deposition of metals	ISO ASTM 52902-19	Additive manufacturing—test artifacts—geometric capability assessment of additive manufacturing systems
ASTM F3301-18a	Standard for additive manufacturing—post processing methods—standard specification for thermal post-processing metal parts made via powder bed fusion	ISO ASTM 52904-2019	Additive manufacturing—process characteristics and performance—practice for the metal powder bed fusion process to meet critical applications
ASTM F3529-21	Guide for additive manufacturing—design—material extrusion of polymers	ISO ASTM 52911-1-2019	Additive manufacturing—design—part 1: laser-based powder bed fusion of metals
ASTM F3530-22	Standard guide for additive manufacturing—design—post-processing for metal PBF-LB	ISO ASTM 52911-2-2019	Additive manufacturing—design—part 2: laser-based powder bed fusion of polymers
ASTM F3624-23	Standard guide for additive manufacturing of metals—powder bed fusion—measurement and characterization of surface texture	ISO ASTM 52911-3-2023	Additive manufacturing—design—part 3: PBF-EB of metallic materials

Table 7.8 US 3D-printed product standards

Standard number	Standard name
ASTM F3302-18	Standard for additive manufacturing—finished part properties—standard specification for titanium alloys via powder bed fusion
ASTM F3318-18	Standard for additive manufacturing—finished part properties—specification for AlSi10Mg with powder bed fusion—laser beam
ASTM F3637-23	Standard guide for additive manufacturing of metal—finished part properties—methods for relative density measurement
ISO ASTM 52909-2022	Additive manufacturing of metals—finished part properties—orientation and location dependence of mechanical properties for metal powder bed fusion

References

Min Y, Liu B. Study of regulatory requirements of customized device in the U.S. Chin J Med Instrum. 2017;41(1):43–7.

U.S. Food and Drug Administration. Custom device exemption. In: Contains nonbinding recommendations. U.S. Department of Health and Human Services Food and Drug administration Center for Devices and Radiological Health; 2014. Available via Baidu. https://www.fda.gov/media/89897/download. Accessed 24 Sept 2014.

U.S. Food and Drug Administration. Technical considerations for additive manufactured medical devices. In: Contains nonbinding recommendations. U.S. Department of Health and Human Services Food and Drug administration, Center for Devices and Radiological Health, Center for Biologics Evaluation and Research; 2017. Available via Baidu. https://www.fda.gov/media/97633/download. Accessed 5 Dec 2017.

U.S. Food and Drug Administration. Device classification panels. In: Medical devices. U.S. Food and Drug Administration; 2018. Available via Baidu. https://www.fda.gov/medical-devices/classify-your-medical-device/device-classification-panels. Accessed 31 Aug 2018.

U.S. Food and Drug Administration. Premarket approval (PMA). In: Medical devices. U.S. Food and Drug Administration; 2019. Available via Baidu. https://www.fda.gov/medical-devices/premarket-submissions-selecting-and-preparing-correct-submission/premarket-approval-pma. Accessed 16 May 2019.

U.S. Food and Drug Administration. Premarket notification 510(k). In: Medical devices. U.S. Food and Drug Administration; 2023. Available via Baidu. https://www.fda.gov/medical-devices/premarket-submissions-selecting-and-preparing-correct-submission/premarket-notification-510k. Accessed 12 May 2023.

Yu X, Mu R, Yu X. A comparative study on the standard management of medical devices between China and the United States. Chin Pharm Aff. 2020;34(8):877–81.

European Regulations and Standards

8

Dan Han, Jintao Gao, Xiaoqi Lian, Xiangmei Zhang, Yanchi Li, Yibei Chen, and Bin Liu

8.1 Introduction

As the world's second-largest manufacturer and consumer of medical devices, the EU has a long history and substantial experience in the management of medical devices. In the early 1990s, EU countries, represented by the UK, France, and Germany, preliminarily formed their own medical device management systems. These included the British Good Manufacturing Practice (GMP) requirements and adverse event reporting system, French clinical trial requirements, and German drug law and medical device safety regulations. With the announcement of the EU Single Market Treaty, the unified and coordinated European Medical Devices Directive (MDD) was officially released in 1993. Its purpose was to remove trade barriers, obtain mutual recognition, and perform technical coordination among EU member states. The MDD is one of the most important legislative tools of the EU, and its purpose is to ensure the consistency of laws within the EU. As a part of the unified market plan, the MDD has formulated a unified regulatory system for the management of medical devices in the EU, which is composed of three main directives: the Active Implantable Medical Devices Directive, the Medical Devices Directive, and the In Vitro Diagnostic Directive. The MDD is also the most influential medical device regulation thus far. It has been implemented in all EU member states and has achieved good results. This directive is hailed as a model that reflects the global unification of medical device regulations. The MDD introduced the following important concepts and requirements. Medical devices are divided into four categories according to the classification rules and follow different compliance review pathways. The MDD proposed the management of drug-device combination

D. Han · J. Gao · X. Lian · X. Zhang · Y. Li · Y. Chen · B. Liu (✉)
GBA Center for Medical Device Evaluation and Inspection, NMPA, Shenzhen, China
e-mail: handan@mdei.org.cn; gaojt@mdei.org.cn; lianxq@mdei.org.cn; zhangxm@mdei.org.cn; liyc@mdei.org.cn; chenyb@mdei.org.cn; liubin@mdei.org.cn

Z. Guo et al. (eds.), *3D-Printed Prosthesis in Orthopedic Oncology*,
https://doi.org/10.1007/978-981-95-1454-0_8

products, and basic requirements to ensure basic conditions for the safety and performance of medical devices were proposed and are used in cooperation with medical device standards to detail the technical indicators of the products. The MDD also includes the requirements for assessing the risk of medical devices and the requirements for clinical data related to the safety and effectiveness of medical devices. The MDD elucidated the obligation of manufacturers to report adverse events and test their marketed medical devices, proposed the concept of a third-party review agency, and implemented decentralized management (Ministry of Commerce of the People's Republic of China 2015).

8.2 Regulations and Guidance for Custom-Made Medical Devices

8.2.1 Regulatory Laws and Regulatory Pathways of Medical Devices

Europe has a complete medical device regulatory system to ensure the safety and effectiveness of all medical devices that are sold in the market, and this system includes the European Union Medical Devices Regulation, implementation rules and standards. Medical devices need to be approved for marketing after they are subjected to research and development, internal validation, conformity assessment, Conformité Européenne (CE) certification, registration application, and review by regulatory agencies. CE certification is the core link. The certification body conducts document review and on-site inspection before issuing the certificate. In addition to EU regulation, there are state-level supervision, industry association supervision, and enterprise self-disciplinary supervision. In general, Europe has established a comprehensive and strict medical device regulatory system to ensure product quality and safety and to protect public health. This section will generally analyze the regulatory framework of European medical devices and the approval and registration processes that conventional medical devices need to go through before being marketed in Europe.

8.2.1.1 Regulatory Framework

The EU medical device regulatory framework mainly includes the following:

(a) Regulations

The European Medical Device Regulation (MDR, Regulation (EU) 2017/745) and the In Vitro Diagnostic Medical Device Regulation (IVDR, Regulation (EU) 2017/746) established basic regulatory requirements. These two regulations set clear requirements for medical devices and in vitro diagnostic products that are sold on the European market. Compared with the In Vitro Diagnostic Medical Devices Directive (IVDMDD, 98/79/EC) and the Active Implantable Medical Devices Directive (AIMDD, 90/385/EEC), which are mentioned in the preface of this chapter, the MDR and IVDR are even more stringent, and they are considered to be among the most stringent medical device regulatory systems in the world.

(b) Implementation Rules and Technical Guidance

The European Commission has formulated various implementation rules, recommended guidelines, common specifications, and other documents to cooperate and guide the implementation of medical device regulations.

(c) Standards

European Harmonized Standards provide unified standards for the implementation of medical device regulations.

(d) Supervisory Coordination Mechanism

The Medical Device Coordination Group (MDCG) and the medical device expert panel play important roles in regulatory coordination.

8.2.1.2 Medical Device Approval Process

(a) R&D and Internal Validation Stage

Manufacturers organize product development teams to design products and manage product risks according to the requirements of the MDR. After the completion of R&D, manufacturers need to verify the effectiveness and safety of the product design. This requires the preparation of complete technical documents to record the product design process, design input and output, and specification validation. Moreover, an internal verification test should be carried out, and the verification plan and report should be recorded. These documents are part of the technical documentation of the product.

(b) Conformity Assessment Stage

Manufacturers select the appropriate assessment process based on the risk classification of the medical device. The new MDR simplified evaluation process can be used for medium- and low-risk devices, while clinical evaluation is needed for high-risk devices. The assessment activities include proposing an assessment plan, conducting an assessment test, recording data, and generating an assessment report. These documents are also included in the technical files to certify that the products meet the MDR requirements.

(c) CE Certification Stage

Manufacturers submit complete technical documents and evaluation reports to the European authorized medical device certification body. The certification body first reviews the documents to determine their completeness and consistency, and then implements the quality management system review and product sampling test. After confirming that the requirements are met, the certification body issues a certificate of conformity with the CE marking. The material content and process of each step in this process are as follows:

① Submission of Application Materials

Manufacturers prepare application materials according to the classification of different medical devices, which mainly include technical documents (complete product design and validation records), risk management reports (identification of risks and adoption of control measures), conformity assessment reports (simplified or clinical evaluation results), and quality system documents (description of the production and quality control system).

② Document Review

The certification body reviews the application materials and mainly confirms the completeness of the technical documents and the traceability of the design process. The assessment results should fully prove that the product meets the relevant requirements of the MDR. The quality system documents should be complete, and the system should operate effectively.

③ Factory and Product Inspection

The certification body selects key manufacturing links and product samples to conduct spot checks and confirms that the production process meets the quality system requirements, the product samples meet the design and performance requirements specified in the technical documents, and the quality control methods are effectively implemented and recorded.

④ Review and Decision

The certification body comprehensively reviews the documents and on-site audit results, requests supplementary materials if necessary, and finally makes the certification decision.

⑤ Issuance of Certificates

After determining that the requirements are met, the certification body will issue a medical device certificate of conformity containing the CE marking.

(d) Registration Application Stage

After obtaining the CE certificate, manufacturers prepare product samples and registration application documents to submit a registration application to the regulatory authorities of the EU member states. The application materials include the CE certificate, product manual, and manufacturer qualification certificate.

(e) Review by Regulatory Agency Stage

After accepting the application, the regulatory agency will conduct a comprehensive review, including reexamining the technical documents, confirming compliance with the product design process, and checking the strictness of the evaluation process of the certification body. The review may propose requirements for supplementary data, and on-site inspections will also be implemented.

(f) Approved Marketing Stage

Ultimately, the regulatory agency decides whether to approve or reject the registration application based on the conclusion of the review. After approval, a registration certificate is issued, and the manufacturer can officially launch the product on the market.

(g) Postmarketing Monitoring Stage
After marketing, products will receive continuous supervision of regulatory agencies. Manufacturers need to carry out production quality control and actively report adverse product events. Regulatory agencies regularly inspect the compliance of manufacturers.

8.2.1.3 Other Regulatory Pathways

National Regulation: At the level of the EU member states, each country has established corresponding medical device regulatory agencies that are responsible for the approval and registration of medical devices in their own countries. These agencies usually work according to the MDR to ensure the safety and effectiveness of medical devices. These national regulatory agencies and the European Medicines Agency (EMA) work closely to safeguard the order of the EU medical device market and the rights and interests of patients.

Supervision of Industry Associations: Industry organizations, such as the European Medical Device Industry Association, play an important role in the supervision of medical devices. These organizations work closely with governmental departments, academia, and manufacturers to jointly promote the development of the medical device industry and the improvement of the regulatory system. Industry associations usually focus on technological development, policy formulation, and market dynamics in the industry and provide guidance and support to manufacturers.

Self-Disciplinary Supervision: Medical device manufacturers also need to establish a complete quality management system to ensure the safety and effectiveness of their products. These manufacturers need to follow the requirements of the MDR and implement the principle of quality first throughout the entire process of product development, production, marketing, and after-sales service. Self-disciplinary supervision is very important for the internal management, product quality, and market reputation of manufacturers. Manufacturers need to ensure compliance through self-assessment or third-party audits and actively report major events and adverse events to regulatory authorities.

8.2.2 Regulatory Pathways for Custom-Made Medical Devices

In the previous section, the regulations and the approval and registration processes of conventional medical devices that are launched in Europe were introduced. The supervision of custom-made medical devices is similar to that of other medical devices in following the requirements of regulations such as the MDR. However, due to the unique and personalized needs of custom-made devices, the regulatory pathways and requirements of these devices also vary. A custom-made medical device is specially prepared according to the written prescription of a person authorized by national laws. This person is authorized by virtue of his professional qualifications and provides specific design features under the responsibility of that person. A custom-made product is used only by a specific patient to meet their individual conditions and needs. In addition to meeting the specific needs of patients, the safety and efficacy of this type of medical device also need to be ensured. Review agencies are paying more attention to the personalized needs, safety, efficacy, and quality control of products. Moreover, review agencies strictly review the compliance of the manufacturer in terms of technical support capabilities, supply chain management, and document record management. To ensure the safety and effectiveness of custom-made medical devices, manufacturers need to fully understand and comply with relevant regulatory requirements, strengthen internal management, ensure that the design and manufacturing process of products conform to the specifications, and provide necessary support and services. The regulatory requirements, approval process, and review concerns of custom-made medical devices in Europe are described below.

8.2.2.1 Regulations for Custom-Made Medical Devices

The MDR can be applied to custom-made medical devices, and it provides detailed regulatory requirements for custom-made medical devices (Appendix 13). In general, compared with those of conventional medical devices, the premarket registration approval and postmarket supervision of custom-made medical devices are relatively simple. However, due to the particularity and personalization of custom-made medical devices, there are also several special requirements in the MDR.

8.2.2.2 Premarket Approval Process and Review Concerns for Custom-Made Medical Devices

(a) Premarket Approval Process

Pretrial Stage: A prereview is required before a formal application is submitted. The prereview contents should include basic information about the custom-made medical device, such as product name, description, classification, and assess whether it meets the compliance requirements of the MDR. The purpose of this stage is to preliminarily assess the compliance and acceptability of the product.

Technical Document Review: The manufacturer needs to submit detailed technical documents, including documents detailing the product design, manufacturing process, quality management system, etc., for review by the European Medicines Agency (EMA). Technical documents should prove the safety, efficacy, and quality controllability of a product, and focus on personalization needs and specific application scenarios.

On-Site Review: After passing the review of technical documents, the EMA will conduct an on-site review of the manufacturer's production site to verify that the manufacturer's quality management system, production process, and quality control measures meet the regulatory requirements. During a site review, more attention will be given to whether a manufacturer's production capacity and control measures can meet the personalization needs of custom-made medical devices.

Approval Decision: Based on the results of the technical document review and on-site review, the EMA will make an approval decision. If approval is passed, medical devices can be sold in the EU market. However, the manufacturer will need to improve and resubmit the application if the approval is not passed. The approval decision may involve postmarket surveillance requirements for the product.

Postmarket Surveillance: After a medical device is marketed, the EMA will perform continuous surveillance, including the monitoring and reevaluation of adverse events. Manufacturers need to regularly submit postmarketing regulatory reports on products to ensure their continued safety and efficacy. For custom-made medical devices, postmarket supervision should pay special attention to the personalization needs and specific application scenarios of the products.

(b) Review Concerns

During the approval process, the review agency will focus on compliance in the following aspects:

Safety: The safety of custom-made medical devices is the primary consideration in the approval process. The review organization will evaluate whether a product can safely and effectively perform its intended function under the expected use conditions while considering the effects of product design, material selection, manufacturing processes, disinfection processes, and other factors on safety.

Effectiveness: The effectiveness of custom-made medical devices is an important consideration in the approval process. The review organization will evaluate whether the design, function, and usage of the product meet the needs of specific patients or the treatment requirements of specific hospitals.

Quality Controllability: The quality controllability of custom-made medical devices is critical for ensuring the safety and effectiveness of products. The review organization will evaluate whether the manufacturer's quality management system is sound, the production process is standardized, and quality control measures are appropriate. In addition, product traceability and record keeping need to be considered.

Consideration of Personalization Needs: Custom-made medical devices usually need to meet the needs of specific patients or the treatment requirements of specific hospitals. Therefore, review organizations should pay special attention to the personalized design and functional realization of products. For example, a custom-made cardiac pacemaker may need to be personalized based on the specific physiological parameters of the patient, while a custom-made orthopedic device may need to be customized according to the specific bone morphology of the patient.

Risk Assessment and Management: Custom-made medical devices may have additional risks, so the review agency will focus on the assessment and management of the risks of the products. This includes a comprehensive assessment of the expected use, usage methods, potential risk factors for the product, and the development of corresponding risk control measures. Moreover, attention should be given to the arrangements for risk monitoring and reevaluation after the product is launched.

Technical Support Capability: The review organization will also evaluate the manufacturer's technical support capabilities, including whether the technical support capabilities for the installation, commissioning, training, repair, and maintenance of custom-made medical devices are adequate and meet the requirements. For highly specialized custom-made medical devices, manufacturers may need to have specific technical qualifications and certifications to provide corresponding technical support services.

Supply Chain Management: Due to the uniqueness and personalization needs of custom-made medical devices, supply chain management also deserves special attention. The review organization will evaluate the manufacturer's supply chain management capabilities as well as the selection and management of suppliers to ensure that the quality of the raw materials and parts of the products is quality controllable and meets the regulatory requirements. Moreover, attention should be given to product traceability and record keeping.

Document and Record Management: The design, manufacturing, and use of custom-made medical devices involve the management of a large number of documents and records. The review organization will focus on whether the manufacturer's document and record management are standardized, including whether the preparation, review, approval, release, and storage of documents meet the regulatory requirements. Moreover, attention should be given to the accuracy, completeness, and traceability of records as well as the updates and maintenance of documents and records by the manufacturer.

Training and Personnel Qualification: Due to the particularity and professionalism of custom-made medical devices, the review body will pay attention to the manufacturer's training plan and personnel qualifications. Manufacturers should ensure that staff members who have direct contact with and use custom-made medical devices receive adequate training, receive qualification certification, and have the necessary technical capabilities and professional knowledge, and manufacturers should pay attention to the continuous training and skills update of staff.

Contract Management and Customer Support: The review organization will evaluate the contract management and customer support capabilities of the manufacturer and the customer. The manufacturer should formulate reasonable contract terms to clarify the rights and obligations of both parties and provide necessary support and services to customers. For custom-made medical devices, customer support services may include installation and commissioning, use training, repair, and maintenance.

Continuous Improvement and Risk Management: The review organization will focus on whether the manufacturer has mechanisms for continuous improvement and risk management. Manufacturers should regularly evaluate product performance and quality to identify problems and improve product safety and efficacy. Moreover, manufacturers need to develop a risk management plan to identify potential risks and adopt corresponding control measures.

8.2.3 Guidance for Custom-Made Medical Devices

In addition to the requirements of the MDR on custom-made medical devices, the EU MDCG released MDCG 2021-3 Questions and Answers on Custom-Made Devices. This document mainly covers the following ten questions and answers about custom-made medical devices.

(a) What is a custom-made device (CMD)?

MDR Article 2(3) defines a "custom-made device" as any device that is specifically made in accordance with a written prescription of any person authorized by national law by virtue of that person's professional qualifications, which gives specific design characteristics provided under that person's responsibility, and is intended for the sole use of a particular patient exclusively to meet their individual conditions and needs. The file also shows cases that are considered CMDs or not.

Examples of CMDs include the following:

① A dental crown that is manufactured according to a written prescription provided by a dentist that contains design characteristics that are specific to a particular patient's individual condition.

② An orthosis that is made in accordance with a written prescription and contains a specific design characteristic to aid a person with neuromuscular or musculoskeletal impairment of the lower extremity, such as a Knee Ankle Foot Orthosis (KAFO).

③ A hand prosthesis that is intended to replace a lost body part and/or function made in accordance with a written prescription, where the practitioner provides patient-specific design characteristics that are necessary for the manufacturing of the device.

Devices that are not considered CMDs may include the following:

① Devices that are mass-produced and need to be adapted to meet the specific requirements of any professional user; hereafter, these are referred to as adaptable medical devices. (Adaptable medical devices (products that fall under (a) above) are mass-produced medical devices.)
② Devices that are mass-produced by means of industrial manufacturing processes, potentially made in accordance with the written prescriptions of an authorized person.

(b) Can parts, components, or materials that are specifically intended to be used in a custom-made device, adaptable medical device, or patient-matched medical device be placed on the market as medical devices according to the MDR?

In accordance with Article 2(1) MDR, the intended purpose of a medical device can be achieved either alone or in combination with other devices or products. Certain parts, components, or materials may perform a medically intended purpose and can thus fulfill the definition of a medical device. By analogy, parts, components, or materials of custom-made devices, adaptable medical devices, or patient-matched medical devices may be CE-marked medical devices.

Accordingly, it is possible for "intermediate products," which are specifically intended for the manufacture of CMDs, adaptable medical devices or patient-matched medical devices, to also be placed on the market as medical devices, as these products are specifically intended to become a part or component of a final CMD, adaptable medical device (finally adapted) or patient-matched medical device. Instructions for use that are provided by the manufacturer of these CE-marked devices should be followed when performing further preparatory processing, preparation, configuration, installation, assembly, adaptation, or fitting to meet the needs of the user or patient prior to their use.

(c) Are there specific considerations/requirements that must be considered by manufacturers of devices referred to in Question (b)?

Manufacturers of the devices referenced in Question (b) shall fulfill all relevant and applicable requirements of the MDR. To determine the risk classes of those products, it is necessary to consider:

① The intended medical purpose of the final CMD, adaptable medical device, or patient-matched medical device.
② Whether it is an implantable medical device (i.e., whether the part, component, or material is intended to be used in the manufacturing of an implantable CMD, adaptable medical device, or patient-matched medical device).

③ The risks related to the intended contact or interaction of the product as a part, component, or material in the final CMD, adaptable medical device, or patient-matched medical device with the patient's body.

If any of the physical, chemical or biological properties of those products mentioned in Question (b) change during the manufacturing of the CMD, the manufacturing of the patient-matched medical device or the adaptation of the adaptable medical device (e.g., plastics, metallic compounds, ceramic fluids for crowns), compliance of the finished product with the general safety and performance requirements of MDR Annex I must be demonstrated.

It is important to note that the manufacturer must also demonstrate that these products do not create unacceptable risks to the persons performing the relevant preparatory processing (such as preparation, configuration, installation, assembly, adaptation, or fitting) to the needs of the patient prior to their use.

The clinical evaluation conducted by the manufacturer should focus on demonstrating the clinical benefit related to the intended medical purpose of the products when used as parts, components, or materials of custom-made devices, adaptable medical devices, or patient-matched medical devices.

To perform postmarket clinical follow-up (PMCF), liaison with the authorized person responsible for the issuing of the relevant written prescription, CMD manufacturers who have utilized the part, component, or material, and persons adapting the final device is necessary.

Furthermore, the manufacturer of devices mentioned in Question (b) bears the responsibility for these CE-marked medical devices and is responsible for all incumbent MDR obligations, such as postmarket surveillance activities and vigilance reporting for the parts, components, or materials.

(d) Can manufacturers use state-of-the-art industrial manufacturing processes to manufacture CMDs?

As long as the definition of a CMD is fulfilled (refer to Question a) and the device is not mass-produced, manufacturers may use modern state-of-the-art technologies (such as CAD, CAM, or 3D printing) to manufacture CMDs.

(e) Does a 3D-printed device (additive manufacturing) qualify as a CMD?

A 3D-printed device does not qualify as a CMD by default. An assessment should be performed on a case-by-case basis. For a 3D-printed device to qualify as a CMD, the following requirements must be met:

① A written prescription, containing patient-specific design characteristics, is provided by an authorized person and is in compliance with the requirements expressed below (see Question (f)).
② The manufactured device is intended for the sole use of a particular patient, exclusively to meet their individual conditions and needs; and

③ The device is not mass-produced.

(f) What defines a written prescription containing patient-specific design characteristics?

A written prescription must be issued by a qualified person authorized by national law. At a minimum, it should contain:

① The name of the patient (or pseudonym if relevant); and
② Specific design characteristics made by the authorized person that are unique to the patient's anatomic-physiological features and/or pathological condition.

The following (nonexhaustive) additions can accompany a written prescription and, if present, also constitute specific design characteristics: models (physical or 3D model data), molds (e.g., for dental or orthotic purposes), and dental impressions.

Note: Dimensions and/or geometric parameters (such as DICOM files from CT scans) are not considered specific design characteristics on their own. Additional measurement data or information10 must be provided by the prescribing person as part of a written prescription for the CMD to be met.

(g) Should the authorized person mentioned in the definition of a CMD be a health care professional?

No. The Regulation explicitly states that it should be any person authorized by national law. Therefore, it is up to member states to establish who qualifies as an authorized person.

(h) What are the obligations of CMD manufacturers according to the MDR?

In the absence of stated exceptions, CMD manufacturers must meet nearly all of the MDR requirements. Although the authorized person who issues the written prescription primarily determines the design and intended purpose of the CMD, it is the responsibility of the CMD manufacturer to consider which MDR Annex I requirements are applicable to the particular device.

Additionally, as with any other medical device manufacturer, CMD manufacturers should establish, document, implement, maintain, update, and continually improve a quality management system (QMS) that ensures compliance with the MDR in the most effective manner and in a manner that is appropriate for the risk class and the type of device. The QMS must address all the elements described in Article 10(9) of the MDR.

To implement an MDR-compliant postmarket surveillance system, the CMD manufacturer should establish appropriate communication channels with relevant health care providers/professionals or patients to receive feedback on the quality, performance, and, in particular, the clinical performance and safety of the devices in the field.

For risk management, postmarket surveillance, and clinical evaluation life cycle processes as defined by the MDR, CMD manufacturers should apply these obligations to groups of devices with the same intended purpose, materials and processes utilized, principal design, and not to each individual CMD.

In accordance with Article 87(1) of the MDR, CMD manufacturers shall report to the competent authorities any serious incidents and/or corrective actions for field safety as soon as they learn of them.

(i) Which obligations of CMD manufacturers differ from those of other medical device manufacturers?

The conformity assessment procedure for all types of CMDs is described in MDR Annex XIII. In accordance with Section 1 of Annex XIII and in place of a declaration of conformity, CMDs shall be accompanied by an Annex XIII statement. This statement shall be made available to the particular patient or user who is identified by a name, an acronym, or a numerical code.

A conformity assessment procedure including QMS certification by a notified body (in accordance with Chapter I of Annex IX or Part A of Annex XI of the MDR) is applicable to Class III implantable CMDs.11 According to Article 56 (5), the registration of QMS certificates that are issued for Class III implantable CMDs should be entered into EUDAMED. In addition, manufacturers may have to comply with national requirements for the registration of economic operators and devices.

CMD manufacturers are exempt from device UDI registration, assignment, and labeling requirements. As such, although they must appoint a person responsible for regulatory compliance (PRRC) in accordance with Article 15 of the MDR, they are not required to register these persons in EUDAMED.

In addition, Article 32(1) stipulates that a Summary of Safety and Clinical Performance (SSCP) is not required for a custom-made device.

For postmarket surveillance, a report on Class I devices, according to Article 85 of the MDR, and a Periodic Safety Update Report (PSUR) on Class IIa, IIb, and III devices, according to Article 86 of the MDR, must be established by the CMD manufacturer. Both the postmarket surveillance report and the PSUR must be part of the CMD documentation, according to Section 2 of Annex XIII of the MDR.

In the case of Class III implantable CMDs, PSURs are not required to be sent to notified bodies but must be part of the CMD documentation according to Section 2 of Annex XIII of the MDR.

(j) What are the implications for a CMD manufacturer using the CE-marked devices mentioned in Question b instead of non-CE-marked devices?

In both cases, it is the responsibility of the CMD manufacturer to establish full compliance of the CMD with the MDR.

When a CMD manufacturer uses a CE-marked device, part, component, or material (as described in Question b) for the purpose of manufacturing a CMD, the CMD manufacturer may consider the compliance of these CE-marked products with the general safety and performance requirements of the MDR. When performing a clinical evaluation for CMD, the CMD manufacturer can make use of the clinical evaluation performed for these CE-marked products, as this clinical evaluation (refer to the answer to Question c) can support the fulfillment of the general safety and performance requirements and demonstrate the clinical evidence necessary for the final CMD.

When the CMD manufacturer has to perform further preparatory processing, preparation, configuration, installation, assembly, adaptation, or fitting to patient needs prior to the device's use, this process must be performed in accordance with the instructions provided by the manufacturer of the CE-marked device.

It must be noted that it is not possible to presume conformity or to rely on clinical evaluations of non-CE-marked devices. It is also not possible to presume conformity or to rely on clinical evaluations of CE-marked devices when they are being used for purposes other than their intended purpose or without following the instructions provided by the manufacturer.

8.3 Standards and Guidance for Medical 3D-Printing Technology

8.3.1 Medical Device Standards

8.3.1.1 Medical Device Standardization Organizations

The standardization of medical devices in Europe is promoted by two main organizations. The European Committee for Standardization (Comité Européen de Normalisation, CEN) is one of the most important regional standardization organizations in Europe, and it is responsible for the formulation of European standards in various fields. In addition to the electrotechnical field, its members include national standardization organizations from various European countries. The European Committee for Electrotechnical Standardization (CENELEC) is an electrotechnical standardization organization in Europe that is responsible for the development and publication of European electrotechnical standards. Its members are also members of the electrotechnical standardization bodies of different European countries. These two organizations have established a number of technical committees to standardize medical devices. For example, CEN/TC 205 is responsible for general requirements for medical devices, and CLC/TC 62 is responsible for standards for medical electrical equipment. Each technical committee studies and develops relevant standards based on needs.

8.3.1.2 Procedure for Formulating Medical Device Standards

The formulation and revision of European medical device standards must follow transparent and open procedures.

(a) Standard Project Proposal

Based on market and regulatory needs, all parties can propose standardized projects.

(b) Project Approval Review
The relevant technical committees of CEN and CENELEC will review the project and decide whether to approve it.
(c) Working Group Formation
Once the project is established, a standard research working group will be formed. The working group members will represent various interested parties.
(d) Preliminary Draft Preparation
The working group will draft the preliminary draft of standards based on previous studies.
(e) Public Consultation for Opinions
The preliminary draft will be released to the public to receive feedback from people from all walks of life.
(f) Revision and Final Draft
The working group will revise the draft and generate the final draft based on the comments, and then, they will submit it to the technical committee.
(g) Official Release
After approval by the technical committee, the standard will be officially published by CEN/CENELEC as an EN standard.
(h) State Adoption

Each country publishes the approved EN standards as national standards, requiring their implementation in each country. For example, the British Standards Institution (BSI) released the English version of the BS EN standard, the German Institute for Standardization (DIN) released the German version of the DIN EN standard, and the French Association for Standardization (AFNOR) released the French version of the NF EN standard.

8.3.1.3 Major Medical Device Standards

The published European medical device standards cover various aspects (Table 8.1). These standards include quality management, risk management, safety requirements, various evaluation and verification standards, and product standards. The formulation and release of these standards provide a normative basis for the R&D and design, risk management, and regulatory evaluation of medical devices.

Although Europe has formulated a large number of medical device standards, many European manufacturers have directly adopted international standards in R&D and production; in particular, they have adopted ISO standards such as the ISO 13485 Quality Management System and ISO 14971 Risk Management, ASTM standards such as the ASTM F1980 General Safety Requirements and ASTM F2061 Biological Safety Evaluation, and IEC standards such as the IEC 60601-1 General Requirements for Medical Electrical Equipment. This type of international standard is widely used and has strong applicability. By adopting these standards, European manufacturers can adapt to the needs of European and global markets.

Table 8.1 Standard classification of major medical devices in Europe

Type	Standards
Quality management system standards	EN ISO 13485 Quality Management System Requirements for Medical Devices
Risk management standards	EN ISO 14971 Medical Device Risk Management
General safety requirement standards	IEC 60601-1 series General Safety Requirements for Medical Electrical Equipment
Biological evaluation standards	EN ISO 10993 Biological Evaluation of Medical Devices
Software validation standards	EN 62304 Medical Device Software Life Cycle Processes
Usability evaluation standards	IEC 62366 Medical Device Availability Engineering
Product-specific standards	Special standards for various specific medical devices

8.3.1.4 Relevant Standards of Medical 3D-Printing Technology

Europe has established many relevant standards for 3D printing technology, covering multiple dimensions, such as materials, equipment, software, and products. Most of these standards are not unique to the medical field. Rather, these standards also guide the development of the medical 3D printing industry and play an important role in ensuring product quality and promoting technological innovation. Several 3D-printing technology-related standards and their main contents are listed in Table 8.2.

The continuous development and improvement of these standards not only improve the quality and safety of medical 3D-printed products but also promote the continuous innovation and development of medical 3D printing technology. Moreover, these standards have also enhanced consumers' trust in 3D-printed medical products, promoting the growth of market demand. In addition, Europe continues to promote the development and application of medical 3D-printing technology through project funding, R&D, and clinical trials. These efforts have provided strong support for the continuous development of the medical 3D-printing industry and have improved medical services and treatment outcomes.

8.3.2 Relevant Guidance for Medical 3D-Printing Technology

Overall, there is currently no unified or systematic guidance on medical 3D-printing technology in Europe. However, countries and organizations are actively promoting development in this field, and relevant standards and specifications are constantly being improved. Some of the medical device regulatory guidelines that were issued by the European Commission and the European Medicines Agency involve quality control and validation related to 3D-printing technology, and the applicable section can be referenced.

Table 8.2 Examples of European 3D-printing technology-related standards

Theme	Standard number	Main content
Process basis and principle	BS EN ISO 17296-2:2016	This standard describes the basis of the process, existing process types, and process principles of 3D printing technology, including raw material requirements (pretreatment), binding mechanisms, activation sources, and reprocessing processes that are used in each process
Powder bed fusion (PBF) technology	BS EN ISO/ ASTM 52911	This series of standards specifies different terminology and processes related to powder bed fusion (PBF) technology. Each part of the standard describes the guidelines for designing a different 3D printing technology, including process characteristics, structure and material characteristics, anisotropy of materials and parts, model construction, as well as a summary of the advantages and limitations of different processes, and provides clear guidance for the design and manufacturing of 3D printing technology and related products
Metal material	BS EN ISO/ ASTM 52907:2019	This standard provides technical specifications for metal powder raw materials that are used in 3D-printing technology, including requirements and test methods for particle size, chemical composition, density, morphology, and fluidity of metal powder raw materials
	BS EN ISO/ ASTM 52908:2023	This standard specifies the identification, quality requirements, and postprocessing requirements of finished metal powder bed fusion parts, and it describes the methods and procedures for testing and identifying the physical and chemical characteristics of finished parts that are manufactured by 3D-printing technology using metal powder bed fusion
	BS EN ISO/ ASTM 52909:2022	This standard is supplementary guidance for the evaluation of the mechanical properties of metal parts that are manufactured by 3D-printing technology, including static/quasistatic and dynamic tests on finished metal parts. These standards set clear requirements for metal raw materials and metal products, ensuring the quality and safety of 3D-printed products
Equipment	BS PD CEN ISO/ASTM/ TS 52930:2021	This standard describes the steps for process assessment of 3D printers, and it is only applicable to machines that are used for the mass production of metal parts produced by powder bed fusion by laser beam melting (PBF-LB/M). The standard specifies the terms and definitions of this type of 3D printer, as well as related process elements such as installation qualification (IQ), operational qualification (OQ), and performance qualification (PQ). Equipment installation and maintenance, and process validation are key factors for ensuring product quality. This standard ensures the quality and safety of 3D printers that are used in the 3D printing process and provides a reliable basis for the manufacture of 3D-printed products
Medical imaging	BS PD CEN ISO/ASTM/ TR 52916:2022	This standard describes the improvement of medical image data, as well as methods for their acquisition, processing, and optimization, to generate accurate medical models in the field of medical 3D printing technology. The method described in this standard improves the accuracy of the final model, so that high-quality medical image data are obtained

8.3.2.1 MEDDEV 2.1/3 rev 3-Guidelines on Medical Devices, IVD and Postmarket Clinical Follow-Up

This document does not specifically mention 3D printing; however, since most 3D-printed medical devices are custom-made medical devices, the principles and requirements for custom-made medical devices can also be indirectly applied to 3D-printed medical devices.

Custom-made medical devices are specially designed or custom-made according to the needs of a specific patient and according to the professional judgment of the doctor. Custom-made devices need to meet the requirements of the general medical device directive, such as risk management and clinical evaluation. For implantable custom-made devices, if the design is similar to that of existing devices, the clinical data of similar devices can be referenced. If the design is completely different, a new clinical evaluation is needed. Manufacturers of custom-made medical devices need to strengthen quality management to ensure that each product meets specific requirements.

8.3.2.2 MEDDEV 2.7.1 rev 4—Clinical Evaluation: Guide for Manufacturers and Notified Bodies

The document also does not explicitly mention 3D printing or the specific contents of 3D-printed medical devices. However, the relevant steps of clinical evaluation can provide a reference for 3D-printed medical devices. For new medical devices that have been proven to be equivalent to existing medical devices through appropriate validation methods, the clinical data of the existing devices are sufficient, and further clinical trials are not necessary. For new designs that differ from those of existing medical devices, design change management is required to assess the impact of the changes on safety and performance. Major design changes require new clinical evaluation. The clinical evaluation of custom-made medical devices can refer to existing data of similar product categories, but the change in key parameters requires reevaluation. To assess the potential risks, manufacturers need to perform risk analysis on the design features, intended purpose, and indications of new medical devices. Preclinical and clinical evaluations need to determine the design input requirements through appropriate standards.

In summary, in terms of medical 3D-printing technology guidance, Europe still mainly adopts scattered standards, regulatory documents, enterprise white papers, academic papers, etc. Unified and specialized technical guidance documents have not yet been created. With the accumulation and enrichment of relevant content, dedicated technical guidance documents may be generated in Europe in the future.

Reference

Ministry of Commerce of the People's Republic of China. An in-depth analysis of medical device management mechanisms in the United States, the European Union, and China. Ministry of Commerce of the People's Republic of China; 2015. Available via Baidu. http://gpj.mofcom.gov.cn/article/zuixindt/201506/20150601026432.shtml. Accessed 29 June 2015

Chinese Regulations and Standards 9

Jintao Gao, Dan Han, Jinju Ding, Kun Zhang, Minqi Lu, Xuegui Yu, and Bin Liu

9.1 Introduction

Compared with the United States and the European Union, the supervision of medical devices in China began later, but China has always viewed the quality and safety of medical devices as very important. In 1996, China issued the "Medical Device Product Registration Management Measures," which requires that any medical device product that enters the Chinese market after January 1, 1997, must be registered by the Chinese Government Medical Device Registration Authority. The product manufacturer or its authorized agent should submit an application for product registration. In 2000, China issued the Regulations on the Supervision and Administration of Medical Devices to enhance the supervision and management of medical devices, ensure the safety and effectiveness of medical devices, and promote the development of the industry. The regulations were subsequently revised in 2014 and 2021. The latest regulations supplement and improve the aspects of risk management, full-process control, scientific supervision, and social cogovernance, ensuring the safety and effectiveness of medical devices. In the field of 3D-printed custom-made medical devices, although supervision in China began later than that in the United States and the European Union, its development is relatively more complete. China has initially established a systematic medical 3D printing supervision system, including a regulatory system, standard system, guideline system, and product system (Gao et al. 2023a). This chapter will elaborate on the process of establishing the medical 3D printing regulatory system in China, as well as the results of this system.

J. Gao · D. Han · J. Ding · K. Zhang · M. Lu · X. Yu · B. Liu (✉)
GBA Center for Medical Device Evaluation and Inspection, NMPA, Shenzhen, China
e-mail: gaojt@mdei.org.cn; handan@mdei.org.cn; dingjj@mdei.org.cn; zhangkun@mdei.org.cn; lumq@mdei.org.cn; yuxg@mdei.org.cn; liubin@mdei.org.cn

Z. Guo et al. (eds.), *3D-Printed Prosthesis in Orthopedic Oncology*,
https://doi.org/10.1007/978-981-95-1454-0_9

9.2 Regulations and Guidance for Custom-Made Medical Devices

9.2.1 Regulatory Laws and Regulatory Pathways of Medical Devices

9.2.1.1 China's Medical Device Regulatory System

In recent years, China has made a series of major decisions and arrangements to further reform the medical device review and approval system, strengthen the building of regulatory capacity, and build a team of professional inspectors; these changes have contributed to the robust development of the medical device industry and the emergence of innovative products. In the face of the continuous growth of reform, the rapid development of industry, and the growing health care needs of people, the NMPA (National Medical Products Administration) has continued to establish medical device laws and regulatory systems, enhance the supervision of the whole life cycle, promote high-quality development of the industry, and better meet people's needs for high-quality medical devices in this new era (National Medical Products Administration 2022).

The latest "Regulation," which was released in 2021, is composed of eight chapters—general provisions, registration and filing of medical device products, production of medical devices, operation and use of medical devices, handling of adverse events and recall of medical devices, supervisory inspection, legal liability, and supplementary provisions—for a total of 107 articles. The "Regulation" clarifies that the supervision and administration of medical devices should follow the basic principles of risk management, management and control throughout the whole process, scientific regulation, and cogovernance by the entire society; fully absorb the results of the reform of the review and approval system, fully implement the registrant and recorder system, reform the management of clinical evaluation, innovate supervision methods, and increase penalties.

To promote the implementation of the systems that were established in the "Regulation," the NMPA has formulated relevant supporting regulations, including "Measures for the Administration of Registration and Filing of Medical Devices," "Measures for the Supervision and Administration of Medical Device Production," "Measures for the Supervision and Administration of Medical Device Operations," and "The Monitoring and Re-evaluation of Medical Device Adverse Events"; these regulations have led to the formation of a legal system for supervision and management of medical device product life cycles, with laws and regulations as the core and relevant rules for support.

9.2.1.2 China's Medical Device Registration and Marketing Approval Process

Similar to the international supervision model, China implements classified management for medical device supervision. The specific classification can be found in the relevant announcement on the medical device classification catalog released by the NMPA (National Medical Products Administration 2017). Product filing management is implemented for Class I medical devices. Class II and III medical devices are subject to product registration management. For the filing of Class I medical devices in China, the recorder should submit the recording materials to the municipal drug supervision and administration department. The Class II medical devices that are made in China are reviewed by the drug supervision and administration departments of provinces, autonomous regions, and municipalities, and a medical device registration certificate is issued after approval. Class III medical devices made in China are reviewed by the NMPA, and a medical device registration certificate is issued after approval. For the recording of imported Class I medical devices, the recorder should submit the recording materials to the NMPA. Imported Class II and III medical devices will be reviewed by the NMPA, and a medical device registration certificate will be issued after approval. Medical device registration mainly includes acceptance, technical review, administrative approval, and preparation of approval documents. The specific process details and time limit can be found in the Measures for the Administration of Registration and Filing of Medical Devices.

9.2.2 Regulatory Pathways for Custom-Made Medical Devices

9.2.2.1 Regulations for Custom-Made Medical Devices

To meet rare and unique personalized needs in clinical practice, to standardize supervision, and ensure the safety and effectiveness of custom-made medical devices, the National Medical Products Administration and the National Health Commission jointly formulated the "Regulations on the Supervision and Administration of Custom-made Medical Devices (Trial)" (hereafter referred to as the Regulations) in accordance with the "Regulations for the Supervision and Administration of Medical Devices"; the Regulations clarify the requirements for the development, production, use and supervision of custom-made medical devices within the territory of the People's Republic of China (National Medical Products Administration 2019).

The Regulations define custom-made medical devices and patient-matched medical devices separately. Custom-made medical devices are defined as personalized medical devices that are designed and produced by medical device manufacturers based on the special clinical needs of medical institutions to meet the rare and unique medical conditions of designated patients and in situations where the products that are already on the market in China cannot meet the clinical needs. These devices are intended to improve the diagnosis and treatment effectiveness of these particular patients. Patient-matched medical devices are defined as personalized medical devices for designated patients. These devices are designed and manufactured by medical device manufacturers in accordance with standard specifications and based on clinical needs and validated, confirmed processes.

In terms of regulatory pathways, patient-matched medical devices should be registered or filed in accordance with the "Management Measures for Registration and Filing of Medical Devices," in which the product specifications and models are within all possible size ranges for production, while custom-made medical devices are subject to filing management.

9.2.2.2 Premarket Approval Process and Requirements for Custom-Made Medical Devices

(a) Premarket Approval Process

For the filing of custom-made medical devices (Fig. 9.1), the medical device manufacturer and the hospital should file together. Before the manufacture and use of custom-made medical devices, the filing should be submitted to the drug regulatory department of the province, autonomous region, or municipality directly under the Central Government of the location of the medical device manufacturer (or the location of the agent for imported products). When the number of clinical use cases and preliminary studies of a custom-made medical device can meet the requirements for premarket approval, the medical device should be based on the product's profile in accordance with the provisions of the "Measures for the Administration of Medical Device Registration and Filing" application for registration or filing (note: filing is needed for the management of Class I medical devices) under the management category. True, accurate, complete, and traceable clinical use data that meet ethical guidelines can be used as clinical evaluation data for registration.

(b) Requirements

There are corresponding requirements for the qualifications of the recorder, design, processing, use, and supervision of custom-made medical devices in the Regulations, which specify that the production of custom-made medical devices should not be outsourced. These devices are restricted to use by the ordering medical institutions for their specifically designated patients. Nonordering institutions or nondesignated patients are not included.

The Regulations propose specific requirements for the qualifications of manufacturers and for hospitals that use custom-made medical devices. Manufacturers should meet the following conditions: they must have the professional and technical personnel needed for the development and production of custom-made medical devices; they must have the capability and research foundation to develop custom-made medical devices; they must have a registration certificate and manufacturing license for the same type of medical devices that are manufactured according to standard specifications. Overseas manufacturers should hold a qualification certificate that is issued by the medical device regulatory department in the country or region where the registration or production address is located; have the capacity and experience to produce the same type of medical devices that are mass-produced according to the standard specifications; and comply with the corresponding quality

Fig. 9.1 Diagram of the marketing process for custom-made medical devices

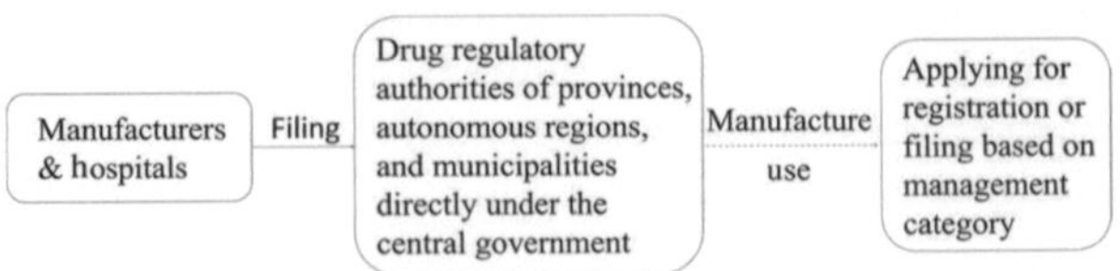

management system. Hospitals that use custom-made medical devices should meet the following conditions: they must be Level 3 general or specialized hospitals (note: China divides hospitals into three levels with a total of ten grades based on hospital size, scientific research direction, personnel and technical strength, medical hardware equipment, etc., with the highest grade being Level 3, special grade) with diagnosis and treatment items that are suitable for the custom-made medical devices that are being used; they must have attending physicians who are registered in hospitals and can use custom-made medical devices; they must have the ability to use similar marketed medical devices and have conducted research on and treated the same disease at advanced clinical professional levels in China; they must have a high level of medical device management; they must have established a complete quality management system for the use of medical devices; and they must have capabilities of evaluating the use of medical devices and monitoring adverse events.

In terms of the design and production of custom-made medical devices, the manufacturer and the hospital should sign an agreement to clarify the rights, obligations, and responsibilities of both parties. The manufacturing order should also be included in this agreement. Additionally, the following information should be provided in the order: information about the manufacturer, hospital, and patient; statements describing the reasons to use custom-made medical devices; unique needs that must be met by the custom-made device; product design requirements; finished product delivery requirements; product acceptance criteria; and product acceptance lists. The authorized attending physician and manufacturer contact person need to sign and date this document. In addition, to meet the requirements of the Medical Device Production Quality Management Specification and its appendixes, the development and production of custom-made medical devices also need to meet special requirements in terms of personnel, design, development, quality control, and traceability management specified in the Regulations. Each year, before the end of January, the filer should submit an annual report that describes the production and use of custom-made medical devices during the previous year to the drug regulatory department and the health administrative department of the province, autonomous region, and municipality directly under the Central Government.

In terms of use management, hospital representatives should inform patients or their guardians of the reasons for and risks of using custom-made medical devices. After patients or their guardians sign an informed consent form, the product filing and other circumstances should be explained to these patients or guardians before the devices are used. Hospital representatives should also negotiate with the manufacturer to create orders. Hospitals should establish a custom-made medical device inspection record system. Custom-made medical devices should be accepted in accordance with the design requirements, product acceptance criteria, and product acceptance checklist as outlined in the agreement and the manufacturing order. Moreover, hospitals should properly maintain production orders; information on product acceptance, modification, use, and return; as well as other information that is closely related to the quality and safety of custom-made medical devices; this documentation is necessary to ensure traceability of the information. The product name and unique identification number of the custom-made medical device should be recorded in medical records. The period for which the relevant information is retained should be no shorter than the lifetime of the medical device that is specified by the manufacturer. Additionally, relevant information about implantable custom-made medical devices should be permanently retained. For custom-made medical devices other than implantation devices, information should be retained for no less than 5 years from the date of product delivery by the manufacturer. After use, hospitals should evaluate custom-made medical devices. The evaluation technical team should be composed of medical, nursing, clinical engineering technology, nosocomial infection control, and manufacturer technicians who analyze and evaluate the actual effect, quality, and safety of the use of custom-made medical devices and who use the evaluation results rationally. Moreover, hospitals should use the evaluation results as an important basis for rational use in later stages. The filer should monitor and reevaluate the occurrence of adverse events associated with custom-made medical devices in accordance with the relevant provisions of the "Administrative Measures for the Monitoring and Re-evaluation of Medical Device Adverse Events." Hospitals should formulate complete safety prevention measures and risk control plans. In the event of an emergency, such as a serious adverse event, the emergency response plan should be immediately activated, prevention and control measures should be adopted, and treatment should be carried out in a timely manner. The Regulations also clarify that custom-made medical devices shall not be advertised in the mass media, and except as permitted by laws and regulations, the use of patient information for purposes other than the production and use of custom-made medical devices is prohibited.

In terms of supervision and management, the drug regulatory departments of provinces, autonomous regions, and municipalities directly under the Central Government should regularly supervise and inspect custom-made medical device manufacturers. The drug supervision and administration departments at the city and county levels should regularly inspect hospitals that use custom-made medical devices. If a hospital uses a custom-made medical device that has not been filed, has exceeded the scope of the filing, or has failed to file, the drug supervision and administration departments at the city and county levels will announce this to the public and include it in the integrity file. Additionally, the drug regulatory departments and health administrative departments of provinces, autonomous regions, and municipalities directly under the Central Government, where hospitals and related manufacturers are located, should be notified. If a hospital is instructed to stop using a device but continues to use the device, consequences should occur in accordance with the "Regulations on the Supervision and Administration of Medical Devices" regarding the situation of nondiscontinuation of medical device use.

9.2.3 Guidance for Custom-Made Medical Devices

9.2.3.1 Relevant Guidance for Custom-Made Medical Devices

In China, class III medical device guidance was developed and issued by the Center for Medical Device Evaluation (CMDE) (NMPA). Guidance about Class II medical devices is provided by the CMDE at provincial-level medical device review institutions, and the CMDE is responsible for relevant organization and coordination, quality control, and release. The guidance is directed toward technical review personnel, registration applicants, and the general public and is used to support the implementation of premarket regulatory policies or clarify the requirements for registration technical review. The guidance is a consensus document that was formulated during the technical review process of medical devices, and it interprets laws and regulations, guides the registration of applications, and adapts to the development of the industry. As a new tool, new method, and new standard for medical device technical review, the guidance is the necessary path to accomplish scientific review, an important output of the scientific action plan for medical device regulation, and a reliable guarantee of high-quality development of the medical device industry (Gao et al. 2023a, b).

Relevant guidance for custom-made medical devices in China is based mainly on the concept of accurate risk control, which is important throughout the full cycle of medical device design and development. According to the requirements of the YY/T 0287 medical device quality management system, a complete design and development process should begin with the design input (clinical needs), continue through the verification and validation process of design and development, and finally reach the design output (product design). In China, regulatory agencies focus on the adequacy and completeness of the design verification and validation process. During this process, physical, chemical, mechanical, biological, and even clinical factors need to be considered. For standardized products, design verification and validation are transient, and there is generally no need for continuous updates unless there is market feedback or changes in regulatory requirements. However, custom-made devices are not the same. According to the definition of custom-made medical devices, compared with standardized medical devices, their particularity lies mainly in the special needs put forward by clinicians and their use for specific patients, and the design needs to be adjusted according to the clinical needs of different users. The input, design verification, and validation processes are also continuously reciprocated and updated. In the original closed-loop design and development process, an important variable was introduced, that is, individualized clinical needs. If these needs are assigned to the responsible body, that person will be a clinician. Therefore, "medicine–engineering interaction quality control" is very important for the confirmation and validation of custom-made product design (Min et al. 2021). At present, the NMPA has also established relevant guidance for the quality control of medicine–engineering interactions involving custom-made medical devices, such as the "Guidance for Medicine–Engineering Interaction Quality Control of Personalized Matching Bone Implants and Ancillary Tools."

In addition, design verification and validation are needed to close the loop of R&D design, and these steps have also been the focus of regulatory agencies. Standardized products can accurately and relatively quickly complete these tasks by selecting the "worst-case" or "typical" model specifications. However, for custom-made products, selecting the "worst case" is difficult; the verification and validation of each design requires considerable material and time, which is not consistent with the fundamental goal of the rapid clinical application of personalized products. Thus, verifying the performance of custom-made, personalized medical devices is a challenge. China proposed the concept of an "equivalent model" for the first time in the validation of custom-made medical device performance, and the concept of an "equivalent model" was further defined in the "Guidance for Custom-made Personalized Bone Implant Equivalence Model," which explained the concept and proposed detailed requirements.

Therefore, the "Guidance for Medicine–Engineering Interaction Quality Control of Personalized Matching Bone Implants and Ancillary Tools" (hereafter referred to as "Medicine–Engineering Interaction Guidance") and "Guidance for Custom-Manufactured Personalized Bone Implants Equivalence Model" (hereafter referred to as "Equivalence Model Guidance") are the two main documents that provide guidance on the supervision of custom-made medical devices in China. Next, the custom-made bone implant is used as an example to elaborate upon the focus of the regulatory agency's technology review on the quality control of medicine–engineering interactions and the construction of an equivalence model.

9.2.3.2 Quality Control of Medicine–Engineering Interactions

The design input of a custom-made medical device begins with the addition of patient imaging data to the requirements given by the attending physician for the structure and specifications of the 3D model of the device, which is followed by an evaluation of product design finalization and performance testing by product engineering and design personnel. "Medicine–Engineering interaction" refers to the cooperation and checks and balances related to the exchange, communication, interaction, and complementarity of clinical information and engineering design information in accordance with the basic principles of "design and development" in YY/T 0287 (ISO 13485). The most important aspect of this interaction is that the responsibilities and authorities of both "doctors" and "engineers" should be clarified first, and "communication" and "interaction" should continue during the entire design and development process (Guo and Liu 2018).

To achieve successful medicine–engineering interaction, the team should have similar knowledge and a good communication foundation. In other words, if engineers cannot understand the needs of clinicians, products cannot truly match individualized needs; if clinicians do not have a basic understanding of product engineering requirements, products may fail the basic bench test. For any team, the fastest way to increase work efficiency is to work together on the same runway. Although the design is personalized, the working process should be solidified to a certain extent to form a standardized operating process to "respond to all changes."

Medicine–engineering interactions are needed in the design of all medical devices, but no standardized medical device is a personalized product; doctors and engineers have high-frequency and high-intensity discussions about each product. Therefore, during the in-design verification and validation of custom-made medical devices, the quality control of medicine–engineering interactions has become particularly important.

Medicine–engineering interactions are important throughout the design and development of custom-made medical devices. The design and development procedures, planning, input, output, review, verification, validation, modification, change, and recording of corresponding documents must be performed by clinical physicians to meet the needs of diagnosis, surgery, and postoperative rehabilitation. Therefore, a large amount of systematic control over the behavior of clinicians is needed to improve the quality of the research and development of custom-made prostheses and instruments. From the perspective of the R&D system of the manufacturing enterprise, engineers (including statisticians) translate the needs of clinicians into engineering content and limit and calibrate the degrees of freedom among clinicians to ensure the stability of product performance. Moreover, medicine–engineering interactions during the design and development of custom-made medical devices affect the characteristics of long-term clinical studies, requiring clinicians to have richer clinical research experience. In the following section, based on the guidance about medicine–engineering interaction that was issued by the NMPA, the relevant requirements for quality control of medicine-engineering interactions are described in detail.

(a) Procedures

The general design program for personalized bone implants includes five main steps: planning, input, output, verification, and validation. When the verification does not meet the requirements, modification is triggered. According to the preamble, based on the results of clinical follow-up of implanted products, design changes are made to the products in the subsequent implementation cases; all steps of the design procedure are performed under reviewer supervision; all processes need to be recorded, and samples are retained. Planning mainly includes qualification verification, planning demonstration, planning and design verification requirements for surgical solutions, and product validation requirements. The input steps mainly include radiological input, 3D reconstruction of the affected bone, and bone implant design and analysis (including hard or soft tissue fixed locations and the number of attachment points). The output steps mainly include the product 3D CAD model, product instruction manual, and final product inspection requirements. The verification steps mainly include back-to-back blind design, cross-retest, and physicochemical property tests of accompanying samples. The validation steps mainly include consistency between the final product and the design results and sterilization confirmation. The conditions that trigger modification and the steps of this work are elucidated in the modification step. The clinical follow-up records and suggested changes are included in the change step. The review content and methods are elucidated in the review step. In the recording and sample retention steps, the recording form and sample retention requirements should be clarified.

(b) Planning

The qualification requirements for medical and engineering personnel who preside over and participate in the design and production of custom-made medical devices include the following. The "medical" side recommends that a doctor with a senior professional title in a tertiary hospital preside over the entire process of custom-made medical device production and use. This doctor should have previous experience in carrying out similar surgeries to treat the same anatomical site and condition with standardized products. Participants on the "engineering" side must have experience in the design of custom-made medical devices or have more than 3 years of experience in the design and development of noncustom-made medical devices with similar implantation procedures. The medicine–engineering interaction includes the following:

1. Jointly demonstrate the feasibility of the design and manufacture of custom-made medical devices. Based on the existing technology reserves (including the raw materials, final product performance, process level, software used, and design capability), the feasibility of implementing custom-made medical devices is determined.
2. Surgical plan interaction. During medicine–engineering interactions for planning personalized implant surgery, the doctor should fully inform the engineers of the details of the surgical plan to prevent cognitive differences due to errors in common sense understanding or differences in professional perspectives, and to prevent errors due to engineering problems. If personnel fail to consider some undisclosed factors, unreasonable factors related to the designed implant may be observed during the operation. Surgical planning should clearly limit the time frame from the acquisition of patient imaging data to the confirmation of the implant and instrument design, and from the design confirmation to the date of surgery, specifically a natural day, to reduce the impact of changes in patient condition on the design validity.
3. Jointly establish the design implementation technical route. The activities necessary for verification, validation, and design transfer at each design stage should be defined, including finite element analysis, fatigue testing, simulated surgery, and the production of component specimens/prototype products.

(c) Input

The input of custom-made medical devices includes the imaging data of the anatomical site, the design of the 3D model of the implant, and the analysis of the use effect after the implantation. The content of medicine–engineering interactions mainly includes the following:

1. Image Input and 3D Reconstruction: The personalized design depends largely on the generation and processing of imaging data as well as the 3D reconstruction of the anatomical and structural component models.
2. Design Criteria and Basis: In the design and analysis of custom-made medical devices, both parties should clarify the requirements for personalized treatment, determine the basis for the design of the substitute tissue structure, and

clarify the relationship between the diseased tissue and the implants (including a hard tissue fixation scheme and a soft tissue fixation scheme). Additionally, the material and mechanical properties of the bone implant, as well as the force-bearing condition of the bone implant in the human body, should be clarified; the goal of design analysis and/or safety factor of the bone implant should be simplified, and the safety and effectiveness of the bone implant design should be clarified.

3. Among personalized matched products with relatively similar expected use and functional performance, sequential and cumulative design information should be generated, and the formatting of input information should reflect the key design information of the previous product, especially for common design areas such as the principal stress area of the entity and the porous area.

(d) Output

The output of custom-made medical devices includes the medical imaging data that are used in the design, the reconstructed 3D model of the diseased area, the 3D CAD model of the final product (should be in a common 3D model format, such as IGES, STEP, and STL), and instructions for product use. The output of custom-made medical device design also includes instructions for the use of each product, and these instructions must clarify the product's design principles, design procedures, design essentials in the input link, design analysis reports, product acceptance criteria, and inspection rules, and product use methods. The content of the medicine–engineering interactions mainly includes the following:

1. The two parties should jointly inspect the implant CAD files.
2. The core quality control parameters should be determined, the quality control parameters related to final product quality should be determined, and the acceptance criteria for the parameters should be clarified. Products that are designed for a certain anatomical region should have a unified design specification, which should clarify the design principles, design procedures, design essentials details in the input link, product acceptance criteria, and corresponding inspection rules for this type of individualized product.
3. Instructions for product use should include clear usage boundaries, including the osteotomy locations and the geometric dimensions of the individualized implant structures. There should be a clear description (coordinate system and coordinate values) of the spatial position of internal fixators, such as screws, in the residual bone tissue, which should clarify the pore size, porosity, and through-porosity of the trabecular bone structure in the osseointegration area, and the anatomical matching filling area should be defined. The 3D point coordinates of the grid structure unit should be clarified. To adapt to possible changes in intraoperative osteotomy and fixation, spare parts with multiple specifications within a certain size gradient should be available.

(e) Review

At each stage of the design and development of custom-made medical devices, systematic review and decision tree construction by doctors and engineers are needed, mainly in the input, output verification, and validation stages. Review records should include a template that allows the review process and results to be recorded at all stages, including the problems that are found in each round of review, corrective measures that are taken, revision results, and adjustments and improvements that are made to the product design specifications. The content of medicine–engineering interactions mainly includes the following. According to the procedural flow and by strictly reviewing the design results at each stage of custom-made medical device design, the review record template should be jointly developed to record the aspects of the review process and results, including the problems, corrective measures, and revision results found in the first round of reviews, especially the adjustment and improvement of product design specifications.

(f) Verification

Different from conventional standardized products that are repeatedly produced in bulk, custom-made medical devices are verified by "personalized processing and manufacturing;" therefore, doctors must be involved, and the design of each custom-made medical device needs to be carried out separately. Therefore, the verification of custom-made medical devices includes the purpose of "ensuring that it can safely and effectively replace the function of the defective site during service." The verification should include a design and development evaluation, a test of the physicochemical properties of the accompanying samples, and an evaluation of the biomechanical properties of the products. Thus, medicine–engineering interactions should mainly include the following:

1. The physical and chemical properties of the accompanying samples should be tested by jointly determining the trigger conditions, test contents, test methods, and test acceptance conditions for testing the physical and chemical properties of the product.
2. The conditions that will trigger new mechanical tests or animal experiments should be clarified. The pathological and physiological characteristics of anatomical locations should be considered when establishing animal models, and attention should be given to the mechanical verification of isolated trabecular bone structures, especially in the osseointegration zone.

(g) Validation

A custom-made medical device is used only for a specific patient, and attention should be given to the sampling statistics for clinical confirmation, the selection of representative products, and the differentiation between clinical evaluation products and released products. Validation of custom-made medical device design relies heavily on treatment data that are collected from similar cases, simulation bench models, and mechanical property tests in animal models, and large-scale clinical studies are necessary before the use of such devices. Validation work should involve more flexible, rigorous, and dynamically adjusted clinical confirmation methods; additionally, validation evidence should be applied throughout the life cycle through statistical control and should be based on iterative data from a series of the same individualized product type with similar biomechanical functions. Thus, medicine–engineering interactions should mainly include the following:

1. Both parties should jointly confirm the match between the implant product and the design model and the reliability and safety of the design of key parts.
2. Sterilization Validation: The implant sterilization process and results should be verified and recorded; for parts with porous structures, conditions that require new sterilization validation should be clearly defined.
3. A biostatistician should work with clinicians to develop long-term clinical study plans and statistical analysis plans (including data statistical step size and cycle), and postmarketing adverse event monitoring and passive traceability should be upgraded to active and planned postmarketing clinical studies.

(h) Modification

For custom-made medical devices, the circumstances under which design modification is needed, the process that is used for design modification, and the verification and validation indicators for the design modification results should be determined. Thus, medicine–engineering interactions should mainly include the following:

1. The acceptance indicators for the final product after the implant design is modified, including the manufacturing accuracy, mechanical properties, surface modification requirements, residual powder cleaning, and sterilization requirements of the product, should be determined.
2. The design modification process should be implemented in accordance with the quality system requirements to ensure traceability.

(i) Change

The design of each product must include the aforementioned processes of design development review, verification, and validation. Compared with the previous product, the new product's main function, soft and hard tissue fixation methods, and cumulative data related to clinical evaluation indicators that exceed predefined acceptance limits or those of previously implanted or used products should be reanalyzed. To avoid the risk associated with the product, follow-up timing, follow-up procedures, preventive intervention measures, and reintervention treatment for previous patients should be increased, and relevant experience should be incorporated into the subsequent design and development of new products. Thus, medicine–engineering interactions should mainly include the following:

1. The two parties should communicate the problems in the follow-up process and use the follow-up questions and data to improve subsequent development and design.
2. The two parties should ensure the traceability of the problems that were discovered during follow-up as well as improvement efforts.

(j) Retaining a Sample for the Record

According to the anatomical location and functional requirements (especially the principal stress areas), custom-made medical devices are divided into different product families, and design and development documents are recorded and archived. Documents should be stored in strict accordance with the time axis of design and development to avoid unintended consequences. Changes to these documents should not delete or cover up the original stored content, and all changes should be made with reviewable tracks. The amount of data used in individualized custom-made design and development is relatively large, and design modifications or subsequent product changes may be made repeatedly as the disease progresses during the medicine–engineering interaction process. These data are closely related to the evaluation of long-term clinical cumulative risk, and records must ensure traceability. Additionally, data owners may include multiple parties across multiple times and spaces; thus, not tampering with data and ensuring information security are particularly important. The use of advanced distributed data management technologies, such as blockchain, is encouraged. Thus, medicine–engineering interactions should mainly include the following:

1. The two parties should jointly verify the changes in the original image data, 3D model, finite element analysis files, and design and development documents during the implant manufacturing process that were determined during the design process.
2. The two parties should jointly determine the changes in the reserve sample.
3. The results of all periodic statistical analyses should be recorded in a timely and accurate manner in the clinical confirmation document, and the validation document should be signed by a physician, engineer, rehabilitation therapist, nurse, and statistician.

9.2.3.3 Construction of the Equivalence Model

A custom-made personalized bone implant equivalence model is a model that is constructed based on clinical expectations to evaluate the anatomical match, biomechanical properties, and expected clinical function of custom-made, personalized bone implant products. Such a model can be used to identify risk factors for implant products in terms of material properties, structural design, geometric dimensions, intended use and use methods, application sites, human mechanical environment, and biological effects of implant products. The model can be constructed based on data from clinical studies of implant products. In brief, these models are digital and physical models that maximize the simulation products and biomechanical environment. Such a model needs to include the structure, size, and material properties of the implant as well as the relationships between the implant and other tissues, such as contact relationships and dynamic or static mechanical relationships. In terms of the temporal dimension, the condition at the beginning of implantation should be considered, and the results should also reflect the long-term stability after implantation. The equivalent model represents a simplification of the actual human skeletal muscle system; however, this model is more complex and complete than the finite element model. A successful "equivalence model" can completely replace multiple in vitro experiments or even human trials. However, at present, the most achievable possibility is in the verification of the mechanical properties of products. Even for personalized medical devices, the boundary values of product structure design are clarified by limiting the use sites and application scenarios. The tissue structure within this boundary can be considered as a whole, and its biomechanical requirements can be determined. In other words, the overall design of a product should serve the overall requirements of the organization and the environment beyond the boundary value. From a microscopic point of view, internal structures, such as the morphology of the product and the pore grid, ultimately determine whether the product can stably support the external environment. A "equivalence model" provides a way to functionally verify complex structures, but traditional performance verification methods, such as biocompatibility tests and animal experiments, are recommended for some general properties. Next, the specific requirements for performance verification and validation of custom-made medical devices in China will be elaborated upon with reference to the guidance for custom-made personalized bone implant equivalence models that was issued by the NMPA.

(a) Structural Characteristics of the Equivalence Model

The construction of an equivalence model should be based on actual clinical needs by elucidating the structure, size, morphology, fixation method, mechanical properties, kinematic properties, biological properties, and other characteristics of the equivalence model with diagrams. This includes but is not limited to the following:

1. Descriptions of the function and applicability of the bone implant, such as the replacement site, patient characteristics, use conditions, expected use environment, and limitations.
2. Descriptions of the overall structural composition of the bone implant, such as its geometry, size, structure, material, and assembly.
3. For implants with a porous structure, descriptions of the structure, morphology, pore characteristics, arrangement (such as porosity, pore diameter, wire diameter, the design and basis for pore size distribution, and open/closed pore ratio), the transition structure change characteristics, and the gradient structure change characteristics.
4. Descriptions of the implant and bone and/or soft tissue interface connection and fixation methods, including initial fixation and long-term considerations.

(b) Functional Evaluation Objective of the Equivalence Model

When evaluating whether the performance and function of custom-made personalized bone implant products meet clinical expectations, the functional evaluation objectives and performance parameters of the equivalence model should be elucidated according to the surgical site and expected clinical use; these include the mechanical properties and stability of the implant, bone reconstruction around the implant, and articulation characteristics of the reconstructed joint.

(c) Methods and Requirements for Equivalence Model Construction

In the construction of an equivalence model, the acquisition requirement and the basis for the determination of each element should be elucidated, and the product risk should be determined. The history of the use of relevant materials in the human body and data from similar or previous generation products that are available on the market should be fully identified, input, and applied. The construction of an equivalence model needs to meet the purpose of functional equivalence. Considering the construction of a numerical model of an implant as an example, equivalence to the clinical application of an implant should be achieved in terms of structural size, material properties, fixation method, and mechanical environment, including the following:

1. The geometrical structure and dimensions should meet the clinical use requirements.
2. The assignment of material properties should include the modulus, anisotropy, and gradient change.
3. The fixation methods, including the fixation position, should be consistent with clinical use.
4. The mechanical environment, including mechanics and kinematic loading conditions, should be consistent with clinical use. Each parameter can be selected according to actual needs. The constitutive relationships of the equivalence model with the implant and human environment in terms of structure, material, fixation method, and mechanical environment should be discussed, and the basis for its selection should be explained.

The construction of equivalence models can involve physical tests, numerical simulation analysis, big data analysis, clinical use data, etc. The methods for the construction of equivalence models should be standardized to meet the repeatability requirements. To elucidate the consistency and rationality of the equivalence model, experimental and numerical simulation analyses should be performed in combination, and the rationality of the construction method should be verified by comparing the relevant results. The registration applicant or filer needs to provide complete research materials and details related to the reliability, rationality, and pertinence of the model.

The registration applicant or filer should clearly define the normal and extreme cases of the equivalence model in terms of geometry, material properties, and loading conditions, and explain the prerequisites for bone implant performance and functional evaluation. The registration applicant or filer should clarify the movement and mechanical strength of the bone implant under extreme conditions based on the clinical use of the relevant products and the risk of application of the bone implant.

(d) Verification of the Equivalence Model Requirement

The verification of the equivalence model includes two stages: verification of the construction method and verification of the model output. The method for constructing the equivalence model must be verified and validated. The registration applicant or filer is required to provide discussion materials regarding the relevant methods to explain the reliability, rationality, and pertinence of the method.

1. The registration applicant or filer should demonstrate and explain the input errors of the bone implant, describe the bone and fixtures in the equivalence model of the overall biological system, and verify and confirm the rationality and reliability of the simplification method of structural features. The material properties should also be explained. The rationality and reliability of the fixed constraint and loading conditions should be demonstrated and explained. For example, given the use of fresh cadaveric bone, animal bone, or artificial bone in physical models, the rationale for material selection should be explained.
2. The input parameters in the model should be subjected to sensitivity analysis to illustrate the impact of the input parameters, for example, the rationalization of loading time and test frequency, as well as mesh size and element type in the computer finite element model, on the model results.
3. The registration applicant or filer should explain the evaluation criteria and acceptability of model equivalence, and the extent of the difference between the equivalence model and the expected clinical use should be explained.

The output of the equivalence model can be verified by physical tests, clinical data, numerical simulation analyses, literature reports, etc., or with a combination of these data with reference to corresponding standards to verify the evaluation ability of the equivalence model, including but not limited to the following situations:

1. Based on physical tests and numerical models, the reliability of the output of the equivalence model can be verified by comparing the same input parameters under the same mounting fixation and mechanical loading conditions.
2. Based on similar marketed products with existing clinical data, other products can be constructed, and the equivalence model demonstrates the rationality of the output of the equivalence model.
3. The output results of physical tests or numerical models are within the reference ranges reported in the literature under similar conditions.

(e) Regular Review and Continuous Improvement of the Equivalence Model

The equivalence model should be used to evaluate products, postmarketing clinical application data, and study data from similar products should be collected, and the equivalence data from the models should be verified by clinical application. Additionally, adverse events caused by insufficient model construction and other information that can be used in the evaluation should be considered. Clinical application data with improved models should be used for the evaluation, improvement, and continuous improvement of the equivalence models.

9.3 Standards and Guidance for Medical 3D-Printing Technology

9.3.1 Medical Device Standards

9.3.1.1 Introduction to Standardization Work

In China, the basic structure of the standards system follows the "Standardization Law of the People's Republic of China" (The National People's Congress of the People's Republic of China 2017), which specifies that standards include national standards, industry standards, local standards, association standards, and enterprise standards. National standards are divided into mandatory standards and voluntary standards. Mandatory standards must be implemented, and the state encourages the use of voluntary standards. The technical requirements of voluntary national standards, industry standards, and group standards should not be lower than those of mandatory national standards. National standards are technical requirements that are very important for national economic and technological development and must be unified nationwide. Once a national standard is announced, the industrial standards that overlap with it will be abolished.

Standards at each level are formulated and revised by different bodies. The relevant administrative departments of the State Council are responsible for the proposal, draft organization, solicitation of opinions, and technical review of projects related to mandatory national standards according to their duties. The standardization administrative department of the State Council is responsible for project approval, numbering, and external notification of mandatory national standards. Voluntary national standards may be formulated for technical requirements that meet the needs of basic universality and compatibility with mandatory national standards and that play a leading role in each relevant industry. Industrial standards can be formulated for technical requirements that do not have recommended national standards and need to be unified within a certain nation. The industry standards are formulated by the relevant administrative department of the State Council and reported to the standardization administrative department of the State Council for the record.

The state encourages social groups, such as societies, associations, chambers of commerce, federations, and industrial technology alliances, to coordinate relevant market entities to jointly develop voluntary standards that meet the needs of the market and innovation. The adoption of voluntary standards is agreed upon by the members of the group or made available for voluntary adoption by societies in accordance with the regulations of the group. The formulation of voluntary standards should follow the principles of openness, transparency, and fairness. Additionally, it should be ensured that all participants obtain relevant information, and the common needs of all participants should be reflected. The investigation, analysis, experimentation, and demonstration of standard-related matters should be organized.

9.3.1.2 Classification and Application of Medical Device Standards

Medical device standards are defined as the unified technical requirements that are followed during the development, production, operation, use, and supervision of medical devices (State Administration for Market Regulation 2017). Medical device standards include mandatory national standards, voluntary national standards, mandatory industry standards, voluntary industry standards, and association standards. International standards are also applied in China.

Compared with national standards, there are more types and quantities of industry standards for medical devices, and they are often more targeted toward specific products. The development and release cycles of association standards are relatively short, and these cycles are coordinated with the participation of social organizations in market entities. Therefore, association standards have stronger market supply power and a faster response to industry demand. Association standards are effective supplements to blank industry standards and are very important for encouraging innovation, promoting technological progress, and laying a foundation for the formulation and revision of relevant industry standards in the future. National standards and industry standards are the main reference and basis documents in the R&D and registration of medical devices. The collaborative development and coordinated support of medical device standard systems, which are developed via government-led and market-dependent mechanisms, are important guarantees for meeting the development needs of the industry.

9.3.1.3 Construction of a Standardized System for Medical 3D-Printing

Medical device standards are an important part of ensuring the safety and effectiveness of medical devices. Usually, standards determine quality, and high-quality standards can result in the production of high-quality medical devices. However, before 2019, China had not established dedicated national standards or industry standards related to medical 3D printing, and the development of the industry was uneven. There is an urgent need to establish a standard system to support the rapid development of medical 3D printing technology.

The construction of a standard system for medical 3D printing is accompanied by the process of medical device standardization reform in China. Before 2016, the adoption of medical device standards in the Chinese industry usually focused on government-led standards, such as national standards or industry standards, as well as some international standards. Since 2016, the reform process of medical device standardization in China has accelerated. One of the important measures is the cultivation and development of association standards (Zheng and Sun 2015; Wang 2017; Li 2017). Because of their market genes and consistency with the interests of market players, association standards closely follow the demand of the market, accelerate the speed of standard formulation, increase the effective supply of standards, solve the problem of nonstandard production, and promote the development of the industry. Moreover, the main body that formulates association standards includes professional organizations in the industry with corresponding standardization capabilities, and these standards are formulated in accordance with standardized processes. These association standards can protect technological innovation achievements, increase industry access thresholds, enhance industry competitiveness, and stimulate enthusiasm for innovation. In the context of medical device standardization reform, the overall purpose of constructing China's medical 3D printing standards system is to establish a new standard system in which the national or industry standards led by the government and the association standards led by the market are coordinated and developed. Currently, China has established a relatively complete standard system for medical 3D printing (Fig. 9.2). The standard system covers raw materials, process validation methods, equipment, data transmission, risk management, and products, with a focus on quality control throughout the entire life cycle of medical 3D printing technology.

9.3.1.4 Relevant Standards of Medical 3D Printing Technology

Medical 3D printing technology includes seven processes: image acquisition, product design, format conversion, material control, printing processing, postprocessing, and detection and verification. Each link has a decisive impact on the final product, and standards must be established around the quality control priorities of such products (Mao and Han 2022). According to the control focus, the medical 3D printing standard system is constructed around six levels: basic standards, data/software, equipment, materials, processes, and products.

(a) Basic Standards of Medical 3D Printing Technology

The part involved the terminology and classification of medical 3D printing technology. The relevant national standards GB/T 35351-2017 and GB/T 35021-2018 provide definitions of the terminology, basic process principles, classifications, and types of raw materials that are involved in 3D printing technology, which are also applicable to the medical 3D printing field. Research and development of special terminology and classification in the medical 3D printing field are conducive to the development of follow-up work to meet the needs of industry development and regulation.

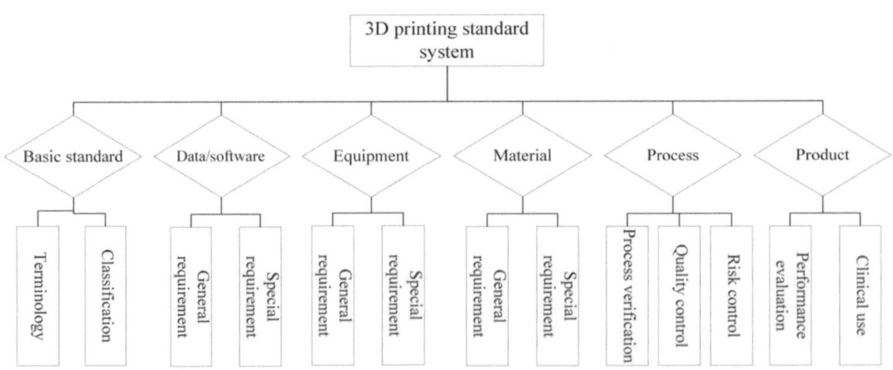

Fig. 9.2 Architecture of the Chinese medical 3D printing standard system

(b) Data/Software Standards of Medical 3D Printing Technology

The establishment of standards should focus on the methods of controlling software and data transmission that are required for the data analysis and modeling of medical 3D printing technology, including the safety and validity of data transmission, the accuracy of data processing methods, the stability and accuracy of modeling methods, the reliability and stability of related software, and the basic requirements for the construction of medicine–engineering interaction platforms. Attention should also be given to the conversion of file formats and the design from digital devices to physical devices, such as the placement position, direction, and distance between components, materials, and the selection of layer thickness. Tests should be performed on the transmission and processing of data to ensure its performance. China has established relevant standards for medical 3D printing data/software (Table 9.1).

(c) Equipment Standards for Medical 3D Printing Technology

Medical 3D printing technology involves a variety of manufacturing processes, such as stereolithography, material extrusion, electron beam melting, and selective laser melting. The use of different printing raw materials requires the selection of suitable printing processes. According to the requirements of different processes, the general requirement and special requirement standards for printing equipment, the verification method standards of operation stability and accuracy of equipment parameters, and the control method standards of equipment modification need to be studied and established. Currently, China has established the relevant association standard "T/CAMDI 073-2021 Powder Bed Electron Beam Additive Manufacturing Equipment for Medical Devices."

(d) Material Standards of Medical 3D Printing Technology

The materials that are commonly used in medical 3D printing processes include metals, ceramics, photosensitive resins, polymers, and biomaterials. The physical and chemical properties of materials have a great impact on the performance and quality of printed parts. Special attention should be given to the shape stability of materials during the processing and forming processes, as well as changes in physicochemical properties during manufacturing processes. Different performance

Table 9.1 Data/software standards for medical 3D printing technology in China

Standard number	Standard name
T/CAMDI 028-2019	General Requirements for Internet Implementation of Custom Additive Manufactured (3D Printing) Medical Devices
T/CAMDI 045-2020	Finite Element Analysis of 3D Printed Metal Implants
T/CAMDI 062-2021	Special Requirements for 3D Modeling Software in Additive Manufactured Personalized Medical Devices
T/CAMDI 090-2022	Technical Requirements for Automatic 3D Reconstruction of Medical Image Processing

indicators can be set for different types of raw materials according to the printing process. For recyclable raw materials, environmental factors (such as temperature, oxygen, humidity, and UV light) may cause changes in the properties of the raw materials. Therefore, the material recycling process should be described, and whether recycling affects material biocompatibility should be demonstrated. The quality of the final products is also directly or indirectly affected by the material. Only when the selection and use of materials are fully evaluated and the biocompatibility of the materials, processing aids, and finished products is ensured can the entire manufacturing process and products be safe and reliable. Therefore, emphasis should be placed on the research and development of material standards that meet the special requirements of medical devices using 3D printing technology, such as general requirements for raw materials, special requirements for different types of materials, and technical considerations for material reuse. China has established relevant material standards for medical 3D printing (Table 9.2).

(e) Process Standards of Medical 3D Printing Technology

The 3D printing process is roughly divided into three steps: Printing, postprocessing, and sterilization and cleaning. There are many printing processes, and each process has its corresponding range of process parameters. To ensure that the batch-to-batch difference remains within a controllable range, it is necessary to ensure the stability of the process parameters during the printing process (Fan and Xie 2018). Certain manufacturing processes require postprocessing of the product, such as heat treatment or mechanical polishing, which also affect the performance of the materials used and the final device. Since 3D printing products usually have complex structural features including porous structures, which increases the difficulty of product cleaning and sterilization, the influence of complex structures should be

Table 9.2 Material standards for medical 3D printing in China

Standard number	Standard name
YY/T 1701-2020	Medical Grade Ti-6Al-4V/Ti-6Al-4V ELI Powder used for Additive Manufacturing
YY/T 1702-2020	Dentistry-Additive Manufacturing-Selective Laser Melting Metallic Materials for Fixed and Removable Restorations and Appliances
YY/T 1851-2022	Medical Pure Tantalum Powder for Additive Manufacturing
YY/T 1910-2023	Medical Grade Beta-Tricalcium Phosphate Powder for Additive Manufacturing
T/CAMDI 042-2020	The Biomedical Tantalum Powder Used for Additive Manufacturing
T/CAMDI 059-2021	Control Standard for the Reuse of Medical Metal Powder in Additive Manufacturing
T/CAMDI 088-2022	Dentistry-Requirements for Additive Manufacturing (Vat photopolymerization) of Zirconia Ceramic Materials
T/CAMDI 097-2022	Poly-ether-ether-ketone (PEEK) Materials for the Additive Manufacturing of Implantable Medical Device

fully considered and the sterilization and cleaning process parameters should be determined according to the specific structural shape; moreover, cleaning should be performed and sterilization should be verified, and, if necessary, the effectiveness of the sterilization and cleaning processes may be demonstrated by conducting destructive tests. Process parameters include software, materials, and processes. Any change in any parameter needs to be verified. In addition, the methods of controlling quality and risk under different processes should be considered. Therefore, research on process verification methods, quality control methods, and risk control methods is needed. Based on these analyses, the overall idea of standard system design research is to consider all aspects of the manufacturing process as the starting point and to conduct a comprehensive evaluation from commonality to individuality, from hardware to software, from materials to methods. China has established relevant process standards for medical 3D printing (Table 9.3).

(f) Product Standards of Medical 3D Printing Technology

Product standards of 3D printing technology can be considered the standards for evaluating the performance of the final product, and the standards for clinical use can also be included to provide technical support for product design as well as for development, supervision, and clinical application. Product standards provide a basis for government supervision and industry development, helping to improve the quality of end products, raise the industry threshold, maintain market order, and protect the rights and interests of patients. Moreover, product standards help to improve the recognition of Chinese products in the international market, promote product exports, and enhance international competitiveness. Therefore, the construction of a standard medical 3D printing system should include the construction of product standards. China has established relevant product standards for medical 3D printing technology (Table 9.4).

Table 9.3 Process standards of Chinese medical 3D printing technology

Standard number	Standard name
YY/T 1809-2021	Additive Manufacturing for Medical Applications: Verification Methods of Cleaning and Cleaning Effectiveness of Metal Powder used in Powder-Bed Fusion Process
YY/T 1909-2023	Additive Manufacturing for Medical Applications: Requirements for Control and Validation of Metal Powder-Bed Electron Beam Fusion Process
T/CAMDI 093-2022	Additive Manufacturing for Medical Applications: Requirements for Control and Validation of Light-Curing Process

Table 9.4 Product standards for medical 3D printing in China

Standard number	Standard name	Standard number	Standard name
YY/T 1802-2021	Additive Manufacturing Medical Product—3D Printing Titanium Alloy Implant Metal Ion Precipitation Evaluation Method	T/CAMDI 066-2021	Additive Manufacturing of Customized Tantalum Bone Defect Filler
YY/T 1845-2022	General Requirements of Guides for Orthopaedic Surgery	T/CAMDI 067-2021	Additive Manufacturing Tantalum Spinal Prosthesis
T/CAMDI 025-2019	Mechanical Equivalent Model of Customized Medical Devices	T/CAMDI 068-2021	Additive Manufacturing Auricle Pressure Orthotic Device
T/CAMDI 026-2019	Special Requirements of Customized Medical Device Quality System	T/CAMDI 069-2021	Additive-Manufactured Patient-Matched Wrist-Hand Orthoses
T/CAMDI 027-2019	Matched Artificial Temporomandibular Joint	T/CAMDI 070-2021	Customized Additive-Manufactured Polyetheretherketone (PEEK) Craniomaxillofacial Implants
T/CAMDI 029-2019	The Whole Process Monitoring, Judgment Index and Acceptance Conditions of Customized Medical Device Medical-industrial Interaction	T/CAMDI 071-2021	Personalized Metal Additive Manufacturing Chest Wall Deformity Orthosis Device
T/CAMDI 037-2020	Clinical Application Standard of 3D Printed Tantalum	T/CAMDI 072-2021	Customized Additive Manufactured Scoliosis Orthosis
T/CAMDI 038-2020	Additive Manufacturing (3D Printing) of Dental Implant Surgical Guides	T/CAMDI 083-2022	Bracketless for Orthodontic Appliance
T/CAMDI 039-2020	Bioprinting Medical Devices-Special Requirements for Quality Management System	T/CAMDI 084-2022	Additive Manufacturing of Tantalum Jaw Repair Implants
T/CAMDI 040-2020	Special Requirements of Quality Management System for Metal Additive Manufactured Medical Devices	T/CAMDI 085-2022	Additive Manufacturing of Custom-made Titanium Mesh for Alveolar Bone Augmentation
T/CAMDI 041-2020	Additive Manufacturing (3D Printing) of Customized Guide plates for Orthopedic Surgery	T/CAMDI 086-2022	Additive Manufactured (light curing) Temporary Crown and Bridge Resin
T/CAMDI 043-2020	Additive Manufacturing (3D Printing) of Custom-made Dental Implant	T/CAMDI 087-2022	Additive Manufactured (light-curing) Denture Base Resin
T/CAMDI 044-2020	Additive Manufactured (3D Printed) Metal Dental Implant	T/CAMDI 089-2022	Customized Additive Manufactured Plantar Orthosis
T/CAMDI 046-2020	Evaluation Method and Criterion of 3D Printing Metal Implants Quality Uniformity	T/CAMDI 091-2022	Additive Manufacturing of Metal Modular Segmental prostheses of the extremity

(continued)

Table 9.4 (continued)

Standard number	Standard name	Standard number	Standard name
T/CAMDI 060-2021	Test Standard for Fatigue Performance of Additive Manufacturing Femoral Stem	T/CAMDI 092-2022	Additive Manufacturing Metal Shoulder Prosthesis
T/CAMDI 061-2021	Standard for Evaluating the Biological Hazards of Residual Particles in the Additive Manufactured Metal Implant	T/CAMDI 094-2022	Additive Manufacturing of Zirconia Dental Implant
T/CAMDI 063-2021	Personalized Additive Manufacturing Occlusal Splint	T/CAMDI 095-2022	General Requirements for Skin Repair Products Produced by Additive Manufacturing
T/CAMDI 064-2021	Additive Manufacturing Tantalum Hip Joint Prosthesis	T/CAMDI 096-2022	Input Requirements for Additive Manufacturing Implant Design
T/CAMDI 065-2021	Additive Manufacturing Tantalum Knee Joint Prosthesis		

9.3.2 Relevant Guidance for Medical 3D Printing Technology

9.3.2.1 Construction of a Guidance Document System for Medical 3D Printing

With the continuous development of medical 3D printing technology and the clarification of the regulatory channels for personalized medical devices, the industry's demand for the transformation of related products is increasing. While intensive standardization work is being carried out, relevant guidance for device products is being gradually introduced. This guidance directly guides the R&D, production, quality control, registration, and technical reviews of 3D printing standard products and personalized products by regulatory agencies. Although the scope of application of some guidance clearly excludes custom-made products, the applicable sections can also be used as references for custom-made devices.

A guidance document system for medical 3D printing has been efficiently constructed and applied in the context of accelerated industrial and regulatory development. This system is an important carrier of regulatory science research achievements related to medical 3D printing. It focuses on advantageous areas in medical 3D printing research and clinical application research, exploring unique regulatory tools, standards, and approaches. Compared with laws and standards, guidance is more specific and flexible and can be used to comprehensively identify specific risks.

In the generation of a guidance document system for medical 3D printing, China has used innovative and exploratory approaches, including compilation methods, collaboration models, and evaluation thinking. In the process of formulating the guidance, the NMPA organized domestic advantageous units in the medical 3D printing field to carry out joint tackling. This model of collaboration, harnessing the respective strengths of industry, academia, research, medicine, inspection, and government, has accelerated progress in the field. Based on the concept of accurate risk control, the core of risk identification and control runs through the full life cycle of medical devices. It covers various stages, including design, R&D, production, testing, registration, and marketing for clinical application. The construction of this guidance document system has improved the evaluation process and enhanced the supervision of 3D-printed medical devices. This guidance promotes the transformation of scientific research achievements and the healthy and rapid development of the industry in this field. In addition, it better meets the safety, effectiveness, and accessibility requirements for the clinical use of 3D-printed medical devices.

9.3.2.2 Relevant Guidance for Medical 3D Printing

The guidance for medical 3D printing is more advanced than the guidance for conventional approaches, as reflected by several aspects. First, this type of guidance belongs to the category of new process application and is forward-looking. The release of some guidance occurs prior to the launch of products, which fills regulatory gaps. It also accelerates the transformation and application of advantageous achievements. Second, compared with the conventional registration guidance of registration applications and technical reviews, this type of guidance also focuses on key risks in design, R&D, production, and other stages, which effectively guides manufacturers to improve risk identification and control throughout the entire life cycle.

The first application of 3D printing technology in high-risk medical device products involved the use of bone, joints, and oral hard tissues. Therefore, the earliest guidance was the "Guidance for Technical Review of Registration of Medical Devices for Personalized Additive Manufacturing of Passive Implantable Bones, Joints, and Oral Hard Tissues," which was issued by the regulatory department in 2019. This guidance was formulated to better promote and standardize the innovative development of personalized, additive manufacturing medical devices, to guide applicants in the registration of personalized, additive manufacturing medical devices, and to provide guidance for the CMDE in reviewing registration application dossiers. This approach provides general guidance with comprehensive content coverage and has become the basis for the subsequent construction of a guidance document system for medical 3D printing. To more specifically guide the registration and technical review of some 3D-printed products that can be quickly transformed into clinical treatments and have significant application advantages, the regulatory department successively released guidance for multiple product categories in 2020. In addition, due to the special requirements of 3D printing technology for materials and the great influence of material quality on the performance of 3D-printed products, the regulatory department has issued corresponding guidance with a focus on materials. The relevant guidance used for medical 3D printing is shown in Table 9.5.

In the following section, the key contents of the general guidance will be the focus, and the main characteristics of the other guidance will be outlined.

Table 9.5 Classification of relevant guidance for medical 3D printing

Category	File name	Release time
General	Guidance for Technical Review of Registration of Medical Devices for Personalized Additive Manufacturing of Passive Implantable Bone, Joint, and Oral Hard Tissues	2019
	Guidance for the Study on the Uniformity of Physico-Chemical Properties of Metal Implants During Additive Manufacturing	2022
Product	Guidance for the Registration Technology Review of 3D Printed Artificial Vertebral Bodies	2020
	Guidance for the Technical Review of the Registration of 3D Printed Acetabular Cup Products	2020
	Guidance for the Registration Review of Additively Manufactured Intervertebral Fusion Cages	2020
	Guidance for the Registration Review of 3D Printed Patient-Matched Mandibular Prostheses	2020
Material	Guidance for the Registration Technical Review of Additively Manufactured Polyether Ether Ketone Implants	2022
	Guidance for the Registration Technology Review of Laser Selective Melting Metal Materials for Oral Restorations Using the Additive Manufacturing	2022

(a) General Guidance

The scope of application of the "Guidance for the Registration Technical Review of Medical Devices for Personalized Additive Manufacturing of Passive Implantable Bone, Joint and Oral Hard Tissues" focuses on the personalized, additive manufacturing medical devices that are subject to registration. As stated in the title, the applicable parts of the product are stated, and it is clarified that the product is completely or partially developed by the additive manufacturing process. This guidance emphasizes "Review Focuses" when using the guidelines for technical review. In addition to reviewing product safety and effectiveness, the ability and quality of personalized product design and complete additive manufacturing processing also need to be considered. This is a reflection of the particularity of personalized products and medical 3D-printed products compared to conventional medical devices. The key content of this guidance is the "essential points of technical review," which provides detailed guidance on the relevant contents of the registration application dossiers for the products that are within the scope of application. The following aspects of product research requirements can reflect some special characteristics compared to conventional products. For example, in terms of material characterization, due to the possibility of material changes caused by certain 3D printing processes, this guidance requires the characterization of the chemical composition, microstructure, mechanical properties, etc., of the material based on material properties and process flow before and after printing in order to indicate changes. Second, for porous structures, structural characterization needs to be performed to clarify the key characteristic parameters. Moreover, considering the complexity of the 3D printing process, validation of the cleaning of porous structures should be performed by the registration applicant. If an animal model is used for preclinical evaluation of product performance, the purpose of the test should involve proving that the porous structure can cause osseointegration with the surrounding bone. Third, in terms of mechanical properties, for the first time, this guidance proposed an equivalent model, which requires that products within the scope of application be subjected to mechanical tests using equivalent models. Subsequently, the regulatory department also issued guidance on relevant topics, as detailed in Sect. 9.2.3.3 of this chapter. Fourth, regarding the requirements for product expiration date, it is stipulated that the expiration date of personalized medical devices should also meet the clinical delivery deadline requirements. Fifth, for product manufacturing, the guidance proposes corresponding requirements for medicine–engineering interaction conditions and capability confirmation. The guidance for medicine–engineering interactions was released later, as detailed in the introduction in Sect. 9.2.3.2 of this chapter.

Another general guidance, "Guidance for the Study of the Homogeneity of the Physicochemical Properties of Metal Implants in Additive Manufacturing," focuses on patient-matched medical devices that are manufactured by powder bed melting technology, which is the most widely used technology for manufacturing metal implants in the hard tissue area and includes selective laser melting (SLM) and electron beam melting (EBM). Since the abovementioned process involves the interaction of multiple physical fields, the quality and stability of manufactured products are affected by numerous complicated factors. This guidance proposed the concept of homogeneity for the first time. The homogeneity of the physicochemical properties of metal implants in additive manufacturing refers to the homogeneity of the printing quality of metal implants that are manufactured through additive processes (including heat treatment and surface treatment). It mainly reflects the uniformity of the quality of implants that are produced at different positions in the forming chamber, in different forming directions, and under the same process parameters within the same batch or different batches, as well as the consistency between product quality and design expectations, hereafter referred to as the homogeneity of quality. The guidance states that the purpose of quality uniformity is to ensure that under the same additive manufacturing process parameters, the differences in quality between implant products and between the products and the expected design are within acceptable deviations. In product performance studies, the registration applicant needs to evaluate or compare the consistency of the products in terms of chemical composition, geometric structure, microstructure, and mechanical properties, including size, porous structure, internal quality (defects, metal powder residues, etc.), surface quality (surface defects, surface roughness), dynamic and static mechanical properties (shearing properties, compression properties, tension properties, bending properties, torsion properties), corrosion resistance, and metal ion release. In processing studies, the registration applicant needs to elaborate on the typical factors that may cause inhomogeneity in the quality of the software, equipment, raw powders, process, and postprocessing process used by additive manufacturing, including personnel. Specifically, the influencing factors, possible risks, quality control indicators, and the verified numerical fluctuation range and clinical acceptability should be clarified. The key innovations of the guidance include proposing "homogeneity of quality" and guiding the registration applicant to better identify risk and control product quality inhomogeneity in the R&D and quality control stages before application to facilitate the high-quality innovation and development of these types of products.

(b) Guidance for Other Categories

As introduced earlier, the product guidance that is issued by regulatory authorities is often at the forefront of the application of 3D printing technology in medical devices, the earliest product categories that are transformed, and the first areas to implement product and medical technology iteration. Some guidance has already been issued for the registration review of products that are manufactured by traditional subtractive processes. Compared with the previous requirements, guidance for 3D-printed products has more targeted requirements for the new risks that are introduced by the process, for example, the quality control requirements for raw powders, the clarification of design inputs and outputs for the smallest unit of porous structure, the study of physicochemical properties and the control of defects, which are closely related to the process, and the study of metal ion release.

As mentioned above, the use of raw materials in 3D-printed medical devices is important. The properties and quality of the raw materials are closely related to the performance and quality of the finished products. The properties of materials may change under printing conditions, and the hidden risks may be amplified in finished products. The adaptability of the process and raw materials is also very important. Differences in process parameters will affect the finished products and processing performance. The quality control of the raw materials and the matching of key parameters and processes together determine the performance and quality of the finished products. The "Guidance for the Registration Technical Review of Additive Manufacturing Polyether Ether Ketone (PEEK) Implants" is a representative achievement of regulatory science research. Its release occurred earlier than the marketing of relevant products, providing early guidance for the transformation and marketing of this type of product. 3D-printed PEEK implants are manufactured mainly using fused deposition modeling (FDM) of filamentous raw materials and selective laser sintering (SLS) of powder raw materials. In light of the effect of the processes on the material, the guidance requires a focus on the existence of leachable chemical substances and the acceptability of toxicity in biological characteristic research. Moreover, this guidance provides a reference appendix, which is the "Requirements for Risk Management Information of Additive Manufacturing PEEK Implant Products," for identifying design and development risks as well as production and manufacturing risks. Different manufacturing processes may affect the stability of the physical and chemical properties of the raw materials. Therefore, this guidance emphasizes the need to select PEEK raw materials that match the additive manufacturing process. In response to the risks in the forming process, the guidance points out the requirements related to the matching and stability of the process capability. The "Guidance for the Registration Technology Review of Laser Selective Melting Metal Materials for Oral Restorations Using Additive

Manufacturing" is the first guidance that only targets 3D printing materials. The requirements for metal powder performance research include chemical characterization, morphological characterization, and recycling and reuse verification. The guidance involves requirements for the study of printing equipment parameters and heat treatment processes because of the demand for matching powder and printing processes. In addition, to reflect the powder performance and process matching ability, the guidance also requires that the physicochemical properties and functionality of the printed parts should be studied.

9.3.3 Thoughts on the Transformation of the Medical 3D Printing Industry

9.3.3.1 Thoughts on the Transformation of the Medical 3D Printing Industry in China

Before 3D-printed medical devices, which are a class of innovative products, enter clinical application, the translation from basic research to clinical application is not easy, and the following challenges are encountered:

(a) High Threshold: From the conceptual product to the successful transformation and production of the final product for practical application, innovative devices require a large amount of funds and technical support, as well as strict regulatory approval procedures, before they can be marketed for sale. This makes the research and development of 3D-printed medical devices difficult. The threshold is very high.
(b) High Risk: There are great technical and market risks in the R&D process of 3D-printed medical devices. Once R&D fails or products fail postmarket, enormous economic and reputation losses occur.
(c) Uncertain Market Demand: The market demand for 3D-printed medical devices is often affected by various factors, such as policies, medical insurance, procurement decisions of medical institutions, and acceptance by doctors, which makes the market demand for medical devices uncertain. Moreover, many 3D-printed medical devices are "slow in clinical acceptance."
(d) High R&D Costs: The medical device industry covers multiple disciplines and is knowledge-intensive. 3D-printed medical devices are characterized by diversification and complexity. Inventing or improving a device based on new materials is a complex systems engineering process, and the R&D cost is relatively high. Once the capital chain breaks at a certain stage, the transformation of product R&D may fail.
(e) Imperfect Industrial Support Facilities: The transformation of 3D-printed medical devices is inseparable from complete industrial support facilities. Currently, the transformation of innovative devices faces the problem of immature industrial support facilities, and all stages related to "people, machines, materials, methods, and the environment" face many challenges.

(f) Conceptual Differences Between Basic Research and Industrial Transformation: Basic research focuses on innovation, more so at the stage of laboratory research, while industrial transformation focuses on product safety, effectiveness, and product stability. These efforts focus on different areas, which makes it difficult for some basic research results to be transformed into clinical applications.
(g) Imperfect Regulatory System: The methods for evaluating or testing conventional materials and processes are not necessarily suitable for 3D-printed medical devices, and the transformation path of innovative devices is unclear, which is also an important reason for the slow transformation speed.

9.3.3.2 Construction of a 3D-Printed Medical Device System in China

R&D is the basis of transformation, while transformation is the sublimation and social realization of R&D. Together, the two constitute translational science. At the beginning of the establishment of China's medical 3D printing regulatory system, the goal was to promote the innovation leadership of China's 3D printing regulatory system and achieve the innovative development of the medical 3D printing industry. Therefore, the product system is also an important part of China's medical 3D printing regulatory system; it directly reflects the development level of the industry and is closely related to the scale of industrial development. In the early stages of promoting the transformation of China's medical 3D printing industry, orthopedic and oral implant devices in the implant field and assistive devices in the nonimplant field were the first options for achieving innovative development, followed by other medical directions. At present, the number of 3D-printed medical devices being transformed into products in China is increasing each year, and these products, which can meet the specific clinical needs of patients, are entering the clinical application stage.

As the patterns of translational sciences continue to be revealed and regulatory models in advanced fields are constantly being introduced, China has preliminarily established a product transformation system, which is reflected mainly in the following two aspects. First, through the establishment of convenient paths for scientific transformation, generic products have been created. At present, several Chinese medical 3D printing technologies have entered the leading stage worldwide. Second, with the continuous improvements of the regulatory system, standard system, and guidance system, China has gradually established a convenient path for the scientific transformation of 3D-printed medical devices, the efficiency of industrial transformation has greatly increased, and the number of products that are available for registration is constantly increasing. According to incomplete statistics, as of November 2023, approximately 40 3D-printed orthopedic implants, including titanium alloys, pure tantalum, cobalt-chromium-molybdenum alloys, and polyether ether ketone, have been approved for registration in China. In addition, more than 100 3D-printed implants have been fabricated as custom-made devices, which has greatly promoted the clinical application of medical 3D printing technology.

At present, China has achieved the industrialization of nondegradable 3D-printed implants in the field of medical 3D printing. In the future, China will rely on joint research on key technologies to continue to promote the construction of a medical 3D printing technology supervision system, constantly enrich its connotation, and achieve the transformation of 3D printing technology to higher levels, such as degradable 3D-printed implants and 3D bioprinting. Through the continuous development of regulatory science research, the construction of new tools, new standards, and new methods will be strengthened to provide technical support for technology development and to build a pathway for the rapid transformation of scientific research achievements into clinical applications. China will take the high-quality development of custom-made medical devices as an opportunity to turn institutional advantage into efficient governance of the medical device industry, providing a typical demonstration of the modernization of industrial governance capability. Additionally, China will continue to create a new sharing and cogovernance supervision model that features government supervision, social collaboration, and the participation of the entire development chain to systematically and proactively increase the vitality of basic research, provide a driving force for the transformation of results, and provide technical support for leading innovation.

9.4 Conclusion

9.4.1 Comparison of the Supervision of Custom-Made Medical Devices

The common feature of the supervision of custom-made medical devices in the United States, Europe, and China is that supervision is conducted under each region's own regulatory framework. However, these regions all issued supplementary documents under their supervision, from the unified understanding of the definitions of relevant terms to the clarification of regulatory requirements then relevant guiding documents were provided. A comparison shows that there are some differences in the supervision of the three countries. In particular, the United States emphasizes stricter postmarket supervision on the premise of requiring custom-made medical devices to meet the requirements of quality system specifications and limits the production quantity of products rather than requiring premarket review and approval; in this regard, China's supervision is also similar to that of the United States. Compared with high-risk medical devices that require premarket registration and approval, custom-made medical devices use the record-filing method; however, to ensure safety and efficacy, regulators have proposed comprehensive restrictive requirements or qualification requirements for the relevant people or items in the full life cycle. The supervision of custom-made devices may be significantly different between Europe and the other two countries. This means that premarket registration approval is also required for these devices, but the approval process and postmarket supervision are relatively simple. It can be seen from the previous review that, similar to those in China, regulatory agencies also have many corresponding requirements according to the particularities of custom-made medical devices.

9.4.2 Comparison of Standards and Guidance Documents

In terms of standardization work, both the United States and Europe started early. Under their respective standard systems, the United States and Europe focus on risk management and full life cycle control, while Chinese standards have relatively basic requirements in these areas. For example, European standards emphasize process control, while Chinese standards place more emphasis on product output requirements. The consistency between the American and European standards and the international standards is greater than that between the Chinese standards and the international standards in some respects. This may more closely match the level of medical technology development and regulatory requirements in China. However, with rapid development in recent years, Chinese standards have given more attention to promoting innovation, and therefore, they are more abundant in product-specific standards. In the medical field of 3D printing, compared to the United States and the European Union, China has established a relatively systematic system of standards and guidance for medical 3D printing, which is exactly what China has done in the fields of regulatory science research and regulatory innovation, and in the development of medical devices in recent years. In China, this effort began later but progressed rapidly. At present, the coverage of China's relevant standards and guidance documents for medical 3D printing has exceeded that of the United States and Europe. Moreover, in the entire medical device field, China is also actively making up for its shortcomings, rapidly absorbing the results of advanced international standards and guidance documents, accelerating the improvement of the medical device standards system, increasing the frequency of standard revisions, and strengthening the issuance of guidance documents to better provide technical support for medical device innovation and development.

References

Fan Z, Xie N. Analysis of technical evaluation for current regulation of 3D printed customized medical devices. Chin J Med Instrum. 2018;42(4):279–281+285.

Gao J, Liu B, Han D, et al. Consideration on the construction of medical additive manufacturing supervision system in China. China Med Device Inform. 2023a;29(21):1–5+35.

Gao G, Zhang Q, Zhang S, et al. Construction of a good guidance practices system for medical devices to strengthen scientific foundation for registration technical evaluation. China Food Drug Adm Mag. 2023b;10:8–19.

Guo X, Liu B. Quality control main point on medicine-engineering interaction during design and development of customized bone implant and instrument. China Med Her. 2018;15(30):160–163+177.

Li Y. Exploration on the development of association standards. In: Proceedings of the 14th China standardization forum. Haikou; 2017;514–17.

Mao X, Han Q. Research on standard system for medical devices of additive manufacturing for medical applications. China Med Her. 2022;19(24):81–5.
Min Y, Zhang J, Liu B, et al. Discussion on technical review guidance for registration of personalized additive manufacturing medical devices of passive implantable bone, joint and oral hard tissues. Chin J Med Instrum. 2021;45(2):200–4.
National Medical Products Administration. Announcement on the issuance of medical device classification catalog (no. 104 of 2017). In: Announcement. National Medical Products Administration; 2017. Available via Baidu. https://www.nmpa.gov.cn/xxgk/ggtg/ylqxggtg/ylqxqtggtg/20170904150301406.html. Accessed 4 Sept 2017.
National Medical Products Administration. Announcement on the issuance of regulations on the supervision and administration of customized medical devices (trial) (no. 53 of 2019). In: Announcement. National Medical Products Administration; 2019. Available via Baidu. https://www.nmpa.gov.cn/directory/web/nmpa/xxgk/ggtg/ylqxggtg/ylqxqtggtg/20190704160701585.html. Accessed 4 July 2019.
National Medical Products Administration. The legal system of medical device supervision in China is becoming more and more perfect. China Pharmaceutical News. 2022.
State Administration for Market Regulation. Medical device standard management. State Administration for Market Regulation; 2017. Available via Baidu. https://www.samr.gov.cn/zw/zfxxgk/fdzdgknr/bgt/art/2023/art_5ab2835958bc467a90271688a0a24897.html. Accessed 17 Apr 2017.
The National People's Congress of the People's Republic of China. Standardization law of the People's Republic of China. The National People's Congress of the People's Republic of China; 2017. Available via Baidu. http://www.npc.gov.cn/npc/c2/c30834/201905/t20190521_278360.html. Accessed 4 Nov 2017.
Wang J. The construction and development of association standards. In: Proceedings of the 14th China standardization forum. Haikou; 2017;529–32.
Zheng X, Sun D. Consideration on the development of association standards under the new situation. In: Proceedings of the 12th China standardization forum. Hangzhou; 2015;86–89.

Part IV

Future Development of 3D-Printed Custom-Made Prostheses

3D-Printed Custom-Made Prostheses Using Nonmetallic Materials

10

Hao Wu, Qi Wu, ChangCheng Chen, and Zheng Guo

10.1 Initial Exploration of Custom-Made Prosthetics Fabricated via 3D Printing Using Nonmetallic Materials in the Clinical Management of Bone Tumors

Bone tumors, which originate in the skeletal system and its surrounding tissues, account for approximately 1% of all human tumors. Bone tumors predominantly occur in the distal femur, proximal tibia, and distal tibia, as well as other long bones of the lower extremities and the spine (Association TGoCO 2019). Primary malignant bone tumors typically present at a young age, are highly malignant, progress rapidly, and have a high mortality rate. Bone tumors are the third most common cause of cancer-related death in individuals under 20 years of age (Xu Hairong et al. 2016). Historically, patients who are diagnosed with bone tumors often face the prospect of amputation. However, with rapid advancements in imaging technology and neoadjuvant chemotherapy, a treatment strategy combining wide resection and limb-salvage reconstruction, with neoadjuvant chemotherapy as a key adjunct, has become the mainstream surgical approach for treating primary malignant bone tumors (Bosma et al. 2018). Nevertheless, the challenge of managing large, irregular bone defects after tumor resection remains a clinical difficulty. Improper management of bone defects can lead to delayed healing or nonunion, adversely affecting the functional recovery of the affected limb.

Methods for repairing bone defects can be categorized into biological reconstruction (Lenze and von Eisenhart-Rothe 2017) (including reimplantation of devitalized tumor segments and allograft bone transplantation) and mechanical reconstruction (Li Jing 2018; Yang Yi et al. 2018) (such as prosthetic joint reconstruction). Biological reconstruction may lead to complications such as fracture of

H. Wu · Q. Wu · C. Chen · Z. Guo (✉)
Department of Orthopedics, Tangdu Hospital, Xi'an, China
e-mail: guozheng@fmmu.edu.cn

Z. Guo et al. (eds.), *3D-Printed Prosthesis in Orthopedic Oncology*,
https://doi.org/10.1007/978-981-95-1454-0_10

the devitalized or transplanted bone, bone resorption, and a high rate of postoperative infection. Moreover, mechanical reconstruction can result in prosthetic loosening or fracture, unequal leg lengths, and poor function. In recent years, the application of 3D printing technology in orthopedics has rapidly advanced. Custom-made prosthetics that are fabricated via 3D printing can not only preserve adjacent joints and improve joint function but also reduce the risk of prosthetic dislocation, promote healing at the prosthetic–bone interface, and decrease the incidence of postoperative infections. Among the available materials, custom-made prosthetics that are fabricated via 3D printing with nonmetallic materials have an elastic modulus that is similar to that of natural bone, reducing the risk of stress shielding. Therefore, nonmetallic, 3D-printed custom prosthetics can overcome the shortcomings of both biological and mechanical reconstruction, offering a new optimized treatment option for repairing bone defects caused by bone tumor resection in non-load-bearing sites. However, due to the limited mechanical strength of nonmetallic materials, the use of high-strength metallic materials, such as titanium alloys, is often required for support in load-bearing areas. Currently, the nonmetallic materials that are used in custom-made prosthetics that are fabricated via 3D printing mainly include polymer materials such as Polyetheretherketone(PEEK), polymeric materials such as polycaprolactone, bioceramics such as calcium phosphate, and their composites such as polycaprolactone/β-tricalcium phosphate composites.

10.1.1 Preliminary Exploration of PEEK Material Prostheses in Clinical Application

PEEK, which has mechanical properties that closely resemble those of natural bone, can effectively prevent stress shielding and bone resorption. PEEK also exhibits good chemical inertness, does not easily cause rejection reactions in the body, and does not produce artifacts in CT and MRI scans, facilitating postoperative patient follow-up. Therefore, PEEK is considered an ideal bone implant material. Traditional injection-molded PEEK intervertebral fusion devices have been widely used in spinal surgery for intervertebral fusion. However, research on the repair of large-volume complex bone defects caused by tumors is still limited. Professor Li Dicheng's team at Xi'an Jiaotong University has conducted in-depth research and established design mechanisms and criteria for PEEK implants for use at different sites, including medical-engineering integration criteria, morphology restoration criteria, reliable fixation criteria, mechanical performance matching criteria, functional recovery criteria, and adaptability criteria. This team developed design methods and performance evaluation systems for personalized PEEK 3D-printed prostheses, developed a 3D-printed manufacturing process with shape/property control, and conducted clinical applications of personalized prostheses for patients in different clinical departments, effectively promoting the functional repair of bone defects (Li Dichen et al. 2018; Wang et al. 2019). Additionally, the team successfully treated a patient with a large chondrosarcoma in the anterior chest wall, with a tumor diameter reaching 25 cm (Fig. 10.1). Based on the patient's CT data, the team

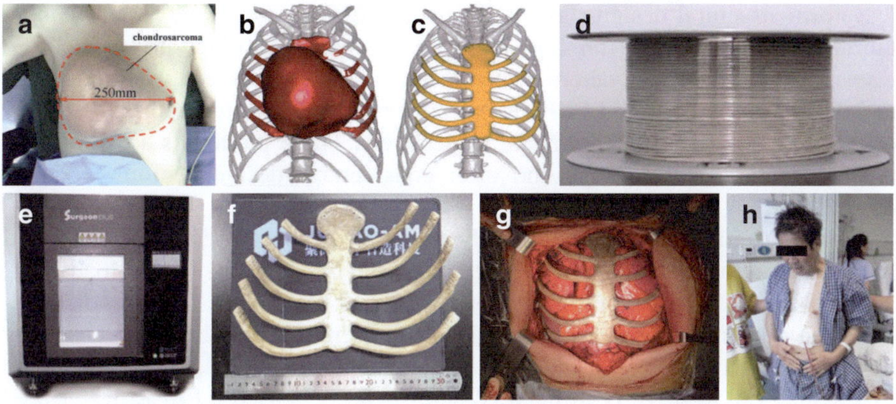

Fig. 10.1 (**a**) Gross view of the tumor. (**b**) Preoperative planning simulation of clinical osteotomy. (**c**) PEEK sternum prosthesis design. (**d**) Self-prepared PEEK filament. (**e**) Self-developed Surgeon 3D printer. (**f**) Physical sternum prosthesis. (**g**) PEEK prosthesis implantation. (**h**) Postoperative recovery effect of the patient (Li et al. 2018)

constructed a three-dimensional model around the tumor, determined a resection range of 5 cm beyond the tumor edge, and designed a personalized PEEK sternum prosthesis for chest wall reconstruction by using software to simulate the resection effect. Subsequently, the team used their self-developed Surgeon 3D printer to prepare the prosthesis and used mechanical performance testing to verify that the printed prosthesis met the requirements for the activities of daily life. During surgery, the anterior chest wall tumor was resected with a margin of more than 5 cm from the tumor edge, and the resected tumor weighed 3.04 kg, resulting in a chest wall defect measuring 32 cm × 30 cm. Then, a 3D-printed PEEK rib sternum prosthesis was implanted and fixed with titanium wires to the clavicle and the remnants of both sides of the ribs. On the second day after surgery, the patient was gradually weaned off mechanical ventilation. Two weeks postoperatively, the patient primarily breathed via abdominal breathing and was able to walk more than 300 m continuously.

To further optimize the mechanical properties of ribs to assist in the recovery of the thoracic breathing function of patients, researchers combined structural design optimization with 3D printing technology to develop a biomimetic prosthetic structure. Kang Jianfeng and others from Xi'an Jiaotong University (Kang et al. 2018) established a centroid trajectory method for designing 3D-printed PEEK rib prostheses. This method involves extracting the centroid trajectory of natural ribs to guide the design of rib prostheses, which are then fabricated using fused deposition modeling technology. Finite element analysis and mechanical testing revealed that the mechanical properties of the fabricated prostheses closely resemble those of natural ribs and surpass those of traditionally designed prostheses. Moreover, after implantation in the human body, not only was the shape of the thorax well restored, but its function was also significantly improved. Additionally, Zhang Chenguang and others simulated the mechanical properties of rib cartilage through waveform structural design (Fig. 10.2), using PEEK material and fused filament fabrication 3D printing technology to create a bionic rib cartilage structure. These researchers found that by altering the design parameters, the equivalent modulus and tensile strength of the PEEK rib cartilage could be adjusted within the ranges of 0.5–17.3 MPa and 0.7–8.3 MPa, respectively. These properties are similar to those of natural rib cartilage and offer considerable design flexibility (Zhang et al. 2020).

Beyond trunk tumors, PEEK prostheses have also been preliminarily applied in reconstruction following the resection of limb bone tumors in non-load-bearing areas, such as the distal radius, scapula, and fibula. The repair and reconstruction of non-load-bearing areas do not require the prosthesis to have very high compressive strength, allowing the advantage of the light weight of the PEEK material to be fully utilized. When researchers used a PEEK 3D-printed prosthesis to treat bone defects after the resection of a giant cell tumor of the distal radius, considering the weak bone integration capability of PEEK material, they utilized a porous titanium alloy transition between the prosthesis and the bone interface. During the design, arc-shaped holes were reserved near the wrist joint according to the attachment positions of the forearm muscles to restore the stability and flexibility of the wrist joint. The PEEK part of the prosthesis was printed using fused deposition modeling technology. The function of the patient's wrist joint was well preserved, and the bone ingrowth and integration of the prosthesis were significantly improved (Fig. 10.3) (Sun et al. 2022). During reconstruction after the resection of scapular tumors, PEEK prostheses also demonstrated good advantages, effectively avoiding the issue of metal prosthesis edges cutting soft tissue. The First Affiliated Hospital of Xinjiang Medical University obtained the data for the prosthesis on the affected side by scanning the scapula on the healthy side via thin-layer CT and three-dimensional reconstruction and then mirroring. The design included soft tissue

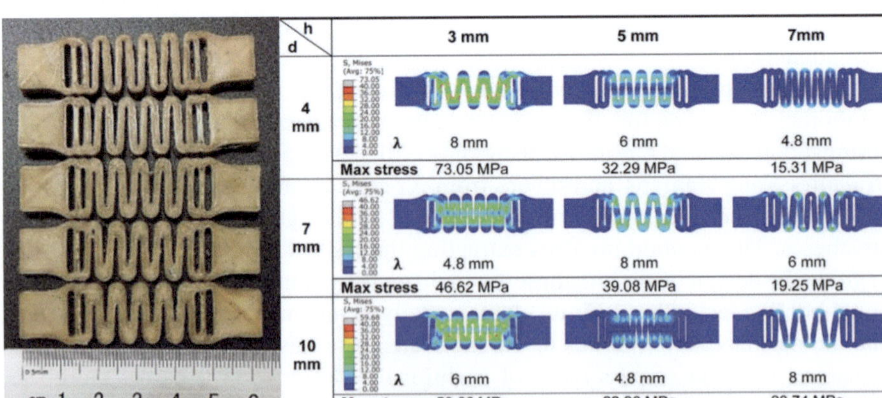

Fig. 10.2 3D-printed rib cartilage structures with different design parameters and finite element analysis (Zhang et al. 2020)

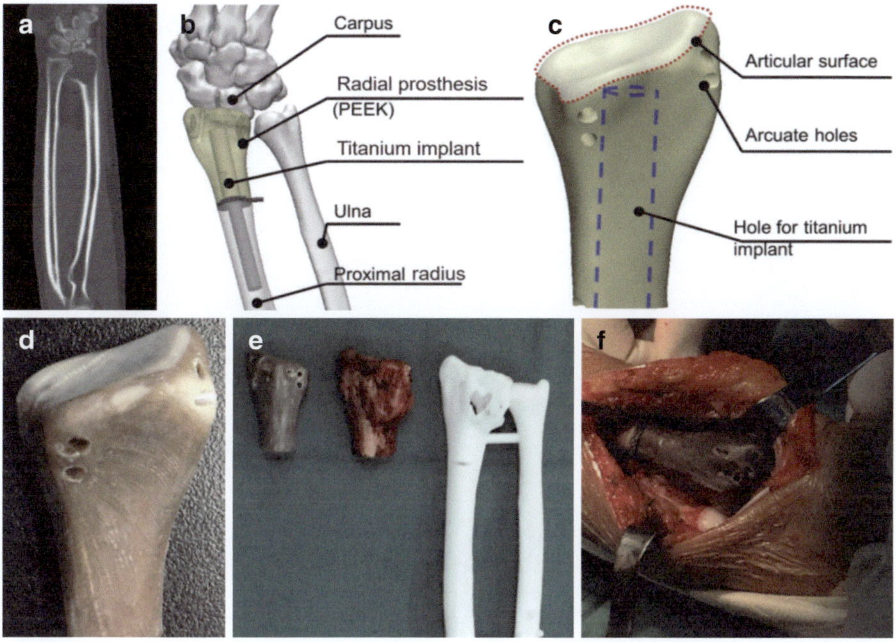

Fig. 10.3 (**a**) CT image. (**b**) Radius reconstruction surgery plan. (**c**) Design of the radius prosthesis. (**d**) Photo of the 3D-printed PEEK radius prosthesis. (**e**) Photo of the prosthesis, tumor, and medical model. (**f**) Intraoperative photo (Sun et al. 2022)

attachment channels according to the reconstruction and fixation scheme. The prosthesis data were imported into a 3D printing device to fabricate a customized PEEK prosthesis. After the scapular and surrounding soft tissue tumors were completely resected, a 3D-printed customized scapular prosthesis was implanted, and a precise fit was achieved. Three months postoperation, the shoulder joint could abduct up to 50°, and the patient was satisfied with the appearance and function. At the last follow-up, the shoulder joint's Constant score was 68 points, with no tumor recurrence or distant metastasis (Wei Xinghui et al. 2021).

Due to the significantly lower compressive strength of PEEK than that of metal materials such as titanium alloys, the application of custom PEEK prostheses in the treatment of load-bearing bone tumors in the lower limbs is less common, often requiring the assistance of metal materials for support. In the case of distal femur tumor resection and reconstruction, researchers designed a PEEK prosthesis based on a healthy femur and validated its safety through finite element analysis. Mechanical performance tests showed that the 3D-printed custom PEEK prosthesis could withstand a vertical load of 1900 N, meeting mechanical requirements. However, surgeons still implant auxiliary fixation steel plates on both sides of the prosthesis to avoid postoperative prosthesis failure (Fig. 10.4) (Sun et al. 2022).

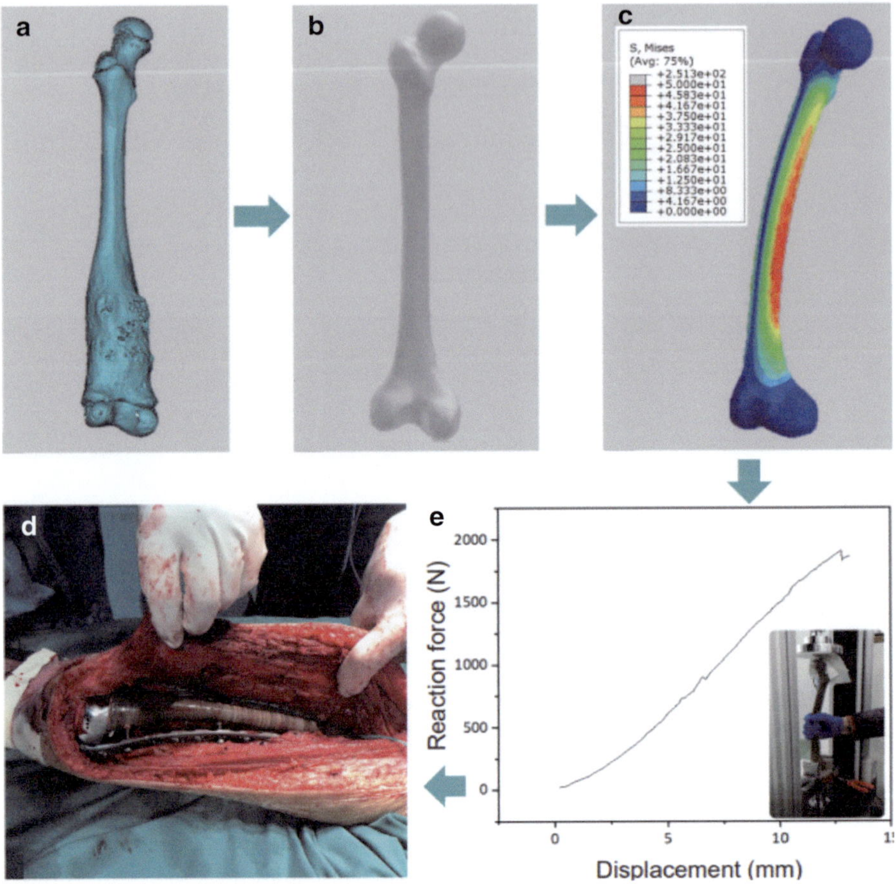

Fig. 10.4 3D-printed PEEK femoral segment prosthesis. (**a**) 3D model of the femoral tumor. (**b**) The healthy femur on the opposite side. (**c**) FEA results of the PEEK femoral prosthesis. (**d**) Force-displacement curve of the 3D-printed PEEK femoral prosthesis. (**e**) Intraoperative photo (Sun et al. 2022)

3D-printed PEEK prostheses are increasingly being applied in clinical settings due to their superior material properties and high degree of customization. However, the specific nature of the 3D printing process results in pronounced mechanical anisotropy in fabricated PEEK prostheses, presenting new challenges for the design of PEEK prostheses and for the evaluation of their stability. Additionally, the high bioinertness of PEEK material makes it difficult for surrounding bone tissue to effectively integrate and connect with the PEEK material, thereby affecting the long-term stability of prosthesis fixation. Surface modification, blending modification, coating modification, and porous structure creation can improve the bioinertness of PEEK materials and enhance the bonding strength between PEEK materials and surrounding bone tissue (Han et al. 2019; Wei et al. 2023). However, current methods for PEEK material modification are still in the research phase and need to be further developed before clinical application.

10.1.2 Preliminary Exploration of Printed Prostheses Fabricated with Bioceramic Materials for Clinical Applications

Bioceramic materials mainly include hydroxyapatite, bioactive glass, and β-tricalcium phosphate (β-TCP), among others. Their main components, calcium and phosphorus, are similar to the natural components of bone tissue. β-TCP, which is a degradable material, is a rich source of calcium and phosphorus for new bone formation; after degradation, it creates a solid–liquid equilibrium of calcium and phosphorus around the scaffold, and it provides sufficient mechanical strength for bone tissue. β-TCP has excellent biocompatibility, can effectively promote and induce bone tissue regeneration, and has significant advantages in terms of degradation rate, making it an ideal 3D printing material for bone tissue research. β-TCP overcomes the limitations of hydroxyapatite and titanium alloy scaffolds, which are difficult to degrade in the body and hinder new bone growth. Currently, the aim of biological tissue development is to replace existing metal prostheses with biomimetic natural bone and cartilage/bone tissue to achieve treatment. The major challenge is how to meet the requirements of structural strength and regenerative function for large tissue segments.

In clinical applications, Professor Pei Guoxian's team from the Air Force Medical University successfully treated a patient with a 12-cm-long tibial bone defect by coculturing the patient's own cells with porous bioceramic materials to form a functional bone composite. They first extracted the patient's bone marrow and isolated and expanded it in vitro in the laboratory to obtain a sufficient number of autologous bone marrow mesenchymal stem cells. Then, based on the patient's bone defect CT data, they prepared a personalized prosthesis using β-TCP and combined the obtained autologous cells with the personalized β-TCP prosthesis. Finally, through open surgery, the personalized bioceramic prosthesis was precisely implanted into the patient's bone defect site. The patient began to walk without crutches 6 months after surgery, the external fixation frame was removed after 12 months, and the patient could walk quickly, climb stairs, and move heavy objects after 22 months. Auxiliary examinations revealed that the bone defect was completely repaired (Gao Yi et al. 2021). Additionally, Lu Jianxi from Shanghai Jiao Tong University and Professor Wang Zhen from the Air Force Medical University used β-TCP in combination with metal materials for bone repair. The results showed that pure porous ceramics could be used to repair bone defects in non-load-bearing areas, and for load-bearing areas such as the spine and lower limbs, other fixed support structures could be combined for repair (Lu Yajie et al. 2019).

By addressing the issues of high brittleness and insufficient mechanical support in single ceramic-based, 3D-printed custom prostheses, many researchers have improved bone repair outcomes by fabricating these prostheses from a composite of polymers and bioactive ceramic-based materials. Seongjae Choi and others designed and fabricated a prosthesis made of polycaprolactone/β-tricalcium phosphate (PCL/β-TCP) composite material for use in the limb-sparing surgical treatment of distal radial osteosarcoma in dogs. Eight weeks postsurgery, local recurrence and lung metastasis occurred in the treated dogs, but there was no displacement or fracture of the prosthesis, and no prosthesis or surgery-related complications were observed (Choi et al. 2019).

Bioceramics possess excellent biocompatibility and osteoinductive properties, facilitating cell proliferation and bone regeneration. In terms of their mechanical properties, these materials also exhibit superior bone conductivity and outstanding wear resistance. However, due to the brittleness of bioceramic materials, it is challenging to use these materials alone to repair load-bearing bone defects. Through the use of composites with polymer materials, the development of bioprinting technologies, and the topological optimization of microstructures (Roohani-Esfahani et al. 2016), the mechanical properties of bioceramic prostheses have been effectively improved. By combining cell-loaded hydrogels and bioactive factors, bioceramics are playing an increasingly important role in bone tissue engineering (Zhu et al. 2017).

10.2 Future Directions for Nonmetal Material Development: New Materials and Technologies

10.2.1 Progress in Nonmetal Material Development

Nonmetal materials are defined as all materials other than metals, mainly including organic polymers and inorganic nonmetal materials.

10.2.1.1 Organic Polymer Materials

Organic polymer materials, which are represented by natural and synthetic polymers, are diverse and exhibit better biological properties than metal materials. Currently developed medical polymer materials possess many excellent physicochemical properties, such as heat resistance, wear resistance, and corrosion resistance. Additionally, the good plasticity and processability of polymer materials allow high precision during the 3D printing process. Natural polymer materials, such as collagen, chitosan, and alginate, have strong biological activity. 3D-printed prostheses that are made from these materials can promote bone tissue repair and regeneration to some extent. However, since most of these materials are derived from biological sources, there is a certain biological risk after implantation. Artificially synthesized polymer materials are divided into inert polymers and degradable polymers. Inert polymers include polyurethanes, polymethyl methacrylate, polyolefins, polycarbonates, and polystyrene. Degradable polymers include polycaprolactone, polylactic acid, polyvinyl alcohol, and polyamino acids. For orthopedic 3D-printed custom prostheses, degradable polymer materials can gradually be replaced by bone tissue in the body, avoiding the risk of secondary surgery and the long-term presence of the prosthesis. This is an important direction for the future development of nonmetal 3D-printed materials.

As mentioned earlier, polyether ether ketone (PEEK) has been widely used in the field of orthopedics. However, the bioinert nature of PEEK tends to result in poor osseointegration at the interface, limiting its efficacy as a material for 3D-printed custom prostheses for use in bone repair. Consequently, significant international research has focused on enhancing the osseointegration capabilities of PEEK through surface modification, coating modification, or mixing with active materials, aiming to expand its application potential as an orthopedic implant. Feng X and others addressed the issue of soft tissue fibrous capsule formation after the implantation of smooth-surfaced PEEK prostheses by creating PEEK prostheses with cross-linked structures of different pore sizes and acid-etched microporous surfaces (Fig. 10.5). In vitro experiments showed that cell adhesion was greater in the group with acid-etched micropores than in the group without these pores. In vivo experiments demonstrated that prostheses with cross-linked structures and acid-etched micropores exhibited tight integration with the tissue. The results confirmed that PEEK prostheses with optimized structures are more beneficial than traditional smooth PEEK prostheses for preventing the formation of soft tissue fibrous capsules after implantation (Feng et al. 2019).

Natural polymer materials have the advantages of good biocompatibility and biodegradability. Natural polymers, such as collagen, alginate, and gelatin, are applied in the fields of tissue engineering and regenerative medicine. However, the mechanical properties of single natural polymers are insufficient, so they are mainly used to prepare hydrogel materials or 3D printing bioinks, showing great potential for future applications in non-load-bearing prosthetic repairs. Zixun Wang and others utilized a novel biomaterial, namely, water-soluble recombinant human collagen

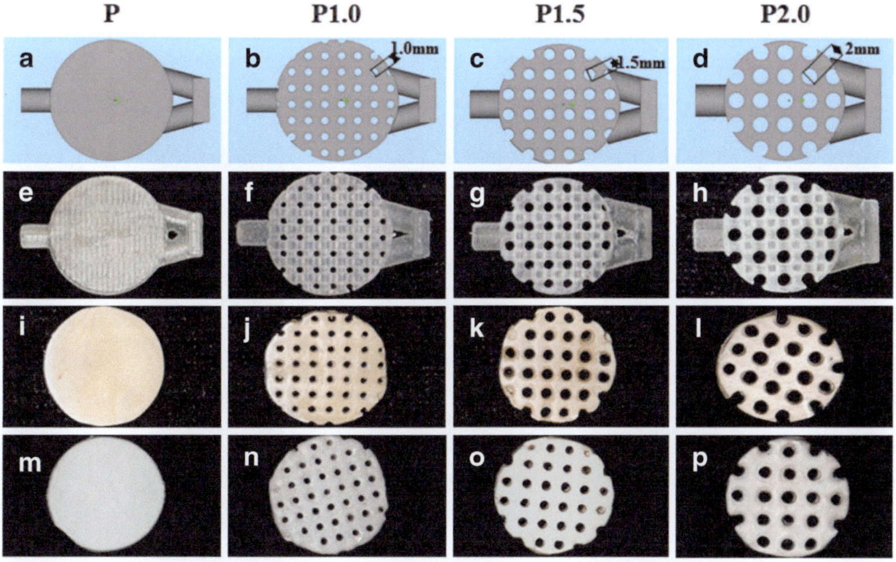

Fig. 10.5 Schematic and photos of PEEK prostheses. Computer-designed images of prostheses with cross-linked structures of different sizes: (**a**) P, (**b**) P1.0, (**c**) P1.5, and (**d**) P2.0. Resin molds of different sizes: (**e**) P, (**f**) P1.0, (**g**) P1.5, and (**h**) P2.0. PEEK samples of different sizes: (**i**) P, (**j**) P1.0, (**k**) P1.5, and (**l**) P2.0. Acid-etched PEEK prostheses of different sizes: (**m**) P, (**n**) P1.0, (**o**) P1.5, and (**p**) P2.0 (Feng et al. 2019)

(RHC), and prepared 3D-printed bioinks through modification with methacrylic anhydride (MAA) and crosslinking with 1-ethyl-3-(3-dimethylaminopropyl) carbodiimide hydrochloride/N-hydroxysuccinimide (EDC/NHS). The experimental results demonstrated that the scaffolds that were prepared with this bioink through UV curing (Fig. 10.6) had good biocompatibility. The scaffolds not only provided a microenvironment for cell diffusion, proliferation, and migration but also promoted the expression of angiogenesis-related proteins (Wang et al. 2022b).

Polycaprolactone (PCL), which belongs to the same category of synthetically produced polymers, is a type of linear aliphatic polyester degradable polymer. The chemical properties of PCL are stable; it degrades slowly, and its degradation products are minimally irritating. It has been approved for clinical use since the 1980s. Compared to PEEK, PCL has better processability and lower manufacturing costs. However, the mechanical properties of PCL are relatively poor, with both strength and hardness lower than those of PEEK materials. Moreover, compared to that of PEEK, the chemical corrosion resistance of PCL is also inferior, and it is susceptible to erosion by acids, bases, salts, and other chemicals. In recent years, as the properties of PCL materials have improved, lipophilic drugs can be uniformly encapsulated within PCL materials, while hydrophilic drugs tend to be distributed on the PCL surface through interfacial adsorption. Therefore, PCL materials have gradually been applied as drug delivery carriers in the preparation of 3D-printed nonmetal prostheses. López-González and others designed and prepared PCL-chitosan hydrogel composite scaffolds loaded with different concentrations of vancomycin to address the issue of bone infection. In vitro experimental results showed

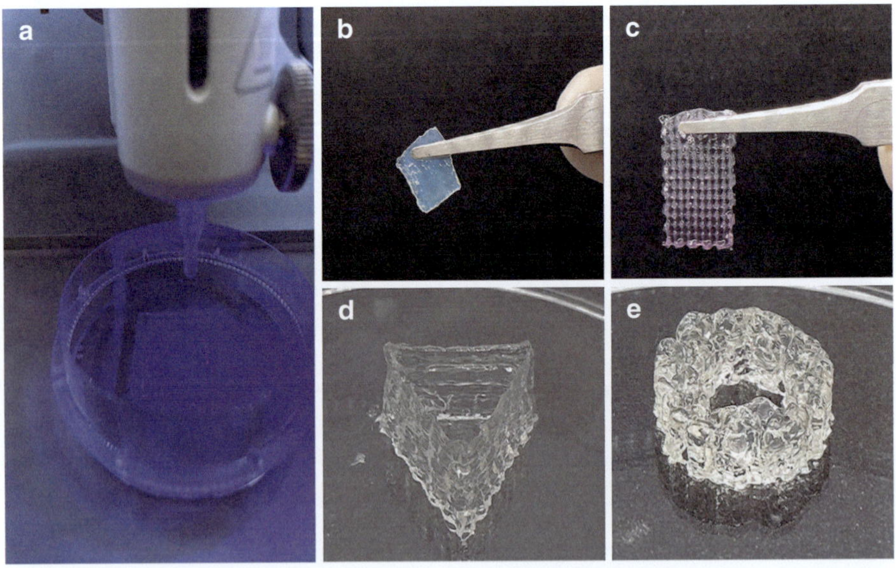

Fig. 10.6 Various complex structures printed in 3D: (**a**) UV-cured 3D-printed bio-ink. (**b**) Slices printed with bio-ink. (**c**) Grid structure printed with bio-ink. (**d**) Equilateral triangles printed with bio-ink. (**e**) Porous cylindrical structures printed with bio-ink (Wang et al. 2022b)

that these composite scaffolds possess good biocompatibility, good biodegradability, and reliable antibacterial effects (López-González et al. 2023).

10.2.1.2 Inorganic Nonmetallic Materials

Inorganic nonmetallic materials include inert ceramics (such as alumina and carbon-based materials) and bioactive ceramics, among which bioactive ceramics are widely used in the field of bone repair. Bioactive ceramics are similar to natural bone and have good biocompatibility, good biodegradability, and strong mechanical properties. Commonly used bioactive ceramics include hydroxyapatite (HA), β-tricalcium phosphate (β-TCP), and bioactive glass. However, bioceramics are highly brittle and have poor toughness and low shear stress, and their mechanical strength significantly decreases during the degradation process. Therefore, bioactive ceramics are often mixed with polymer materials to prepare degradable bone repair scaffolds.

Hydroxyapatite (HA) is currently a widely used inorganic nonmetallic material with good osteogenic activity. However, its disadvantage of being nonbiodegradable limits its clinical application in bone defect repair. Therefore, researchers have mixed degradable polymer materials with hydroxyapatite to prepare 3D-printed nonmetal prostheses to improve their biodegradability. Fengze Wang and others prepared 3D-printed composite scaffolds with PCL as the framework and doped them with different ratios of HA. Compared to the pure PCL scaffold, the addition of HA increased the surface roughness and hydrophilicity, and an increase in the HA content improved the compressive strength and elastic modulus of the scaffolds (Wang et al. 2022a).

A significant feature of bioactive glass (BG) is that when it comes into contact with bodily fluids, a hydroxyapatite-like layer can form on its surface. This layer has a mineral composition similar to that of natural bone, which is beneficial for the integration of bioactive glass with surrounding tissues. However, due to their high brittleness and rapid degradation, the use of bioactive glass scaffolds is limited to the fixation of non-load-bearing bones. Improving the mechanical properties and osteogenic ability of BG scaffolds has become a focus of researchers, with the main direction of improvement being the synthesis of mixed scaffold materials from BG and other materials. Adam C. Marsh and others used fused deposition modeling technology to prepare a novel type of 3D-printed silicate silver-doped bioactive glass (Ag-BG) scaffold (Fig. 10.7). In vitro experimental results indicated that the scaffold has good biocompatibility and antibacterial effects (Marsh et al. 2021). Currently, most research on BG is based on preclinical studies. Only a few clinical studies have reported its application in maxillofacial surgery and spinal fusion surgery. Overall, the clinical application of 3D-printed BG scaffolds in bone defects remains limited.

In addition to organic polymer materials and bioactive ceramics, carbon-based materials have also received widespread attention in the field of materials research in recent years due to their excellent electrical conductivity and thermal conductivity. Carbon-based materials can be classified into zero-dimensional, one-dimensional, two-dimensional, and three-dimensional materials. Zero-dimensional

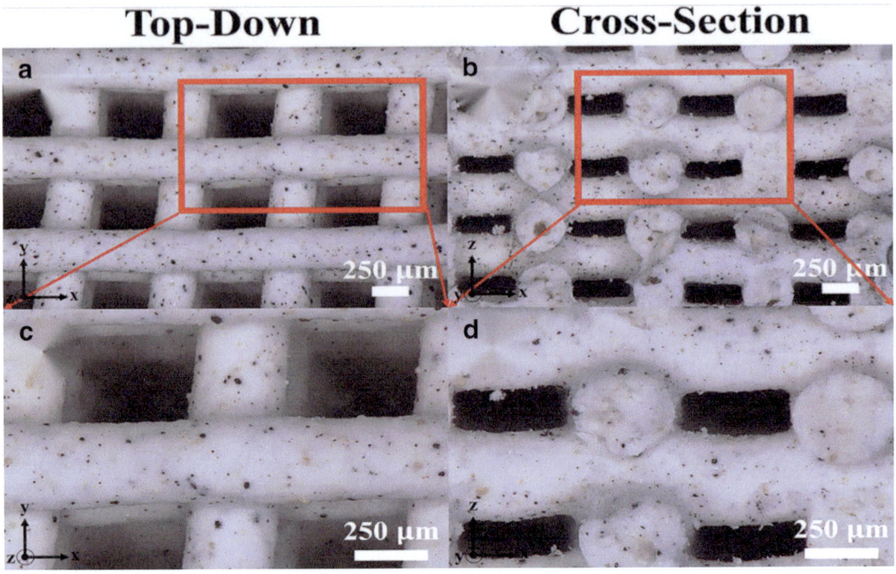

Fig. 10.7 3D-printed Ag-BG scaffold (left image shows the top view, right image shows the cross-sectional view) (Marsh et al. 2021)

materials include carbon quantum dots and fullerenes; one-dimensional materials include carbon nanotubes and nanowires; two-dimensional materials are primarily graphene; and three-dimensional materials, also known as bulk materials, usually refer to structures with a polyatomic three-dimensional structure, including diamond, graphite, and carbon silicon carbide. Currently, carbon-based materials such as graphene, carbon nanotubes, and carbon fibers are often combined with 3D printing technology for application in the field of bone repair.

Graphene (GE/GP) is a honeycomb-shaped 2D material formed by sp2 hybridized carbon atoms and is also known as a single layer of graphite. Because the atomic bonds exist laterally within the 2D structure, once multiple layers of graphene are stacked to form a 3D structure, it results in graphite with relatively poor performance. Therefore, graphene/polymer-based composite materials are often used for 3D printing. Jianfeng Li and others prepared an Alg/Gel hydrogel system doped with graphene oxide (GO) (Fig. 10.8) and cocultured it with adipose-derived stem cells. The cell activity in the Alg/Gel/GO group was greater than that in the Alg/Gel hydrogel group. These results indicate that GO can improve the biocompatibility of Alg/Gel hydrogels (Li et al. 2022).

Similarly, the high production cost and insufficient physicochemical stability of carbon nanotube (CNT) materials have led to their use in the 3D printing field, primarily for the preparation of composite materials rather than pure carbon nanotube materials. Hatice Kaya and others prepared scaffolds of poly(lactic-co-glycolic acid) (PLGA), PLGA/HA, and PLGA/HA/CNT doped with different proportions of multiwalled carbon nanotubes (CNTs) (Fig. 10.9). The introduction of CNTs

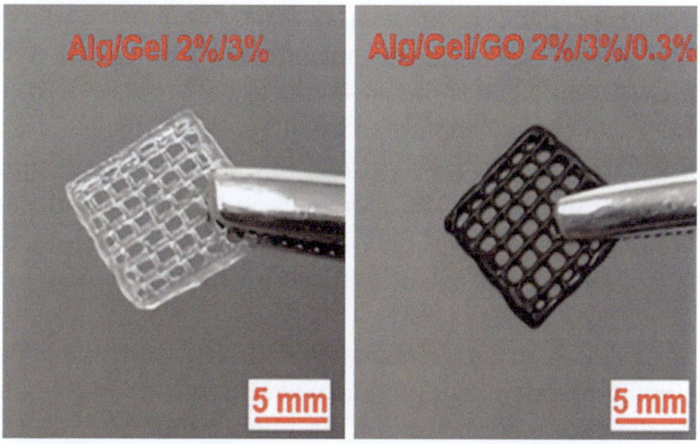

Fig. 10.8 Photos of structures obtained from 3D printing Alg/Gel (2%/3% w/w) and Alg/Gel/GO (2%/3%/0.3% w/w) (Li et al. 2022)

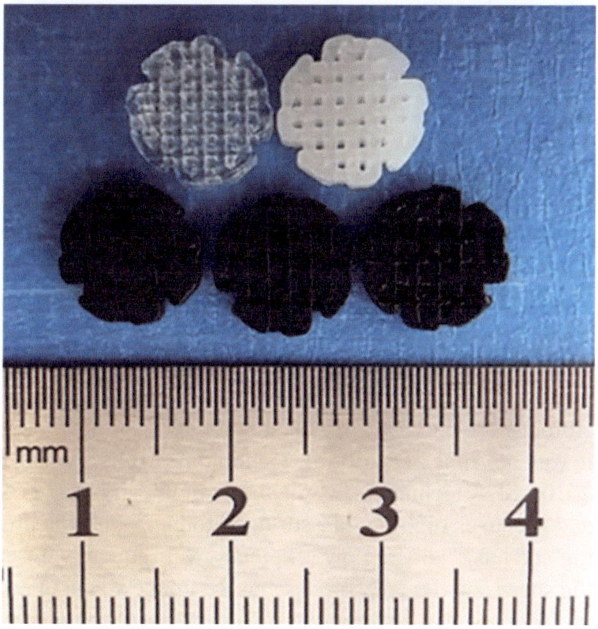

Fig. 10.9 Photo images of porous 3D-printed samples (Kaya et al. 2023)

improved the hydrophilicity and microstructural stability of the scaffolds and significantly enhanced their biocompatibility and osteogenic differentiation ability (Kaya et al. 2023).

10.2.2 Innovations in 3D Printing with Nonmetal Materials

As bone tissue engineering and regenerative medicine drive the continuous development of nonmetal 3D printing materials, significant progress has been made in the corresponding printing processes and precision. On the one hand, some 3D printing technologies based on powder sintering, previously only applicable to metal materials, have been adapted for nonmetal materials through improvements. Techniques such as laser-induced forward transfer (LIFT), selective laser melting (SLM), and electron beam melting (EBM) were initially used only for metals, but LIFT can now be applied to hydrogel-carrying cells (Kim et al. 2016), and SLM and EBM can be used for high-melting-point nonmetal materials, such as bioceramics. On the other hand, the precision and efficiency of commonly used nonmetal 3D printing technologies, such as photopolymerization, extrusion-based printing, and powder melting or sintering-based printing techniques, are continuously improving.

10.2.2.1 Nonmetal Material Photopolymerization Technology

Upon irradiation with specific wavelengths of light, liquid photosensitive resins solidify via photopolymerization, and the method of layer-by-layer manufacturing that is based on this phenomenon is known as photopolymerization technology. The principle of photopolymerization technology was first proposed by Hideo Kodama in 1981 and involves guiding light of a specific wavelength into a vat of photopolymer resin and then solidifying the resin locally layer by layer to achieve printing. Although photopolymerization technology offers fast printing speed, high precision, and smooth surfaces of printed objects, early products were often brittle, prone to deformation, had poor weather resistance, and lacked biocompatibility, making them more suitable for temporary replacement materials. After the discovery of many biologically compatible materials with good photopolymerization capability, such as poly (propylene fumarate) (PPF)-based materials, gelatin-based materials, and trimethylene carbonate (TMC)-based materials, photopolymerization technology has been widely used in bone tissue engineering research due to its ability to be used in coprinting biomaterials with cells, proteins, and growth factors. Stereolithography (SLA), which was the first photopolymerization 3D printing technology to be applied, was invented by Chuck Hull in 1986 and used in 1994 to produce a surgical model for allograft surgery; thus, it was the first 3D printing technology to be applied in medicine (Melchels et al. 2010). SLA technology is mature, simple, and stable; offers high printing precision; and produces high-quality surface products, but it is limited to single-material molding and has relatively low efficiency. Subsequently, researchers achieved faster printing speeds by digitally processing the image signal of each layer of the workpiece and projecting it directly onto the surface of the photosensitive resin using a digital micromirror device (DMD); this approach is known as digital light processing (DLP). Continuous DLP (CDLP) technology further improves printing efficiency by allowing continuous upward movement of the printing platform along the Z-axis (Pagac et al. 2021). However, these technologies can only achieve single-material molding, limiting design flexibility. Material jetting (MJ) technology allows the selective injection of photosensitive materials with different properties and mechanical characteristics into independent print heads according to the sectional data of each layer of the workpiece, with ultraviolet lamps immediately solidifying the ejected droplets, enabling the simultaneous printing of multiple materials (Gülcan et al. 2021).

To meet the increasing demands of scientific research and clinical applications, the precision and efficiency of printing technology continue to evolve. For instance, by reducing the thickness of printing layers, decreasing the size of pixels, and developing algorithms to improve the accuracy of contrast and light dose distribution, the printing precision of currently available stereolithography (SLA) and digital light processing (DLP) photolithography technologies has been rapidly increased. Furthermore, new photocuring molding technologies that are capable of higher resolution and handling more complex structures are continuously emerging. Multiphoton lithography (MPL), which is a high-resolution 3D printing technology that is based on femtosecond lasers, can achieve the best printing precision to date (<1 μm) (Do et al. 2015). This technology enables crosslinking or other structural modifications within cell-containing transparent materials and is expected to play a significant role in organ-on-a-chip devices and highly complex implantable microscaffolds in the future (Do et al. 2015). Volumetric printing (VP), which is another photocuring molding-based 3D printing technology, can rapidly print large-volume structures (tens of cubic centimeters) at an unprecedented speed while ensuring good resolution (40 μm). VP can produce complete large-scale living tissue structures in a matter of seconds, significantly surpassing traditional bioprinting technologies and greatly enhancing printing efficiency (Zandrini et al. 2023).

10.2.2.2 Extrusion-Based Nonmetal Material Printing

Extrusion-based technologies include fused deposition modeling (FDM) and Direct Ink Writing (DIW). FDM is the most typical extrusion-based printing technology, which operates by extruding thermoplastic or composite filaments through a heated nozzle. Due to its simple structure, low usage, and maintenance costs, FDM has become one of the most widely used 3D printing technologies. This method has been applied to various biodegradable materials, such as polycaprolactone (PCL) (Krobot et al. 2023), poly(lactic-co-glycolic acid) (PLGA) (Wubneh et al. 2018), and the composite material PCL/tricalcium phosphate (TCP) (Wang et al. 2021), and the printed products have shown good mechanical properties and biocompatibility. DIW, which is also known as bioplotter, pressure-assisted microsyringe, or pressure-assisted printing, was first patented by Cesarano and Calvert from Sandia National Laboratories in 1997 and became used for printing complex ceramic structures (Yen et al. 2009). DIW differs from other technologies in that it is not limited by materials, requiring only that the precursor ink have the appropriate rheological properties, such as apparent viscosity, yield stress under shear and compression, and viscoelastic properties. Thus, this technology essentially allows any ink to be effectively printed into 3D structures with high-resolution patterning, architectural freedom, and unique material properties. Currently, DIW has become the most common technology for bioprinting cell suspensions, cell-laden hydrogels, and solutions based on the extracellular matrix.

In recent years, several derivative technologies based on extrusion printing have emerged, greatly expanding the application of this technology. These technologies include embedding bioprinting (Lee et al. 2019), microfluidic bioprinting (Colosi et al. 2016), and electrowriting (Reizabal et al. 2023). Embedding bioprinting increases the structural complexity of bioprinted tissue constructs by extruding low-viscosity bioinks into a support bath, thus directly producing 3D volumetric structures and effectively resolving the contradiction between the printability and biocompatibility of materials in traditional extrusion-based bioprinting. Microfluidic bioprinting involves integrating microfluidic systems into extrusion-based bioprinters to facilitate the real-time adjustment of printed cell concentrations, thereby enabling the rapid printing of multicomponent/multicell tissue constructs and providing a reliable approach for future high-cell-density tissue and organ-like printing. Electrowriting achieves micrometer-level printing by applying an electric field between the nozzle and the collector plate, forming (sub)micron-level polymer jets at the tip of the extrusion nozzle to accurately place fibers at predetermined positions in 3D space. Compared to traditional FDM technology, electrowriting not only offers greater printing precision but also can be used for printing highly porous (80%–98% porosity), complex, and biomimetic systems, such as anisotropic networks to simulate cartilage collagen.

In summary, each printing technology has its own advantages and limitations, and each plays an important role in bone tissue engineering. It is crucial to select the appropriate printing technology to achieve effective biomanufacturing. To cater to a broader range of application scenarios, the resolution, speed, and printable volume of existing printing technologies are continuously evolving, significantly advancing the research and clinical applications of bone tissue engineering. Moreover, the concept of environmental protection is gradually being integrated into 3D printing technology. The currently available 3D printing processes often require heating, whereas low-temperature deposition manufacturing (LDM) can fabricate products layer by layer on a cold platform or in a freezer, followed by the removal of solvents through freeze-drying. Although the mechanical properties of scaffolds that are manufactured by LDM are slightly weaker than those of traditional scaffolds at this stage, LDM does not require heating during manufacturing, making it a green and environmentally friendly printing technology (Sun et al. 2023).

10.3 3D-Printed Custom Prosthetics Made with Nonmetal Materials and Regenerative Medicine

As the demand for personalized medicine continues to grow, 3D printing with nonmetal materials is expected to play a significant role. For example, using 3D printing technology, personalized medication doses, medical devices, and biologic implants can be manufactured based on the specific needs and physical conditions of patients. Furthermore, nonmetal scaffolds that are prepared via 3D printing technology can serve as carriers for tissue engineering and biologic 3D printing, offering possibilities for the active repair and replacement of bone tissue in the future. This advance involves transitioning nonmetal, 3D-printed prosthetics from biomimetic replacements to a new phase of regenerative repair.

10.3.1 3D-Printed Custom Prosthetics Made with Nonmetal Materials and Tissue Engineering

3D printing technology development is closely related to tissue engineering progress. Tissue engineering involves depositing high concentrations of autologous cells onto a biologic scaffold to form a cell-material composite, which is then implanted into the body. The in vivo environment induces the formation of the corresponding tissue or organ, thus achieving wound repair and functional reconstruction.

In tissue engineering, 3D printing technology is widely used to manufacture artificial bones, cartilage, muscles, blood vessels, organs, and other tissues. In bone tissue engineering, the selection of seed cells and the construction of biologic scaffolds are of paramount importance. Ideal scaffold materials should not only be biocompatible and biodegradable but also promote cell adhesion, proliferation, and differentiation. The advancement of 3D printing technology allows for the customization of the macroscopic shapes of bone tissue engineering scaffolds and the precise printing of biomimetic porous microstructures, thereby facilitating the adhesion and growth of seed cells. As mentioned in the previous section, Professor Pei Guoxian from the Orthopedics Department of Xijing Hospital demonstrated the feasibility of using 3D printing technology for tissue-engineered bone processing and preparation. This was shown by the excellent therapeutic effects that were observed in the treatment of ultralong segment bone defects using β-TCP ceramic material combined with autologously enriched mesenchymal stem cells, fully proving the viability of 3D printing technology in the fabrication of bone for tissue engineering.

Although 3D printing technology can provide a good spatial structure for seed cells, the osteogenic differentiation of mesenchymal stem cells is not yet mature and may face various problems, such as fibrosis, vascularization, cavitation phenomena, and shrinkage (Xue et al. 2013). Therefore, it is still necessary to continuously search for new seed cells in the future. With the continuous development of artificial intelligence, big data, and other technologies, 3D printing technology may also be combined with these technologies to achieve more intelligent and personalized tissue engineering manufacturing methods. In summary, the application of 3D printing technology in tissue engineering is expected to result in significant changes and progress in the field of medicine.

10.3.2 3D-Printed Custom Prosthetics Made with Nonmetal Materials and Bioprinting

3D bioprinting is a new interdisciplinary and cross-field regenerative medicine engineering technology that utilizes the principles of 3D additive manufacturing. 3D bioprinting uses biomaterials, growth factors, cells, and other active materials as "inks" to reconstruct human tissues and organs.

3D bioprinting requires a series of bioprinting technologies and bioinks. Currently, more mature bioprinting technologies include inkjet-based bioprinting, extrusion-based bioprinting, laser-assisted bioprinting, stereolithography-based bioprinting, and in situ bioprinting. Bioinks that have been widely studied and commonly applied include agarose-based bioinks, alginate-based bioinks, collagen-based bioinks, and hyaluronic acid-based bioinks.

3D bioprinting technology has unique and significant advantages, including high precision, personalized manufacturing, and complex shape construction. 3D bioprinting can produce standard models for surgical simulation, disease diagnosis, and drug testing, as well as tailor-made complex surgical scaffolds for patients. This technology has important research significance and application prospects in the biomedical field. For example, in bone defect repair, 3D bioprinting technology integrates technologies from various related fields, such as mechanics, materials, and cells. 3D bioprinting uses medical imaging technologies, such as CT scans or MRI, to scan the bone defect area of a patient to determine the required scaffold model. Then, a 3D printer is used to print the model, thereby obtaining a precisely matched personalized custom prosthesis. Byambaa and others used extrusion-based direct-write bioprinting technology to mix various GelMA hydrogel bioinks in an attempt to fabricate bone-like tissue with microstructures, including perfusable vascular lumens, thus creating more favorable conditions for bone defect repair (Byambaa et al. 2017).

10.4 Nonmetallic Materials and 4D Printing

4D printing is a novel printing technology that uses smart materials to print structures that are capable of responding to internal or external environmental stimuli, thereby achieving changes in structure and function. Because it endows static printed structures with the ability to change over time, 4D printing has attracted widespread interest among researchers in the biomedical field. Initially, 4D printing was a new technology, but the concept has now expanded to include functionalities or properties that may change over time in response to various external stimuli, such as light, heat, electricity, magnetism, and solutions.

The preparation methods for 4D printing are the same as those for 3D printing, mainly including stereolithography (SLA), digital light processing (DLP), fused deposition modeling (FDM), Direct Ink Writing (DIW), and PolyJet printing. Shape memory polymers (SMPs), liquid crystal elastomers (LCEs), and shape memory hydrogels (SMHs) are among the materials that are most commonly used in 4D printing technology. SMPs are a type of stimulus-responsive smart material that exhibit shape memory; SMPs can transition from a temporary shape to their original shape in response to external stimuli. Thermoresponsive SMPs have become the most extensively studied shape-changing materials due to their high transition temperature, their optical and mechanical properties, and the ease with which their shape memory can be triggered. Baker and others developed self-expanding SMP implants and SMP sleeves that can expand and contract under surgical conditions to assist in stabilizing segmental defects (Fig. 10.10). These authors conducted in vivo evaluations in a mouse model of segmental defects, proving the feasibility of SMP materials for intraoperative delivery and load-bearing in segmental defect transplantation and stabilization. The SMP implants maintained defect stability and were integrated with autologous bone at 12 weeks postsurgery, demonstrating their potential for use as synthetic bone grafts for filling complex bone defects. LCEs are another type of stimulus-responsive smart material that exhibit reversible and anisotropic changes in shape after exposure to stimuli such as heat, light, electricity, and magnetic fields. Although LCEs have been studied for decades, only with the advent of 4D printing in recent years have their potential applications been developed. Shape memory hydrogels (SMHs) are a type of stimulus-responsive hydrophilic soft material with good

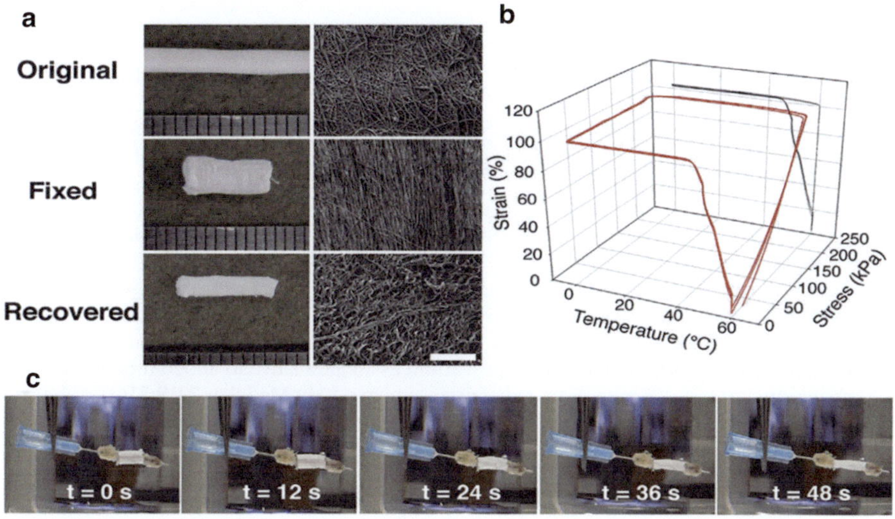

Fig. 10.10 Shape memory behavior of SMP sleeves. (**a**) Macroscopic images and SEM micrographs of the sleeve before fixation, after fixation, and after recovery. The electrospun fibers of the sleeve are randomly oriented before fixation and after recovery, as visible in the SEM images. The electrospun fibers of the sleeve are arranged circumferentially along the temporarily expanded circumference of the sleeve. Scale for macroscopic images: mm, scale for SEM images: 50 mm. (**b**) Quantitative unidirectional shape memory cycle of the SMP sleeve under tension. The sleeve exhibits good fixation and recovery. (**c**) The SMP sleeve contracts around a femur with a 4 mm segmental defect filled with an allograft when immersed in 45 °C saline. The contraction of the sleeve is completed within 50 s (Baker et al. 2016)

biocompatibility that have been rapidly developed in recent decades. SMHs can transition from a temporary shape to their original or permanent shape after exposure to external stimuli, such as heat, light, ultrasound, electric fields, solvents, and magnetic fields. The most well-studied types of SMHs include water-responsive hydrogels, sound-responsive hydrogels, and thermoresponsive hydrogels (Baker et al. 2016).

Although research in the biomedical field using 4D printing technology has made some progress, this technology is still in the early stages of development and faces many challenges that need to be addressed. The most critical issue is that the types of biosmart materials that are currently available for 4D printing are limited, and most are responsive to only a single stimulus. The development of new smart biomaterials that are suitable for complex biological environments and responsive to multiple stimuli is crucial for the application of 4D printing technology in the development of biomedicine. Furthermore, more in-depth research is needed to improve the precision of printed structure deformation control and to enhance the mechanical properties of printed structures.

With the continuous development in the fields of bioengineering, materials science, chemistry, and computer science, there is good reason to believe that 4D printing technology has very broad application prospects in the biomedical field.

References

Association TGoCO. Guidelines for limb salvage treatment of extremity osteosarcoma. Chin J Orthopaed. 2019;39(1):9.

Baker RM, Tseng L-F, Iannolo MT, et al. Self-deploying shape memory polymer scaffolds for grafting and stabilizing complex bone defects: a mouse femoral segmental defect study. Biomaterials. 2016;76:388–98.

Bosma SE, Wong KC, Paul L, et al. A cadaveric comparative study on the surgical accuracy of freehand, computer navigation, and patient-specific instruments in joint-preserving bone tumor resections. Sarcoma. 2018;2018:1–9.

Byambaa B, Annabi N, Yue K, et al. Bioprinted osteogenic and vasculogenic patterns for engineering 3D bone tissue. Adv Healthc Mater. 2017;6(16)

Choi S, Oh YI, Park KH, et al. New clinical application of three-dimensional-printed polycaprolactone/β-tricalcium phosphate scaffold as an alternative to allograft bone for limb-sparing surgery in a dog with distal radial osteosarcoma. J Vet Med Sci. 2019;81(3):434–9.

Colosi C, Shin SR, Manoharan V, et al. Microfluidic bioprinting of heterogeneous 3D tissue constructs using low-viscosity Bioink. Adv Mater. 2016;28(4):677–84.

Do AV, Khorsand B, Geary SM, et al. 3D printing of scaffolds for tissue regeneration applications. Adv Healthc Mater. 2015;4(12):1742–62.

Feng X, Yu H, Liu H, et al. Three-dimensionally-printed polyether-ether-ketone implant with a cross-linked structure and acid-etched microporous surface promotes integration with soft tissue. Int J Mol Sci. 2019;20(15)

Gao Yi FL, Lulu W, et al. Research progress in the application of stem cells in clinical treatment of bone injuries. Chin J Trauma Orthopaed. 2021;23(11):1008–12.

Gülcan O, Günaydın K, Tamer A. The state of the art of material jetting – a critical review. Polymers (Basel). 2021;13(16)

Han X, Yang D, Yang C, et al. Carbon fiber reinforced PEEK composites based on 3D-printing technology for orthopedic and dental applications. J Clin Med. 2019;8(2)

Kang J, Wang L, Yang C, et al. Custom design and biomechanical analysis of 3D-printed PEEK rib prostheses. Biomech Model Mechanobiol. 2018;17(4):1083–92.

Kaya H, Arıcı Ş, Bulut O, et al. CNT incorporation improves the resolution and stability of porous 3D printed PLGA/HA/CNT scaffolds for bone regeneration. Biomed Mater. 2023;18(5)

Kim GB, Lee S, Kim H, et al. Three-dimensional printing: basic principles and applications in medicine and radiology. Korean J Radiol. 2016;17(2):182–97.

Krobot Š, Melčová V, Menčík P, et al. Poly(3-hydroxybutyrate) (PHB) and polycaprolactone (PCL) based blends for tissue engineering and bone medical applications processed by FDM 3D printing. Polymers (Basel). 2023;15(10)

Lee A, Hudson AR, Shiwarski DJ, et al. 3D bioprinting of collagen to rebuild components of the human heart. Science. 2019;365(6452):482–7.

Lenze U, von Eisenhart-Rothe R. Biological reconstruction of bone defects. Orthopade. 2017;46(8):639.

Li Dichen YC, Jianfeng K, et al. Precision design and controlled customization of large-sized individualized PEEK implants. J Mech Eng. 2018;23:121–5.

Li Jing WZ. Progress in surgical reconstruction of bone tumors. Chin J Repar Reconstruct Surg. 2018;32(7):5.

Li J, Liu X, Crook JM, et al. Development of 3D printable graphene oxide based bio-ink for cell support and tissue engineering. Front Bioeng Biotechnol. 2022;10

López-González I, Hernández-Heredia AB, Rodríguez-López MI, et al. Evaluation of the in vitro antimicrobial efficacy against Staphylococcus aureus and epidermidis of a novel 3D-printed degradable drug delivery system based on polycaprolactone/chitosan/vancomycin—preclinical study. Pharmaceutics. 2023;15(6)

Lu Yajie LZ, Minghui L, et al. Reconstruction of large segmental bone defects in patients with lower limb osteosarcoma resection using 3D printed prosthesis combined with β-TCP bioceramics. Chin J Bone Joint. 2019;1:21–6.
Marsh AC, Zhang Y, Poli L, et al. 3D printed bioactive and antibacterial silicate glass-ceramic scaffold by fused filament fabrication. Mater Sci Eng. 2021;C:118.
Melchels FP, Feijen J, Grijpma DW. A review on stereolithography and its applications in biomedical engineering. Biomaterials. 2010;31(24):6121–30.
Pagac M, Hajnys J, Ma QP, et al. A review of vat photopolymerization technology: materials, applications, challenges, and future trends of 3D printing. Polymers (Basel). 2021;13(4)
Reizabal A, Tandon B, Lanceros-Méndez S, et al. Electrohydrodynamic 3D printing of aqueous solutions. Small. 2023;19(7):e2205255.
Roohani-Esfahani SI, Newman P, Zreiqat H. Design and fabrication of 3D printed scaffolds with a mechanical strength comparable to cortical bone to repair large bone defects. Sci Rep. 2016;6:19468.
Sun C, Kang J, Yang C, et al. Additive manufactured polyether-ether-ketone implants for orthopaedic applications: a narrative review. Biomater Transl. 2022;3(2):116–33.
Sun T, Wang J, Huang H, et al. Low-temperature deposition manufacturing technology: a novel 3D printing method for bone scaffolds. Front Bioeng Biotechnol. 2023;11:1222102.
Wang L, Huang L, Li X, et al. Three-dimensional printing PEEK implant: a novel choice for the reconstruction of chest wall defect. Ann Thorac Surg. 2019;107(3):921–8.
Wang Q, Ye W, Ma Z, et al. 3D printed PCL/β-TCP cross-scale scaffold with high-precision fiber for providing cell growth and forming bones in the pores. Mater Sci Eng C Mater Biol Appl. 2021;127:112197.
Wang F, Tankus EB, Santarella F, et al. Fabrication and characterization of PCL/HA filament as a 3D printing material using thermal extrusion technology for bone tissue engineering. Polymers. 2022a;14(4)
Wang Z, Yang Y, Gao Y, et al. Establishing a novel 3D printing bioinks system with recombinant human collagen. Int J Biol Macromol. 2022b;211:400–9.
Wei Xinghui FH, Jun F, et al. Report on five cases of scapular tumor resection and reconstruction with 3D printed polyether ether ketone custom prostheses. China J Orthopaed Traumatol. 2021;10(02):122–7.
Wei X, Zhou W, Tang Z, et al. Magnesium surface-activated 3D printed porous PEEK scaffolds for in vivo osseointegration by promoting angiogenesis and osteogenesis. Bioact Mater. 2023;20:16–28.
Wubneh A, Tsekoura EK, Ayranci C, et al. Current state of fabrication technologies and materials for bone tissue engineering. Acta Biomater. 2018;80:1–30.
Xu Hairong NX, Yuan L, et al. Analysis of 9200 cases of primary bone tumors at Beijing Jishuitan Hospital. J Orthopaed Clin Res. 2016;1(1):5.
Xue K, Qi L, Zhou G, et al. A two-step method of constructing mature cartilage using bone marrow-derived mesenchymal stem cells. Cells Tissues Organs. 2013;197(6):484–95.
Yang Yi GW, Rongli Y, et al. The procedure and common issues of inactivated replantation technology in limb salvage treatment of malignant bone tumors. Orthopaedics. 2018;9(3):6.
Yen HJ, Tseng CS, Hsu SH, et al. Evaluation of chondrocyte growth in the highly porous scaffolds made by fused deposition manufacturing (FDM) filled with type II collagen. Biomed Microdevices. 2009;11(3):615–24.
Zandrini T, Florczak S, Levato R, et al. Breaking the resolution limits of 3D bioprinting: future opportunities and present challenges. Trends Biotechnol. 2023;41(5):604–14.
Zhang C, Wang L, Kang J, et al. Bionic design and verification of 3D printed PEEK costal cartilage prosthesis. J Mech Behav Biomed Mater. 2020;103:103561.
Zhu W, Qu X, Zhu J, et al. Direct 3D bioprinting of prevascularized tissue constructs with complex microarchitecture. Biomaterials. 2017;124:106–15.

3D-Printed, Custom-Made Prostheses with Complex Materials

11

Zhen Tang and Lei Shi

11.1 The Emergence of 3D Printing with Composite Materials

11.1.1 The Purpose and Definition of 3D Printing with Composite Materials

Currently, metal materials are the materials that are most widely used in 3D-printed prostheses, among which titanium alloy (Ti-6Al-4V) and tantalum metal are the most common. The advantages of these materials lie in their excellent biocompatibility and superior mechanical properties, making them the preferred materials for bone tissue repair and replacement therapy. In particular, 3D-printed metal prostheses can form a tight connection with host bone early on, leading to early "bone integration" and allowing the prosthesis to remain stable in the body for a long time, thus preventing revision or surgical failure due to prosthesis loosening and sinking. However, the elastic modulus of metal materials is usually significantly higher than that of normal cortical bone (3–30 GPa) and cancellous bone (0.02–2 GPa), making these materials prone to stress shielding issues due to mismatched elastic moduli at the implant-bone interface, which can affect the lifespan of the implant. Compared to metal materials, polyetheretherketone (PEEK) materials have mechanical properties that are similar to those of natural bone, and these properties effectively prevent stress shielding and bone absorption. Additionally, PEEK materials exhibit good chemical inertness, making them less likely to trigger rejection reactions in the body; thus, PEEK materials are considered ideal bone implant materials (Rendas et al. 2022). However, due to the unique characteristics of the 3D printing process, PEEK prostheses exhibit significant mechanical anisotropy, posing new challenges

Z. Tang
Department of Orthopedics, Tangdu Hospital, Xi'an, China

L. Shi (✉)
Department of Orthopaedics, Xijing Hospital, Xi'an, Shaanxi, People's Republic of China

Z. Guo et al. (eds.), *3D-Printed Prosthesis in Orthopedic Oncology*,
https://doi.org/10.1007/978-981-95-1454-0_11

for the design of PEEK prostheses and for assessing their stability. Furthermore, PEEK materials themselves are highly biologically inert, making it difficult for surrounding bone tissue to effectively integrate and connect with PEEK materials, thereby affecting the long-term stability of PEEK prostheses and limiting their clinical applications.

3D-printed prostheses made with composite materials have emerged as a means by which to improve the mechanical and biological performance of 3D-printed prostheses. There are two main methods. The first is blending modification, which involves mixing different materials in certain proportions to optimize the performance of the blended material and then using this new material for 3D printing to produce a prosthesis. The second method involves separate printing and subsequent assembly, where different materials are used to print different parts of the prosthesis, which are then assembled together to form a complete 3D-printed prosthesis. Regardless of the method that is used, the ultimate goal is to further enhance the characteristics of 3D-printed prostheses, such as the strength of the prosthesis itself, the biological activity of the contact surface, and postoperative X-ray imaging ability.

11.1.2 Methods for 3D Printing with Composite Materials

The direct use of composite materials for 3D printing can involve materials such as PEEK as the base material combined with carbon fiber (CF), hydroxyapatite (HA), magnesium phosphate, graphene, titanium, and other substances.

1. *To Enhance the Strength of PEEK Materials Through 3D Printing with Composite Materials*

Carbon fiber (CF) is the composite material that is most commonly used to increase the strength of PEEK. By adding CF to PEEK, the mechanical properties of PEEK can be significantly improved, increasing its modulus of elasticity within a certain range. Subsequently, through 3D printing technology, implants that meet the requirements for human bone implantation can be produced (Han et al. 2019). Research on CF/PEEK composite 3D printing materials is currently focused mainly on experimental and preclinical studies, and relatively few clinical studies have been conducted. However, implants that are made of CF/PEEK material have begun to be preliminarily studied in clinical practice. Studies have reported that the application of CF/PEEK pedicle screws in the treatment of spinal tumors can significantly reduce metal screw artifacts while ensuring fixation strength, providing favorable conditions for postoperative follow-up imaging evaluation. Additionally, this team reported the preliminary application of the first bone plate made of CF/PEEK in the treatment of humeral metastases in prostate cancer patients. During postoperative follow-up, there was no fracture or displacement of the bone plate, demonstrating the good mechanical performance of the CF/PEEK composite materials (Laux et al. 2018). However, there have been no reports on the use of 3D-printed CF/PEEK prostheses for reconstruction after bone tumor resection. With more in vivo and in vitro studies (Adler et al. 2019), the use of 3D-printed CF/PEEK prostheses is expected to enter clinical practice.

2. *To Enhance the Bioactivity of PEEK Materials Through 3D Printing with Composite Materials*

PEEK composites with hydroxyapatite (HA) are currently a focus of research. The team led by Li Dichen (Zheng et al. 2021) attempted to print PEEK with varying proportions of HA to obtain PEEK composite 3D-printed scaffolds containing 10–30% HA. As the HA content increased, the bioactivity of the scaffolds gradually increased, but the mechanical properties also gradually decreased. In vitro cell experiments showed that scaffolds printed with PEEK/HA composites significantly increased cell ingrowth ability compared to scaffolds printed with pure PEEK. In particular, after being further improved with a porous design, the cell ingrowth ability was further increased, significantly improving the biocompatibility of the material. Building upon PEEK/HA composite materials, several scholars (Kumar et al. 2023) have proposed mixing and printing three materials: PEEK-HA-Mg2SiO4. Research results showed that new products that are printed with this mixture exhibited excellent biomechanics, biocompatibility, and osteogenic cell inductivity compared to those printed with pure PEEK and PEEK/HA-printed implants. The excellent mechanical and biological properties of these products make this mixture a potential candidate for future clinical applications. Professor Bhaduri's (Sikder et al. 2020) team attempted to mix and print PEEK with amorphous magnesium phosphate (AMP), and through in vivo and in vitro studies, they showed that the AMP-PEEK group exhibited significantly better cell proliferation and differentiation capabilities than did the pure PEEK group. Additionally, in animal implantation experiments, implants in the AMP-PEEK group showed significantly better bone contact rates and bone ingrowth than those in the pure PEEK group. Through in vivo and in vitro studies, it was confirmed that printing with an AMP-PEEK mixture improved the biological performance of implants while maintaining their mechanical strength. Zhu et al. (2021) designed and developed a PEEK composite graphene 3D-printed scaffold with an HA coating that could release drugs on its surface. In vivo and in vitro experimental studies showed that this new scaffold material demonstrated good bone ingrowth capabilities. When the material was loaded with antibacterial and antitumor drugs, the drug release capability allowed the material to exert certain inhibitory effects on infection and tumor growth. This novel composite 3D-printed scaffold with a drug-releasing HA coating not only enhanced its own biological properties but also exerted anti-inflammatory and tumor therapeutic effects, highlighting the advantages of composite 3D printing and providing a theoretical basis for its future application in the repair of bone defects caused by tumors and inflammation.

3. *3D Printing of Composite Materials Other Than PEEK*

Additionally, some composite materials have also been used for producing customized prostheses through 3D printing. For example, Seongjae Choi et al. (2019) used customized polycaprolactone/β-tricalcium phosphate (PCL/β-TCP) prostheses for limb-salvage surgery in dogs with distal radial osteosarcoma. Eight weeks after the operation, local recurrence and lung metastasis were observed in the affected dogs, while no displacement of the prosthesis and no prosthesis- or surgery-related complications were observed during this period (Fig. 11.1).

However, such research is currently focused mainly on basic and preclinical studies, including animal experiments. There are very few in vivo studies on the 3D printing of composite materials (see Sect. 11.2 of this Chapter). The safety and effectiveness of these materials in the human body still need to be confirmed with further clinical studies.

For the assembly of 3D-printed prostheses for which different materials are used to print different parts that are later assembled, the materials that are used mainly include PEEK and titanium alloy. PEEK material is utilized for printing joint surfaces or the central parts of modular prostheses due to its light weight, high strength, and low modulus. In areas that require bone integration with the surrounding bone, titanium alloy is used for printing due to its excellent biocompatibility and bioactivity, facilitating early bone ingrowth and integration. By fully leveraging the advantages of PEEK and titanium alloy, both short- and long-term prosthesis stability can be achieved, maximizing the lifespan of the 3D-printed prosthesis. This technology has already been applied in clinical treatment for the repair of bone defects after distal radial and midshaft bone tumor resection and has shown satisfactory results in early postoperative follow-up (see Sect. 11.2 of this Chapter).

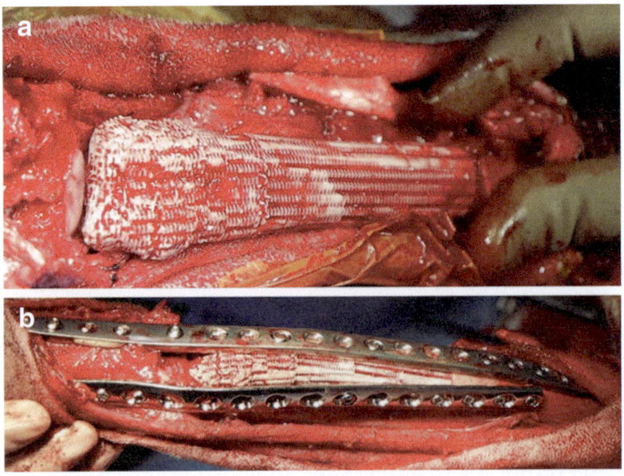

Fig. 11.1 Intraoperative images of a 3D-printed PCL/β-TCP scaffold in distal radial limb salvage surgery. Positioning of the 3D-printed scaffold at the distal radius where the osteosarcoma (OSA) was removed (**a**). Fixation of the entire wrist joint with double steel plates (**b**) (Choi et al. 2019)

11.2 Exploration of Customized 3D-Printed Prostheses Made with Composite Materials

In recent years, 3D-printed prostheses have been clinically applied in various fields, such as orthopedics, maxillofacial surgery, and thoracic surgery, and have achieved satisfactory therapeutic outcomes. Particularly in the bone tumor field, with the continuous advancement of digital technology, precise tumor resection during surgery and accurate repair of defects after tumor excision using 3D-printed prostheses have significantly improved postoperative functionality for patients.

For giant cell tumors and malignant tumors with better prognoses, as the effectiveness of radiotherapy, chemotherapy, and targeted therapy continues to improve, patients' expected survival times have greatly increased, increasing the demand for long-term survival of prostheses within the body. Unlike custom 3D-printed prostheses made with single materials, composite materials can theoretically provide 3D-printed prostheses with superior biological and mechanical properties, enhancing their biological performance in the body and promoting their long-term survival within the body.

However, clinical research on 3D-printed custom prostheses made with composite materials is still in its early stages, and no large-scale studies have been reported. Our team has performed some preliminary work in this area, hoping to provide insights into the future development of 3D-printed custom prostheses made with composite materials.

11.2.1 The Clinical Application of Radiopaque 3D-Printed Custom Prostheses Made with PEEK and Composite Materials

The nonradiopacity of PEEK material itself poses challenges in evaluating the postoperative position, function, and stability of PEEK prostheses that are used for bone tumor resection and reconstruction. Therefore, incorporating an appropriate amount of BaSO4 into the PEEK material before composite printing can effectively address these issues, providing convenience for postoperative prosthetic evaluation in clinical settings.

1. *Radiopaque 3D-Printed Scapular Prostheses* (Wei et al. 2021)

Scapular malignant tumors account for approximately 3% of all bone tumors in the body, with chondrosarcoma, osteosarcoma, and metastatic tumors being the primary types. Due to the unique anatomical structure of the scapula, early-stage scapular tumors often present with no obvious symptoms, leading to a greater extent of invasion by the time they are detected. For malignant or benign highly invasive tumors of the scapula, total scapulectomy is often necessary. After scapulectomy, the options for reconstruction include leaving the space empty (hanging the humerus) or performing reconstruction. Current reconstruction methods include tumor bone devitalization replantation, allogeneic scapular bone transplantation, and scapular prosthesis replacement. Among these options, scapular prosthesis replacement has become the main method that is used in clinical practice due to its ability to achieve a certain shape and function.

Our team utilized a composite material that was prepared by adding radiopaque BaSO4 to PEEK and used 3D printing to create customized scapular prostheses to repair bone defects after total scapulectomy. With this novel 3D printing material, the prosthesis that was produced retained the excellent mechanical properties of PEEK and transformed the originally nonradiopaque PEEK prosthesis into one that is clearly visible under X-ray. This modification allowed real-time observation of the prosthesis during surgery under fluoroscopy, enabling timely adjustments to ensure precise reconstruction according to preoperative planning. Additionally, postoperative follow-up examinations provide a more intuitive understanding of the prosthesis's survival in the body, including its position and stability, facilitating clinical follow-up.

Satisfactory clinical outcomes have been achieved with the current clinical use of this technology. This technique is described below using a typical case study.

Typical Case

An 18-year-old male patient presented to the hospital with right shoulder pain and swelling that had lasted for 3 months. Upon completion of relevant examinations, MRI findings indicated tumor invasion of the scapula and surrounding muscle and soft tissue, showing infiltrative growth and bone destruction of the scapula. A local biopsy that was performed before surgery revealed a small, round cell malignant tumor, suggestive of chondrosarcoma. The patient received three cycles of preoperative chemotherapy with cisplatin, doxorubicin, and ifosfamide, followed by six cycles of neoadjuvant chemotherapy. Postchemotherapy, the lesion size was significantly decreased compared to that before chemotherapy (Figs. 11.2 and 11.3).

Subsequently, three-dimensional data of the affected scapula were obtained through three-dimensional CT reconstruction and image processing, and a prosthesis was designed based on the surgical reconstruction and fixation plan. Soft tissue attachment channels were designed around the prosthesis (Fig. 11.4). Ultimately, a customized PEEK composite with a barium filler prosthesis was created.

Before chemotherapy, the tumor had invaded the scapula and surrounding muscle and soft tissue, showing infiltrative growth and bone destruction of the scapula. The biopsy results indicated a small, round cell malignant tumor, suggestive of chondrosarcoma.

After three cycles of preoperative chemotherapy with cisplatin, doxorubicin, and ifosfamide, the tumor volume was significantly decreased, and the surrounding tissues became less affected. The chemotherapy results were satisfactory.

Based on the attachment positions of the muscles around the scapula, attachment channels were designed around the 3D-printed scapular prosthesis to prepare for intraoperative reconstruction of the muscles around the scapula.

Surgical Procedure: A posterior shoulder arc incision was made. After complete resection of the scapular tumor, a 3D-printed customized PEEK composite prosthesis with barium filler was accurately implanted. By utilizing the preoperatively designed channels, the prosthesis was reattached to the surrounding muscles to

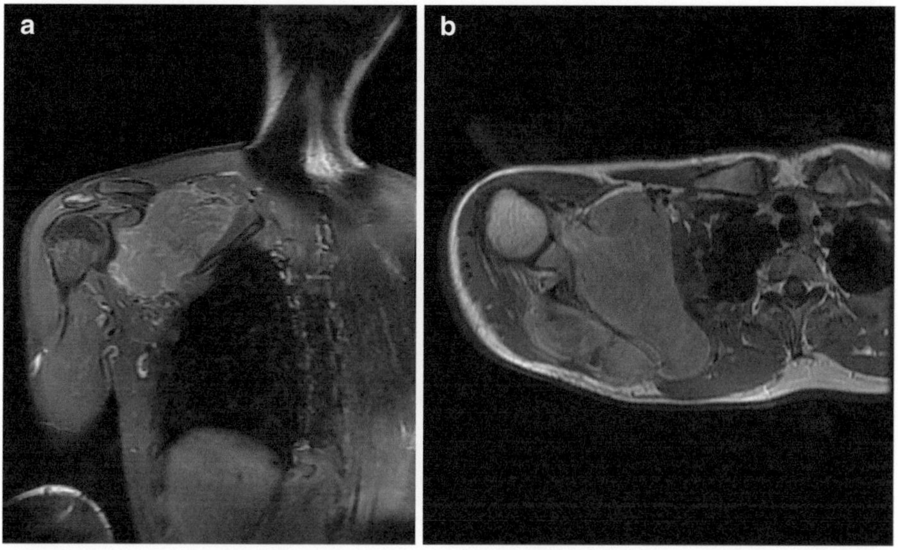

Fig. 11.2 Coronal (**a**) and horizontal (**b**) planes of cross-sectional MR images (Wei et al. 2021)

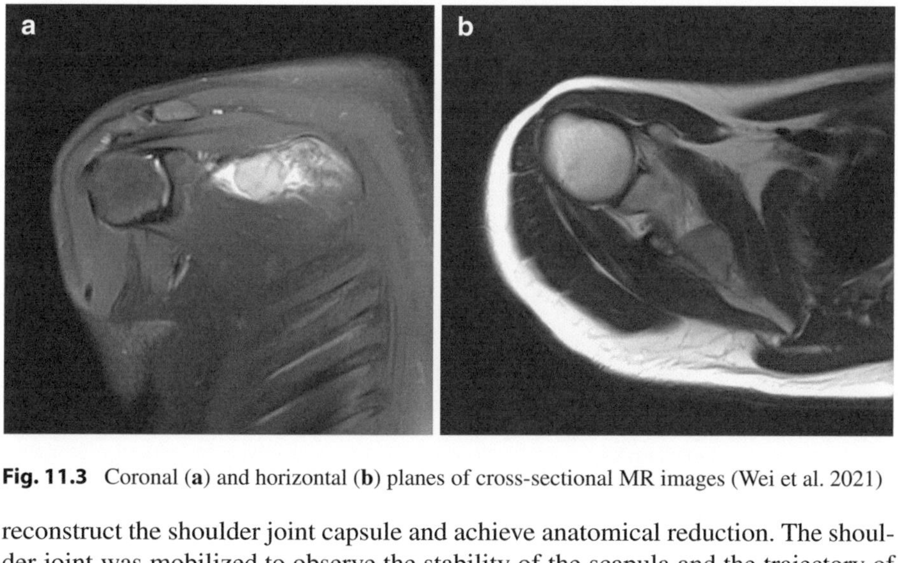

Fig. 11.3 Coronal (**a**) and horizontal (**b**) planes of cross-sectional MR images (Wei et al. 2021)

reconstruct the shoulder joint capsule and achieve anatomical reduction. The shoulder joint was mobilized to observe the stability of the scapula and the trajectory of movement (Fig. 11.5).

According to the preoperative plan, the scapula and surrounding tumor tissues were completely resected during surgery. By utilizing the preoperatively designed attachment channels around the 3D-printed scapular prosthesis, the surrounding muscles were adequately sutured to the scapula, restoring the stability of the scapula.

The scapular prosthesis, which was printed using a PEEK composite material with barium added, overcame the limitation of PEEK prostheses not being visible on X-rays. During surgery, the prosthesis could be clearly visualized in real time

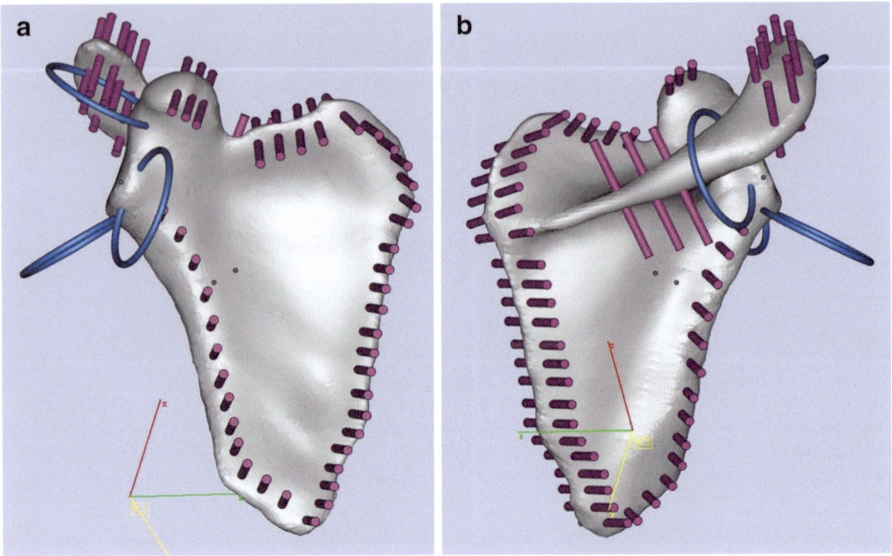

Fig. 11.4 Design of soft tissue attachment channels in the prosthesis. Front view (**a**) and back view (**b**) (Wei et al. 2021)

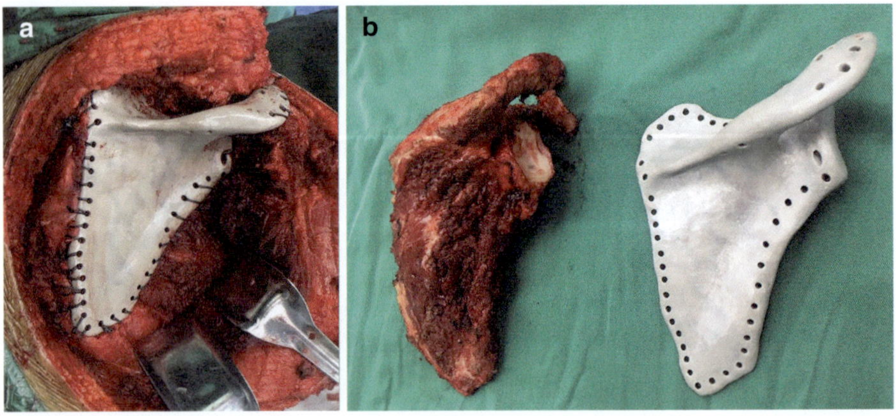

Fig. 11.5 Intraoperative implantation of a 3D-printed scapular prosthesis (**a**). 3D-printed scapular prosthesis and scapula (**b**) (Wei et al. 2021)

under fluoroscopy, allowing adjustments to be made promptly to ensure proper placement according to the preoperative design. The postoperative X-ray and CT reconstruction results showed that the prosthesis achieved near-anatomical reconstruction of the scapula after tumor resection, with good positioning and satisfactory stability (Fig. 11.6). Postoperative follow-up revealed that the patient could externally rotate the shoulder joint to 50°, with a good shoulder appearance and satisfactory function (Fig. 11.7). At the last follow-up, the shoulder joint constant functional score was 68, and no tumor recurrence or distant metastasis was observed.

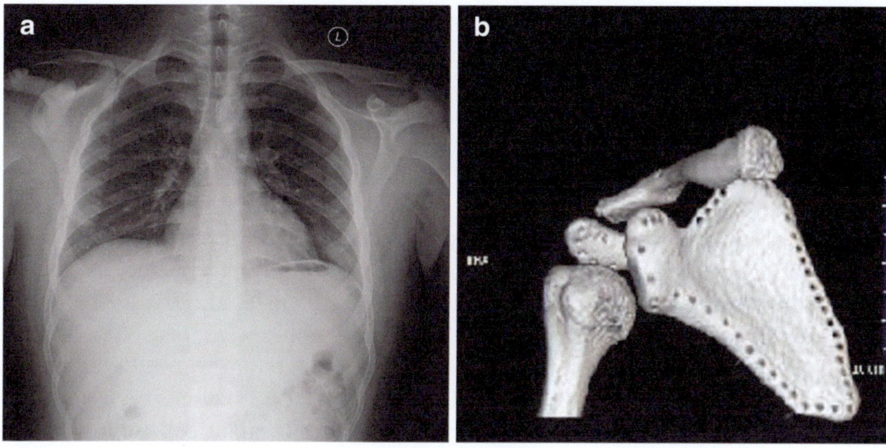

Fig. 11.6 Postoperative X-ray (**a**) and 3D CT reconstruction (**b**) (Wei et al. 2021)

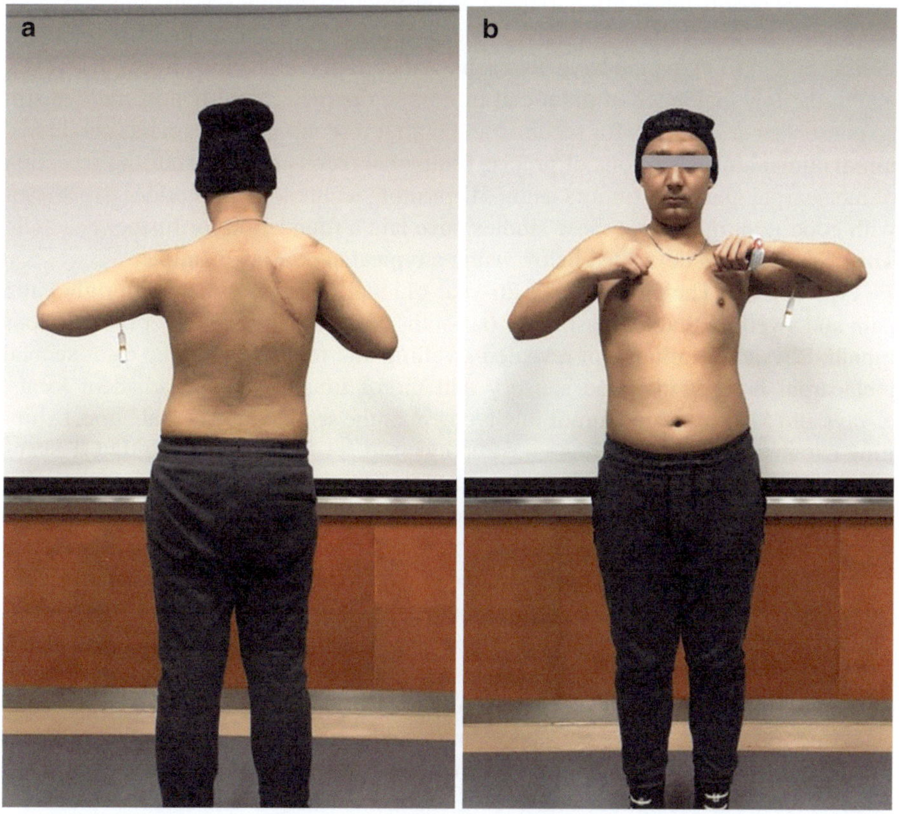

Fig. 11.7 Patient functional photo at 3 months after surgery at the 3-month follow-up after surgery, the patient's shoulder joint could be externally rotated to 50°, and it had satisfactory appearance and function. Back view (**a**) and front view (**b**) (Wei et al. 2021)

After 3D printing with a PEEK + barium composite material, the PEEK prosthesis, which itself would not be radiopaque, was clearly visible on postoperative X-rays. This visibility aided in evaluating the position, function, and stability of the 3D-printed prosthesis, facilitating the assessment of clinical outcomes after surgery.

2. *Radiopaque 3D-Printed Metacarpal Prosthesis*

Giant cell tumors in the hand are very rare, accounting for only approximately 4% of all giant cell tumors in the body, and those that occur in the metacarpal bones represent only approximately 1.5% of all cases (Williams et al. 2010). Therefore, current reports on giant cell tumors of the metacarpal bones have focused mainly on individual case reports. The largest case series in the literature was reported by the Indian scholar Kotwal (Kotwal et al. 2020), who reported 11 patients with metacarpal giant cell tumors. Due to the high recurrence rate of giant cell tumors in the metacarpal bones, all the patients in this series underwent en bloc resection, followed by reconstruction using the fibula, iliac bone, and vascularized toe to achieve satisfactory results. In addition to these reconstruction methods, some scholars have used artificial bone filling (Yadav et al. 2022) and direct abandonment methods (Saikia et al. 2011), which have also achieved certain therapeutic effects. However, due to the low incidence of giant cell tumors in the metacarpal bones, there is still no consensus on methods for reconstruction after resection. Our team has conducted initial clinical investigations of precise biological reconstruction after the resection of metacarpal giant cell tumors using 3D printing technology to produce prostheses with good joint matching; these studies have laid a foundation for further research. This technology is described below using a typical case as an example.

Typical Case: The patient was a 26-year-old male who presented with right palm pain and swelling that had lasted for 6 months and had worsened over the previous month. Physical examination revealed swelling and tenderness in the right second metacarpal bone, with good sensory and motor function in the adjacent joints. X-rays and MRI indicated tumor involvement of the second metacarpal bone, exhibiting expansile growth and bone destruction (Fig. 11.8). SPECT and 3D CT scans suggested expansile bone destruction of the second metacarpal bone with active bone metabolism and peripheral sclerotic margins, highly suggestive of a giant cell tumor. The preoperative local needle biopsy results indicated a probable giant cell tumor. The patient received subcutaneous injections of 120 mg denosumab four times, leading to significant pain relief and a reduction in lesion size.

The preoperative X-ray indicated expansile lytic bone destruction of the second metacarpal bone. MRI revealed bone destruction at the proximal end of the second metacarpal bone, extending distally along the medullary cavity.

Based on 3D CT reconstruction and subsequent image processing, three-dimensional data of the second metacarpal bone of the affected side were obtained. A prosthesis was designed, and a surgical reconstruction and fixation plan was developed. The prosthesis was designed with soft tissue attachment channels at the distal end and screw fixation holes at the proximal end (Fig. 11.9). Ultimately, a custom-made PEEK/$BaSO_4$ prosthesis was created.

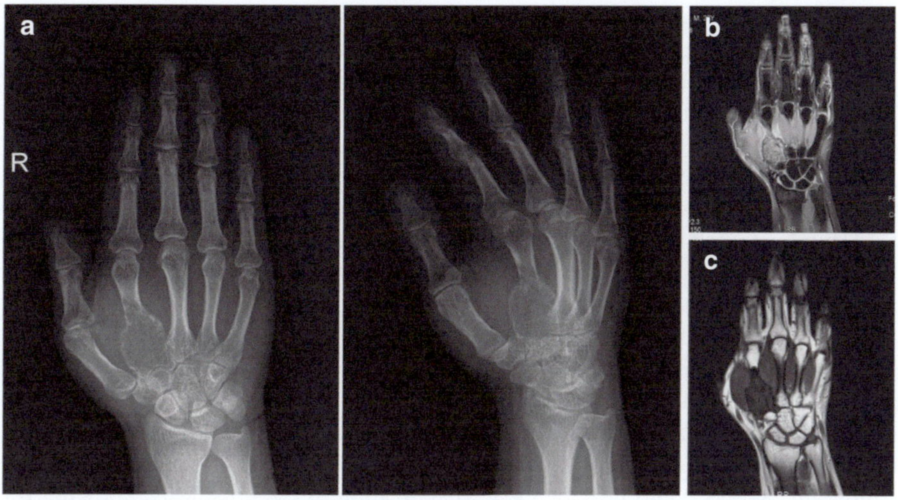

Fig. 11.8 Preoperative X-ray (**a**) and MRI examinations (**b**, **c**)

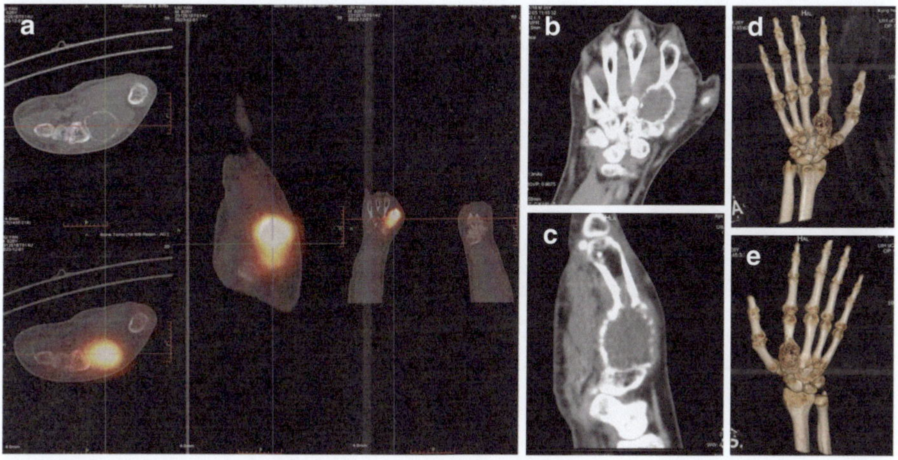

Fig. 11.9 Preoperative SPECT (**a**) and 3D CT reconstruction (**b**–**e**)

SPECT indicated expansile bone destruction of the second metacarpal bone with active bone metabolism, highly suggestive of a giant cell tumor. 3D CT reconstruction revealed lytic expansile bone destruction of the second metacarpal bone, with sclerotic margins around the lesion.

Surgical Procedure: A dorsal curved incision was made over the second metacarpal bone. The second metacarpal bone was completely separated and excised, and the tumor was removed en bloc. Subsequently, the custom-made PEEK/$BaSO_4$ prosthesis for the second metacarpal bone was precisely implanted. The preoperatively prepared channels were used to reattach the prosthesis distal joint capsule, which was reinforced with suture ligaments. The proximal end was fixed with a 3.5-mm screw to the base of the proximal phalanx and metacarpal head, and the joint capsule was reinforced with suture ligaments to achieve anatomical reduction. The passive range of motion of the metacarpophalangeal joint was good (Figs. 11.10 and 11.11).

Postoperative X-ray and 3D CT reconstructions demonstrated that the metacarpal prosthesis was well positioned and securely fixed.

The tumor resection during surgery was complete, and the prosthesis installation was well matched. Intraoperative fluoroscopy confirmed that the prosthesis was accurately positioned and securely fixed.

Our team utilized a PEEK composite material with $BaSO_4$ added for 3D printing, transforming the PEEK prosthesis, which would not have been visible via X-ray, into a prosthesis that could be directly observed via X-ray. This innovation allowed surgeons to observe the prosthesis in real time under fluoroscopy during surgery, enabling prompt corrections to ensure accurate placement. During postoperative follow-up, X-rays could provide clear visualization of the prosthesis, allowing for

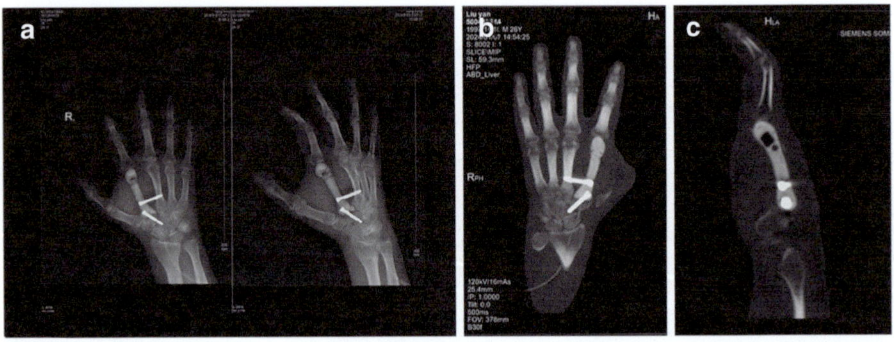

Fig. 11.10 Postoperative X ray (**a**) and 3D reconstructed CT images (**b-c**) Postoperative X-ray and 3D CT reconstructions demonstrated that the metacarpal prosthesis was well positioned and securely fixed

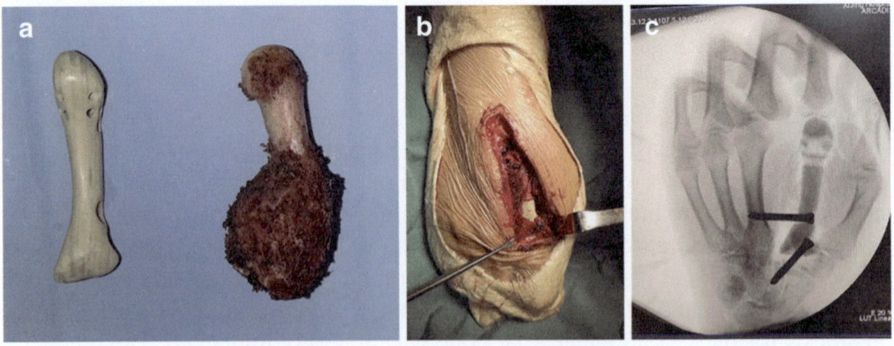

Fig. 11.11 Intraoperative tumor resection (**a**), prosthesis installation (**b**) and X-ray (**c**)

dynamic assessment of its morphology, position, and stability. This significantly enhanced the convenience and observability of postoperative follow-up. For prostheses that are made with PEEK material using 3D printing, this approach has important clinical significance and application value.

11.2.2 The Clinical Application of Custom Prostheses Assembled from 3D-Printed PEEK Components and 3D-Printed Titanium Alloy Components with Bone Integration Capabilities

To combine the excellent biocompatibility and osseointegration capabilities of titanium alloy with the superior mechanical properties and chemical inertness of PEEK, different parts of the prostheses can be separately printed and then assembled for use. This approach allows manufacturers to maximize the strengths of the materials that are used for each part of the 3D-printed prosthesis, enhancing the biological and mechanical performance of the assembled prosthesis within the body and laying a solid foundation for long-term survival. Our team has achieved satisfactory therapeutic effects in clinical practice.

1. *An Individualized Custom Prosthesis for the Distal Radius Using 3D-Printed Titanium Alloy with Bone Integration Capability +3D-Printed PEEK Components*

In addition to the distal femur and proximal tibia, the distal radius is the third most common site for giant cell tumors, accounting for approximately 10% of cases (Hess et al. 2023). Patients in Campanacci stages I and II are usually treated with curettage and bone grafting or bone cement filling. However, for patients with Campanacci stage III tumors or recurrent tumors, en bloc resection surgery followed by reconstruction using 3D-printed custom prostheses is often necessary (Wysocki et al. 2015). Professor Tu Zhongqi's team (Wang et al. 2020) at West China Hospital has achieved satisfactory clinical outcomes in treating distal radius giant cell tumors with biomimetic intramedullary fixation with 3D-printed custom prostheses. Our team has also achieved satisfactory results in clinical practice using 3D-printed PEEK prostheses combined with 3D-printed titanium alloy intramedullary fixation rods to repair bone defects after the resection of distal radius giant cell tumors. This technique is described below using a typical case.

Typical Case

A 25-year-old male patient presented with right wrist pain that had worsened over the previous year, and the pain had intensified over the previous 2 months, leading to his admission to the hospital. Upon examination, there was mild swelling in the right wrist, with slight restriction of movement due to pain. The local skin temperature was not elevated. A firm, hard lump measuring approximately 2.0 cm × 2.0 cm × 2.0 cm was palpable, with poor local mobility and mild tenderness on palpation. Following comprehensive investigations postadmission, X-rays, CT scans, and MRIs revealed eccentrically expanding bone destruction at the distal end of the right radius, suggesting a giant cell tumor (Figs. 11.12 and 11.13). A diagnostic incisional biopsy of the right distal radius lesion was performed, and the postoperative pathological findings strongly indicated a diagnosis of a giant cell tumor. The patient was treated with 120 mg of denosumab

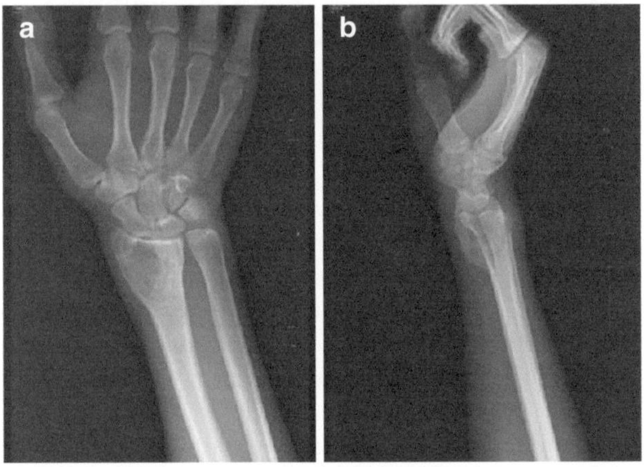

Fig. 11.12 Anteroposterior (**a**) and lateral (**b**) view of X-ray examination results

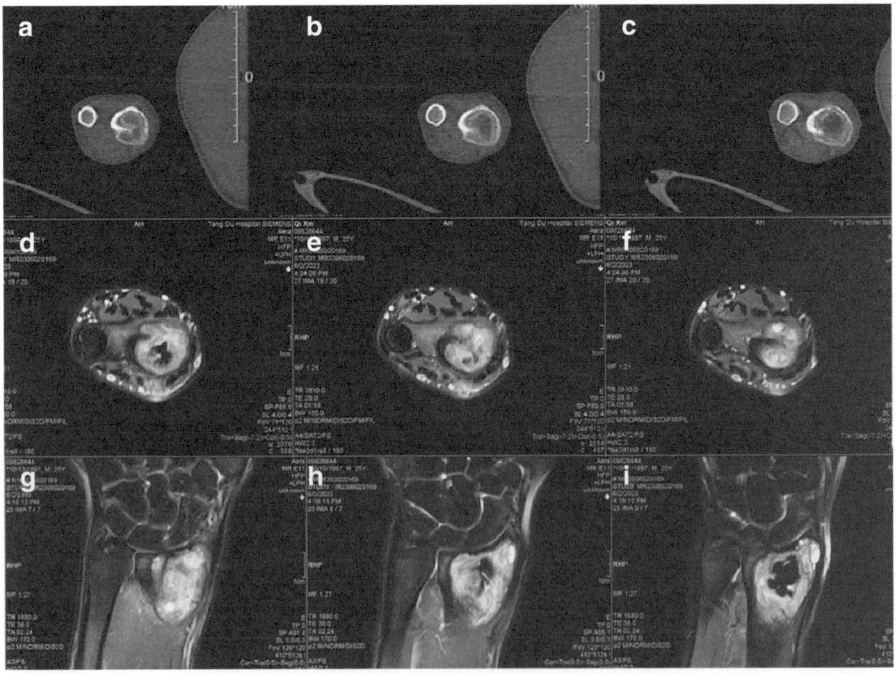

Fig. 11.13 CT (**a**–**c**) and MRI (**d**–**i**) examination results

administered on Days 1, 8, and 14, which resulted in a significant reduction in tumor size, as observed on MRI.

Prior to surgery, thin-section CT scans of the distal radius of the affected side were obtained to generate three-dimensional data to simulate reconstruction with a distal radius prosthesis. The prosthesis was segmented into two parts: one part comprised the distal radius prosthesis body that interfaced with the wrist joint surface and was designed with holes around the joint surface to accommodate soft tissue attachments during the reconstruction fixation procedure; the other part was the intramedullary fixation portion of the prosthesis that interfaced with the proximal radius. The segmented data were input into 3D printing devices, with the distal radius prosthesis body printed using PEEK material and the intramedullary fixation portion printed using titanium alloy material. These two components were then assembled to obtain the final distal radius prosthesis (Fig. 11.14).

X-ray revealed eccentric lytic bone destruction at the distal end of the radius, with the formation of a local mass.

CT/MR images revealed osteolytic destruction at the distal end of the radius, with a soft tissue mass extending through the bone cortex, leading to a local pathological bone fracture.

Surgical Procedure: A curved incision was made on the dorsal side of the right wrist joint, tilted toward the radial side, and a shuttle-shaped excision biopsy channel was created to sequentially open and separate, exposing the distal radius. Intraoperatively, the tumor was observed to be expanding toward the dorsal and radial sides at the distal end of the radius, with a complete pseudocapsule. The extensor tendons on the dorsal side were protected and pulled to the sides to fully expose the distal radius. According to the preoperative plan, an intraoperative bone-cutting guide was installed, the radius was cut, and the tumor segment bone was completely removed after freeing the surrounding tissues, ensuring that the

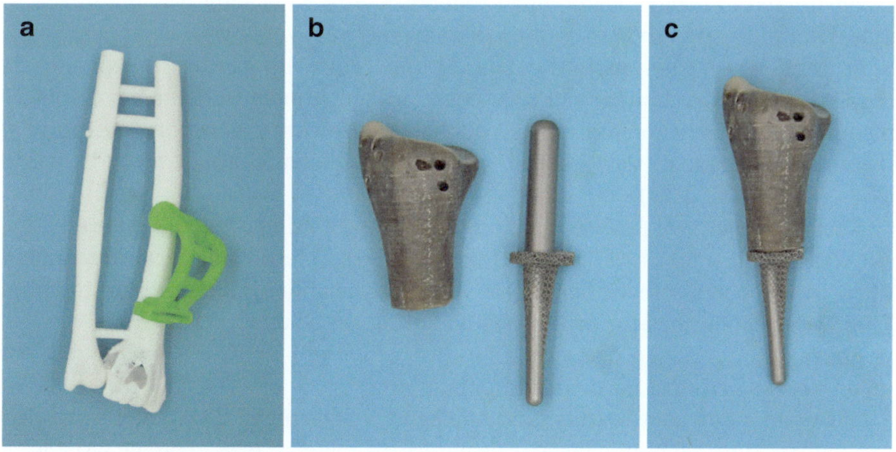

Fig. 11.14 3D-printed the right distal radius lesion (**a**). 3D-printed PEEK +3D-printed titanium alloy composite prosthesis (**b**, **c**)

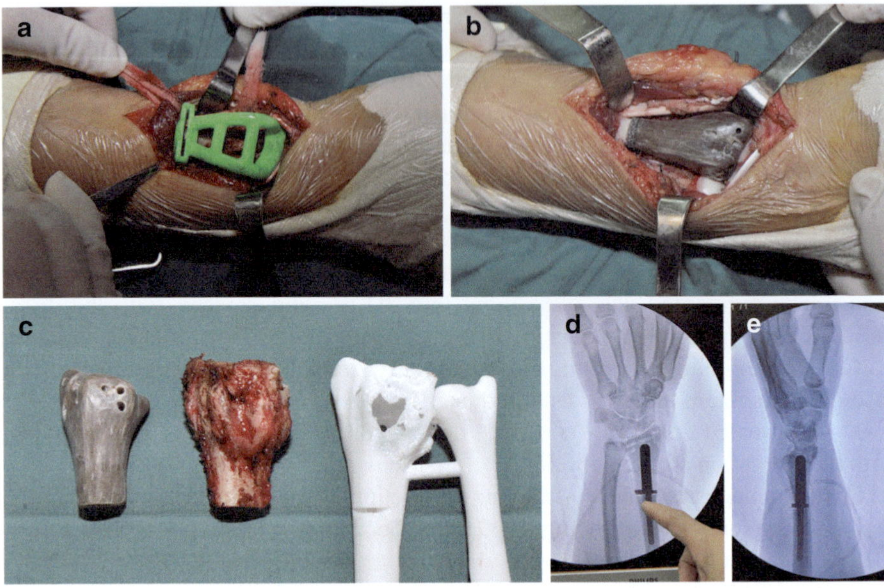

Fig. 11.15 Intraoperative Conditions. Intraoperative prosthesis installation (**a**, **b**), tumor resection (**c**) and X-ray (**d**, **e**)

length of the excised bone segment was appropriate compared to the prosthesis (Fig. 11.15). The residual proximal radius was fixed, the medullary canal was sequentially expanded, and the prosthesis was inserted and secured. Intraoperative fluoroscopy confirmed the proper position of the prosthesis, and it had good alignment with the various parts of the radiocarpal joint. The wrist joint could flex, extend, and laterally deviate passively with ease. The wrist joint capsule was reconstructed to achieve anatomical reduction. The wrist joint was mobilized to assess stability and range of motion. The patient recovered well postoperatively, with good wrist joint mobility. During the follow-up period, the prosthesis remained in a good position and was securely fixed without loosening or displacement, and local bone integration was confirmed. However, there was separation at the distal radioulnar joint, but it did not significantly affect wrist function (Figs. 11.16 and 11.17).

During the surgery, precise excision was achieved using a cutting guide, and the excised specimen matched the size of the prosthesis. The prosthesis was accurately fitted to the bone defect after tumor resection, enabling precise reconstruction. Fluoroscopy confirmed the proper position of the prosthesis.

During the follow-up period, the position of the prosthesis remained good, but there was separation at the distal radioulnar joint.

When adopting an assembly based design for 3D-printed distal radius prostheses, low-friction and highly wear-resistant PEEK material is used on the wrist joint surface, which, compared to traditional titanium alloy prostheses, reduces the wear between the radius prosthesis and carpal bones, slows wrist joint degeneration due

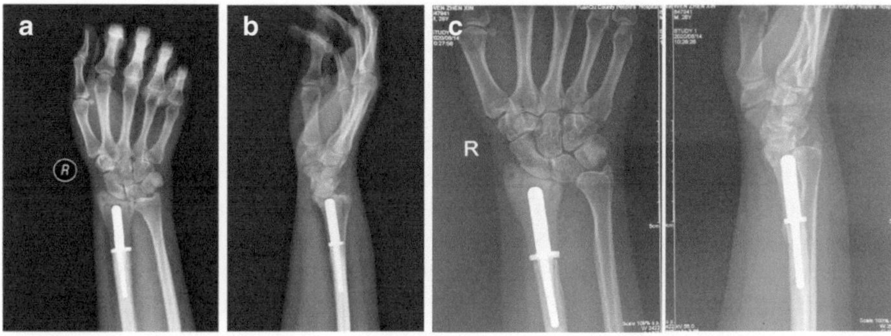

Fig. 11.16 Postoperative follow-up. Anteroposterior (**a**, **c**) and lateral (**b**, **d**) view of X-ray examination results

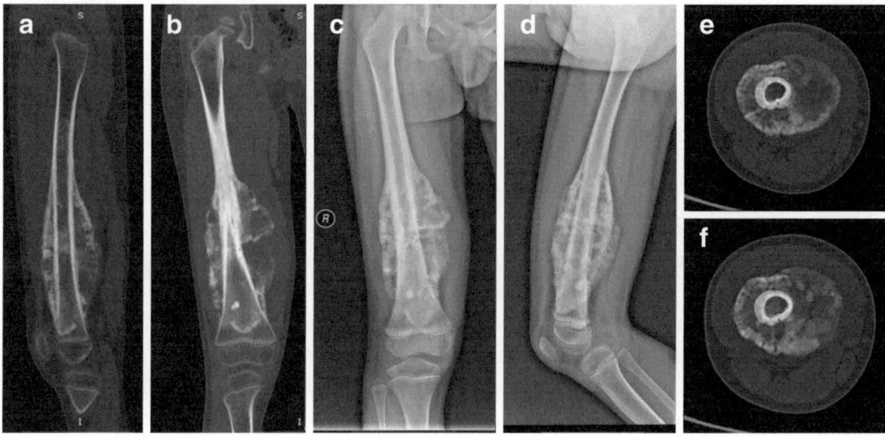

Fig. 11.17 Lateral (**a**) and anteroposterior (**b**) view of preoperative X-ray. Anteroposterior (**c**), lateral (**d**) and axial (**e**, **f**) view of 3D CT images

to wear, and reduces the wear of tendons around the wrist joint during flexion and extension, thereby decreasing the risk of tendon injury and adhesion and improving the long-term survival of the prosthesis in the body. Due to the lightweight design of 3D-printed PEEK prostheses, patients experience a greater sense of comfort during use, which helps them accept the presence of internal prostheses both physically and psychologically, ultimately improving their quality of life. However, if a prosthesis is printed with PEEK material alone, bone ingrowth and integration in the medullary cavity are inevitably affected, leading to poor prosthesis stability in the body, which may result in loosening, displacement, or even fracture. Therefore, for medullary fixation, our team has used a 3D-printed titanium alloy medullary fixation rod, combining a medullary fixation rod with a PEEK prosthesis at the distal end of the radius to achieve PEEK prosthesis fixation in the medullary cavity; this approach replaces the purely mechanical fixation of the PEEK material with the mechanical and biological fixation of the titanium alloy, significantly increasing the strength of prosthesis fixation in the medullary cavity and avoiding the inert biological performance of the PEEK material in the medullary cavity. The use of 3D-printed titanium alloy medullary fixation is conducive to early bone ingrowth and integration in the medullary cavity, achieving prosthesis stability in the medullary cavity and promoting long-term use of the prosthesis in the body. The theoretical survival period of the prosthesis and the probability of fracture or loosening are lower in upper limb prostheses that are subjected to less weight bearing than in lower limb prostheses that are subjected to greater stress. Therefore, if the prosthesis can remain stable for a long time and function well, it will greatly improve the quality of life of patients. In the follow-up of this patient, the prosthesis was well positioned, the medullary fixation was reliable, the wrist function was good, and the postoperative efficacy was satisfactory. However, separation of the distal radioulnar joint was still observed, indicating that further improvement is needed in the design and application of prostheses to increase the stability of the distal radioulnar joint.

2. *An Individualized, Custom Femoral Prosthesis Assembled from Titanium Alloy with Bone Integration Ability +3D-Printed PEEK Components*

The area around the knee joint is the most common site of osteosarcoma, which often occurs in adolescents and has a higher incidence in males than in females. With advances in neoadjuvant chemotherapy, radiotherapy, and targeted therapy, limb-salvage surgery is now commonly used for treatment (Beird et al. 2022). In limb-salvage procedures, successfully preserving the joint surface can greatly improve patient outcomes. Previously, the most common method for reconstructing the preserved joint surface involved the use of large allograft bones. However, due to limitations in allograft availability, an increasing number of researchers are considering alternative solutions.

The emergence of 3D printing technology has provided new ideas and methods for addressing this challenge. Our team has attempted to use 3D-printed titanium alloy prostheses to replace the part that contacts the joint surface and 3D-printed PEEK prostheses to replace traditional allograft bones. By assembling and joining these two types of prostheses, a new type of 3D-printed composite prosthesis can be produced, with the aim of enhancing the in vivo biocompatibility and stability of the prosthesis. This technology is currently in the clinical exploration stage, and we share our experience below by describing a typical case for reference.

Typical Case: A 7-year-old male presented with pain in the right thigh that had lasted for more than 4 months. Physical examination revealed a hard, poorly defined, immobile mass measuring approximately 5 × 7 cm at the distal end of the right thigh. There were no abnormalities in the movement or sensation of the right lower limb, and the degree of dorsalis pedis artery pulsation was good. X-ray findings revealed bone destruction in the mid-lower segment of the right femur, with indistinct contours, triangular periosteal reaction, sunburst-like bone formation, and a soft tissue mass, suggestive of osteosarcoma. CT scans indicated bone destruction in the mid-lower segment of the right femur surrounded by extensive osteogenic formation.

After an incisional biopsy, the pathological diagnosis was conventional osteosarcoma. The patient received cisplatin-doxorubicin and ifosfamide as neoadjuvant chemotherapy for two cycles, with four sessions in total. Preoperative thin-section CT scans of the femur of the affected side were performed to obtain three-dimensional data to simulate the reconstruction of the affected femoral prosthesis. The prosthesis was segmented into two parts: one for contacting the residual distal femoral bone and the other for replacing the femoral shaft and proximal femur for intramedullary fixation.

The segmented data were input into 3D printing devices, with the distal femoral prosthesis body and intramedullary fixation part printed using PEEK material and the intramedullary fixation part treated with titanium alloy surface spray. The component that contacted the residual distal femoral bone was printed using titanium alloy material. The two parts were then assembled to produce the distal femoral prosthesis (Fig. 11.18).

Findings from the X-ray/CT revealed bone destruction in the mid-lower segment of the femur, a triangular periosteal reaction, and extensive osteogenic formation.

The application of a 3D-printed PEEK +3D titanium alloy composite prosthesis in reconstruction after femoral osteosarcoma resection.

Surgical Procedure: A medial incision was made in the right thigh, and the scar from the previous biopsy surgery was excised in a spindle shape. Layer-by-layer dissection was performed down to the muscle layer, and the tumor in the lower segment of the femur was exposed by separating it from the posterior aspect of the

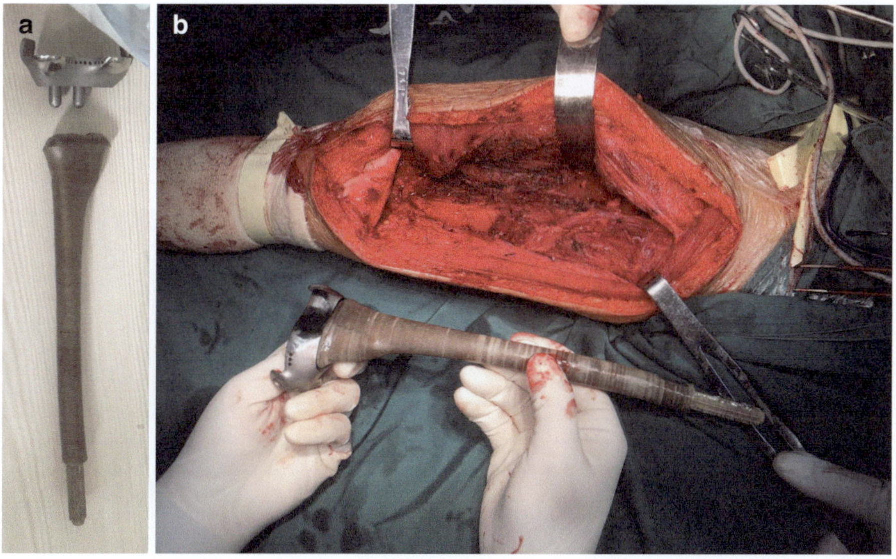

Fig. 11.18 Assembled prosthesis (**a**) and application of the assembled prosthesis in surgery (**b**)

medial thigh muscles. The segment of the tumor above the normal bone shaft was separated, and the femoral artery and vein were carefully protected. The middle thigh muscle, along with some of the medial thigh muscles, was dissected together with the tumor. The distal femoral growth plate was exposed, and an osteotomy guide plate was installed to cut the femur at the proximal end of the normal bone shaft and the growth plate.

The tumor was completely excised after separating it from the surrounding normal muscle layers. After the assembly of the metal prosthesis with the femoral PEEK prosthesis, the 3D-printed assembled prosthesis was installed. The fit of the prosthesis was good, the alignment was satisfactory, and the lengths of both lower limbs were consistent. Support plates were used on the medial and lateral sides to reinforce fixation. Intraoperatively, fluoroscopy revealed that the 3D-printed prosthesis was in a good position, and the steel plates were securely fixed. The passive movement of the knee and hip joints was good.

Postoperatively, the patient recovered well, and during follow-up, the position of the prosthesis remained good without any signs of loosening, displacement, or fracture. By the third month, the patient was able to resume normal daily activities, and the postoperative recovery was satisfactory (Fig. 11.19).

During the follow-up period, the prosthesis was in a good position, it was in close contact with the adjacent bone, it was securely fixed, and there was no loosening or displacement.

Through the design of an assembled 3D-printed prosthesis in the mid-distal part of the femur, a 3D-printed PEEK prosthesis with good mechanical properties and biocompatibility was used in the femoral shaft. Compared to traditional metal prostheses, the light weight of PEEK reduced the weight of the long segment prosthesis, enhancing patient comfort during prosthesis use and improving quality of life. Additionally, its biostability in the body helps avoid adverse reactions, such as the electrolysis of metal debris, reducing the risk of aseptic prosthesis loosening and creating a more stable biological environment around the prosthesis for its long-term survival inside the body. To increase the fixation strength in the medullary

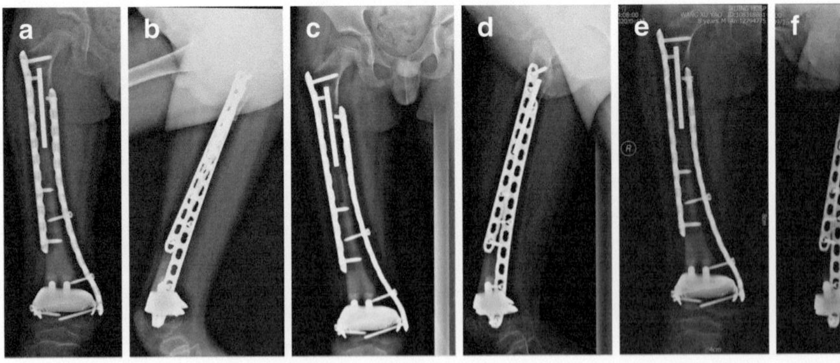

Fig. 11.19 Postoperative follow-up (**a**–**f**)

cavity, the surface of the PEEK medullary fixation rod was treated with titanium alloy coating, improving its biological activity, facilitating early bone ingrowth and integration, and achieving prosthesis stability.

However, if the entire residual bone portion of the prosthesis near the proximal end of the femur is also printed with PEEK, the biologically inert nature of the PEEK material would likely affect bone integration, leading to poor prosthesis stability in the body, potentially causing loosening, displacement, or even fracture. Therefore, in the area that contacts the residual bone at the distal end of the femur, our team used a 3D-printed titanium alloy prosthesis design. By combining the metal prosthesis at the distal end of the femur with the PEEK prosthesis at the femoral shaft, the prosthesis achieves mechanical and biological fixation with the 3D-printed titanium alloy interface through early screw plate-assisted fixation, bone ingrowth, and creeping, thus increasing the fixation strength of the prosthesis. Particularly in weight-bearing areas of the lower limbs, prosthesis stability is crucial. Once bone integration occurs between the prosthesis and the residual bone, the prosthesis may remain stable and survive in the body in the long term. Especially with the preservation of joint surfaces, if the prosthesis can survive long-term, patients can achieve better joint function, significantly improving their quality of life. During the follow-up of this patient, the prosthesis was in a good position and securely fixed, the hip and knee functions were good, and the postoperative outcomes were satisfactory.

3. *Advantages and Disadvantages of Assembled 3D-Printed Custom Prostheses in Clinical Practice*

The research team innovatively combined and assembled 3D-printed prostheses made of two different materials, namely, PEEK and titanium alloy, for use in areas that require bone integration and early stability of the portion of the prosthesis that contacts bone. Titanium alloy was used in the design of 3D-printed prostheses to maximize its excellent biological performance when in contact with bone to promote bone integration. Additionally, PEEK was used in the design of 3D-printed prostheses in areas where reduced friction and wear around joints or tendons were needed, taking advantage of the lightweight and biologically inert properties of PEEK. This approach fully leveraged the unique characteristics of each material, creating a novel multifunctional prosthesis where the combination was greater than the sum of its parts. In initial clinical applications, this approach has achieved satisfactory therapeutic effects.

However, this technology also has many shortcomings. For example, the precision requirements for 3D-printed prostheses are higher, printing with composite materials increases costs, and manufacturing time is longer. Additionally, this technology is still in its early stages of clinical application, and its long-term efficacy is not yet clear. Further research and observation are needed to study the long-term effects of these prostheses on the body. Due to the presence of secondary interfaces in these newly assembled prostheses, whether instability or fracture will occur during use also needs to be verified in additional clinical applications.

11.3 The Future of Custom 3D-Printed Prostheses Made with Composite Materials

The current materials that are used in 3D-printed prostheses made with composite materials can be divided into two main categories: metals and nonmetals. Metal materials, especially titanium alloys and tantalum metals, are the materials that are most commonly used in clinical 3D-printed custom prostheses. Therefore, the application of composite materials, such as composite HA, composite bioactive glass, and composite PEEK, in 3D printing can enhance the biological activity of prostheses, reduce the elastic modulus of prostheses, and decrease stress concentration effects, making such prostheses very promising for clinical applications. Additionally, printing titanium alloy combined with tantalum metal can further improve the biological activity of prostheses, which is particularly valuable for patients with osteoporosis and poor bone conditions for prosthesis revision. The combination of titanium alloy with magnesium metal in 3D printing may enhance the resistance of the prosthesis to infection to some extent. If successful, this could allow for the use of 3D-printed prostheses in specific scenarios.

Furthermore, the development of 3D-printed prostheses made with cobalt-chromium alloy may have a significant impact on weight-bearing prosthetic reconstruction. Implantation experiments in sheep have shown that cobalt-chromium alloy prostheses printed using 3D technology exhibited better bone integration capabilities than titanium alloy prostheses, although the bone-prosthesis contact rate was lower than that of titanium alloy prostheses. The combination of cobalt-chromium alloy with titanium alloy or tantalum materials for printing to improve the biological performance of the bone-prosthesis interface may lead to a transition from bone cement fixation to biological fixation in joint replacement surgeries.

3D printing of nonmetal composite materials is mainly used for constructing tissue engineering scaffolds, with research primarily focused on bone defect repair. However, current research is predominantly based on cellular and animal biological studies, and clinical research is limited. Nonmetal materials can be further classified into degradable and nondegradable materials. In the degradable materials category, the team has explored the use of PCL/β-TCP composite materials for printing degradable intervertebral fusion devices, and the initial clinical research results are promising. However, factors such as uncontrollable in vivo degradation rates remain uncertain. As material technology advances in the future, these materials have the potential to become viable options for clinical applications.

Nonetheless, the 3D-printed prostheses made with nondegradable composites that show the greatest promise for future clinical applications may be based on PEEK materials. Among these materials, PEEK/HA has been extensively studied in preclinical research, showing satisfactory results in cell and animal experiments. The team has begun exploring its use in preliminary clinical research on bone repair in humans, and if successful, PEEK/HA may partially replace allogeneic bone in clinical applications, addressing the clinical challenge of insufficient allogeneic bone sources.

3D-printed prostheses made with composite materials can be applied in various clinical scenarios, such as cranial reconstruction, maxillofacial reconstruction, and sternum and rib reconstruction, and the most common application is defect repair in long bones and axial bones. In the future, if weight-bearing sites, such as pelvic tumor resection and lower limb joint tumor resection sites, can be reconstructed with 3D-printed prostheses made with PEEK composites, the weight of the prostheses could be significantly reduced, the biological activity of the prostheses could be enhanced, and patient comfort could be improved without compromising the mechanical strength. This advance could greatly promote the further development of 3D-printed artificial prostheses.

References

Adler D, Akbar M, Spicher A, et al. Biomechanical study of a novel, expandable, non-metallic and radiolucent CF/PEEK vertebral body replacement (VBR). Materials. 2019;12(17):1–11.

Beird HC, Bielack SS, Flanagan AM, et al. Osteosarcoma. Nat Rev Dis Primers. 2022;8(1):1–19.

Choi S, Oh Y-I, Park K-H, et al. New clinical application of three-dimensional-printed polycaprolactone/β-tricalcium phosphate scaffold as an alternative to allograft bone for limb-sparing surgery in a dog with distal radial osteosarcoma. J Vet Med Sci. 2019;81(3):434–9.

Han X, Yang D, Yang C, et al. Carbon fiber reinforced PEEK composites based on 3D-printing technology for orthopedic and dental applications. J Clin Med. 2019;8(2):1–17.

Hess MC, Kafchinski L, Ransom E. Giant cell tumor of the distal radius. Orthop Clin N Am. 2023;54(1):75–88.

Kotwal PP, Ansari MT, Mahmood A, et al. A management strategy for giant cell tumor of the metacarpal: a single-center series of 11 cases. J Clin Orthop Trauma. 2020;11(4):657–61.

Kumar N, Alathur Ramakrishnan S, Lopez KG, et al. Novel 3D printable PEEK-HA-Mg2SiO4 composite material for spine implants: biocompatibility and imaging compatibility assessments. Eur Spine J. 2023;32(7):2255–65.

Laux CJ, Hodel SM, Farshad M, et al. Carbon fibre/polyether ether ketone (CF/PEEK) implants in orthopaedic oncology. World J Surg Oncol. 2018;16(1):1–6.

Rendas P, Figueiredo L, Machado C, et al. Mechanical performance and bioactivation of 3D-printed PEEK for high-performance implant manufacture: a review. Prog Biomater. 2022;12(2):89–111.

Saikia KC, Bhuyan SK, Ahmed F, et al. Giant cell tumor of the metacarpal bones. Indian J Orthop. 2011;45(5):475–8.

Sikder P, Ferreira JA, Fakhrabadi EA, et al. Bioactive amorphous magnesium phosphate-polyetheretherketone composite filaments for 3D printing. Dent Mater. 2020;36(7):865–83.

Wang Y, Min L, Lu M, et al. The functional outcomes and complications of different reconstruction methods for giant cell tumor of the distal radius: comparison of osteoarticular allograft and three-dimensional-printed prosthesis. BMC Musculoskelet Disord. 2020;21(1):1–15.

Wei X, Fan H, Fu J, et al. Reconstruction with 3D printed polyetheretherketone customized prosthesis after scapular tumor resection: a report of 5 cases. Chin J Bone Joint. 2021;10(2):122–7.

Williams J, Hodari A, Janevski P, et al. Recurrence of giant cell tumors in the hand: a prospective study. J Hand Surg Am. 2010;35(3):451–6.

Wysocki RW, Soni E, Virkus WW, et al. Is intralesional treatment of giant cell tumor of the distal radius comparable to resection with respect to local control and functional outcome? Clin Orthop Relat Res. 2015;473(2):706–15.

Yadav S, Singhal S, Patel S, et al. A rare case of giant-cell tumor of hand in a young male. Cureus. 2022;14(1):2–7.

Zheng J, Kang J, Sun C, et al. Effects of printing path and material components on mechanical properties of 3D-printed polyether-ether-ketone/hydroxyapatite composites. J Mech Behav Biomed Mater. 2021;118(2021):1–9.

Zhu C, He M, Sun D, et al. 3D-printed multifunctional polyetheretherketone bone scaffold for multimodal treatment of osteosarcoma and osteomyelitis. ACS Appl Mater Interfaces. 2021;13(40):47327–40.

Surface Modification of 3D-Printed Custom-Made Prostheses

12

Dongmei Yu, Hao Wu, Zhen Tang, Shusen Bao, and Qiong Ma

Due to their widespread application, high fabrication precision, and personalized matching degree, customized 3D-printed prostheses have attracted increased amounts of attention from clinical surgeons. Compared with traditional orthopedic metal implants, these prostheses have three-dimensional porous structures, which promote the growth of bone tissue, and a low elastic modulus, which effectively mitigates stress shielding effects, thereby decreasing the incidence of complications such as bone resorption and implant displacement or collapse (Ahn et al. 2018). Currently, customized 3D-printed prostheses are extensively used as artificial joints, spinal fusion cages, dental implants, and bone repair products (Lal and Patralekh 2018). However, titanium alloy is the most common material that is used to produce these prostheses, meeting the various clinical demands but lacking diverse biological functions. Therefore, the surface modification of customized, 3D-printed prostheses endows these prostheses with a surface morphology and chemical composition that exhibits excellent antibacterial, osteogenic, and wear and corrosion resistance properties. Thus, surface modification plays a significant role in promoting the clinical application of customized 3D-printed prostheses.

12.1 Clinical Applications of Customized 3D-Printed Prostheses Made with Surface Modification Technology

3D printing technology has the advantages of rapid modeling, high precision, and personalized customization on the basis of individual requirements. In the fabrication of porous titanium alloys, 3D printing can achieve the accurate control of porous structures and facilitate the formation of complex shapes through precise

D. Yu · H. Wu · Z. Tang · S. Bao · Q. Ma (✉)
Department of Orthopedics, Tangdu Hospital, Xi'an, China
e-mail: maqiong@fmmu.edu.cn

Z. Guo et al. (eds.), *3D-Printed Prosthesis in Orthopedic Oncology*,
https://doi.org/10.1007/978-981-95-1454-0_12

control of printing parameters and template design. Three-dimensional porous structures have been introduced into the design of titanium alloy implants, which significantly enhance the mechanical properties of these implants and their integration with bone tissue. Porous titanium alloys, which are new biomaterials with excellent mechanical properties, have been extensively used in the production of orthopedic medical devices, such as artificial joints, spinal fusion cages, dental implants, and bone repair substitutes (Lim et al. 2021). However, 3D-printed prostheses, which are increasing in clinical demand, require additional functions, such as osteoinduction, antibacterial sterilization, and wear and corrosion resistance (Overmann and Forsberg 2020). Therefore, surface modification of 3D-printed prostheses via physical or chemical methods plays a crucial role in improving the functions of the materials that are used by altering their surface morphology and properties.

Customized 3D-printed prostheses are commonly made of titanium alloys, but they lack inherent bioactivity, and the inert oxide layers on their surface reduce the integration between the implant and the bone tissue, thereby leading to loosening, displacement, or even implant failure. The surface modification of customized 3D-printed prostheses is a pivotal area of research for promoting osteogenesis at the surface interface. The surface roughness and micro/nanostructure of titanium alloys significantly influence the adhesion, proliferation, and differentiation of osteoblasts. The surface morphology of implants resulting from sandblasting, acid etching, and alkali-thermal treatments can effectively improve the surface hydrophilicity and roughness of prostheses, consequently enhancing their osteogenic performance. From the perspective of surface bioactive coatings, bioactive coatings (such as growth factor, metal ion, and active ceramic coatings) with osteoinductivity that are established on prosthesis surfaces via physical adsorption or chemical crosslinking can also effectively increase the osteoinductivity and integration of customized, 3D-printed prostheses. Therefore, the osteogenic capability on the surfaces of customized 3D-printed prostheses, which can be increased by surface modification techniques, is a focal issue in current research and future clinical applications.

In the field of orthopedics, the risk of infection associated with implant prostheses ranges from 2% to 5%, usually resulting in severe complications; this is a significant challenge that orthopedic surgeons cannot ignore (Miller et al. 2020). A three-dimensional porous structure of customized 3D-printed prostheses can prevent exudate accumulation, thus decreasing the incidence of postoperative infections; however, materials that are used in prostheses and lack antimicrobial activity have difficulty in preventing implant-related infections. Currently, customized 3D-printed prostheses are not capable to resist bacterial adhesion, colonization, or biofilm formation. Therefore, surface modification techniques, which are promising strategies for preventing implant-related infections in the use of customized 3D-printed prostheses, can mitigate early bacterial attachment, kill subsequently adherent bacteria, and prevent biofilm formation. Recently, researchers have conducted extensive work to understand the basis of antimicrobial modifications through ion implantation, nanomorphology, and coating on the surface of titanium alloys. This has significantly promoted the development and preparation of new antimicrobial 3D-printed titanium alloy prostheses, which have great potential for clinical application.

Currently, the surface friction and wear resistance of customized 3D-printed titanium alloy prostheses are scarce. Implant materials remain in the body for an extended period, and the debris that is produced and the harmful elements that are released, such as aluminum and vanadium, can trigger tissue inflammation, resulting in the failure of implant integration. Moreover, it is difficult for medical implants to achieve long-term service within the body. Additionally, the surfaces of titanium alloys exhibit weak fatigue resistance due to their high fatigue sensitivity, and fatigue fractures occur over time. The progression of fatigue fracture can be divided into three stages: crack initiation and subcritical and unstable crack propagation. Surface treatment of titanium alloys can cause nano-crystalline microstructure to emerge on the surface while maintaining a coarse-grain microstructure on the inside, with a gradient variation in grain size from their surface to the interior; this increases the wear and fatigue resistance of the titanium alloy surface. Long-term exposure of titanium alloy prostheses to bodily fluids can lead to corrosion, which is closely related to fatigue fracture. Customized 3D-printed prostheses that are susceptible to corrosive media often fail due to the interaction between fatigue and corrosion. Therefore, surface nanocrystallization and interior coarse-grain coating on customized, 3D-printed prostheses can ameliorate the long-term fatigue and wear and corrosion resistance of clinical implants. This approach not only extends the service life of customized 3D-printed prostheses but also prevents prosthesis fracture and surgical revision.

12.2 Development and Application of New Bioactive Coatings for Customized 3D-Printed Prostheses

12.2.1 Progress in the Development of New Bioactive Osteogenic Coatings

The inert nature and low bioactivity of 3D-printed, porous, customized titanium alloy prostheses pose major challenges in the development of bone tissue engineering. To address these issues, researchers have introduced various surface modifications to enhance bioactivity and osseointegration and further facilitate their clinical application. These technologies are primarily divided into two categories: biomaterial coating and surface treatment (Overmann et al. 2020).

Biomaterial coating is a common surface modification technique that alters the surface properties of porous titanium alloy prostheses by applying an additional layer on their surface. These coatings, which include bioactive substances, drugs, and cytokines, provide better cell attachment and osteoinductive capability. Common coating materials include hydroxyapatite (HAP), tricalcium phosphate (CaP), poly-ε-caprolactone (PCL), and polylactic acid (PLA). These coatings improve the biocompatibility, bioactivity, and osseointegration of porous titanium alloy prostheses, resulting in bone defect repair (Ehrensberger et al. 2020).

Surface treatment, which involves physical or chemical processes, is another common technique for the surface modification of porous titanium alloy prostheses. Popular surface treatment techniques, including anodization, acid etching, solvent treatment, and plasma treatment, can alter the surface morphology, roughness, pore size, and surface energy of porous tantalum, thereby reinforcing its interaction with surrounding tissues and cells. Surface treatments can improve the cell attachment, osteogenic capability, and bone integration performance of porous titanium alloy prostheses. These biomaterial coatings and surface treatment techniques provide a variety of surface modifications for porous titanium alloy prostheses to meet different clinical needs and application scenarios. However, the selection and optimization of each technique require in-depth exploration and evaluation to ensure the excellent biocompatibility, bioactivity, and long-term stability of modified porous titanium alloy prostheses in clinical applications (Zheng et al. 2020).

12.2.2 Progress in the Development of New Bioactive Antimicrobial Coatings

Infections that are related to orthopedic implants, including prostheses fixed within artificial joints, represent one of the most severe complications after the clinical application of metal orthopedic implants, and such infections also occur in clinical applications related to customized, 3D-printed orthopedic prostheses. Once infection occurs, it can not only lead to the failure of customized 3D-printed orthopedic prostheses but also possibly cause infectious bone defects and limb dysfunction in patients. Therefore, surface modification of customized 3D-printed orthopedic prostheses can endow them with excellent biological functions to prevent or treat infection, which is very important for enhancing their clinical effectiveness. Currently, the production of antibacterial coatings based on the specific characteristics of orthopedic implant infections has become an important orientation in the further development of techniques for the surface modification of 3D-printed customized prostheses.

Regarding characteristic infections that are related to orthopedic implants, bacteria adhere to the surface of the implant during the initial stage of infection, which is the most crucial stage of infection. Consequently, current efforts in developing antibacterial coatings on customized 3D-printed prostheses primarily focus on the prevention of early bacterial adhesion and colonization. Additionally, sustained antibacterial action is equally important for the prevention of delayed and mid- to late-stage infections. Hence, surface antibacterial coatings that are designed for customized 3D-printed prostheses are divided into antibacterial adhesion coatings, coatings with slow release of antimicrobial agents, and other types of antibacterial coatings. These antibacterial coatings can be categorized into two types based on their chemical composition: organic and inorganic antibacterial coatings.

Antibiotic-loaded coatings, which are organic antibacterial layers, are currently the most widely used type of bio-antibacterial coating. Broad-spectrum antibiotics, such as gentamicin, vancomycin, and amoxicillin, are favored by most researchers. The application of antibiotic coatings has significantly decreased the incidence of implant-related infections, as well as the side effects and dysbiosis that are associated with systemic medication. Xu Cui et al. developed an antibacterial coating on the surface of 3D-printed titanium alloy scaffolds by mixing vancomycin with polyvinyl alcohol (PVA). This coating showed excellent antibacterial performance in both in vitro and in vivo experiments and unique advantages in infection prevention after spinal surgery (Li et al. 2020). However, limitations in the effectiveness of antibiotic coatings have increasingly emerged as in-depth research has been conducted. On one hand, the burst release of antibiotic coatings during in vivo processes often results in unsustainable release. On the other hand, antibiotic resistance and biofilm formation on the implant surface can lead to latent and chronic infections. Therefore, when developing antibiotic coatings, it is necessary to combine various sensitive antibiotics and select lipophilic antibiotics that can penetrate biofilms to eradicate latent bacteria, thereby achieving infection control. In addition to antibiotics, organic polymer materials, such as quaternized chitosan and polyethyleneimine with nitrogen, along with antimicrobial peptides (AMPs), are frequently used as surface antibacterial coatings. The team of academician Yingjun Wang developed an antibacterial coating on the surface of titanium implants by immobilizing mesoporous silica nanoparticles (MSNs) that were loaded with the antimicrobial peptide HHC36. The in vitro results showed that the antibacterial effects of this coating against four clinically common bacteria, namely, *Staphylococcus aureus* (*S. aureus*), *Escherichia coli*, *Pseudomonas aeruginosa*, and MRSA, exceeded 95.71% (Chen et al. 2021). Takashi and colleagues demonstrated that antibacterial spinal fusion cages that were constructed by coating quaternized chitosan on a titanium cage surface resulted in improved wound healing, decreased infection symptoms, and reduced bacterial quantity during *S. aureus* spinal infection and simultaneously promoted osseointegration (Kodama et al. 2021). However, the development of organic antibacterial coatings on the surface of 3D-printed customized prostheses has rarely been reported, indicating that their therapeutic effects further need to be confirmed.

Metallic antibacterial coatings, which are inorganic antibacterial coatings, have recently received increasing domestic and international attention, and significant progress has been made in surface modification. Metal antibacterial agents, including metallic ions (such as Ag, Cu, and Zn) and photocatalytic metal oxides (such as TiO_2 and Fe_2O_3), have strong antibacterial activity against a broad spectrum of microbes, and little antibiotic resistance, and these agents are suitable for use as antibacterial coatings. Silver ions, which are typical metal ionic antibacterial agents, are the most widely and effectively used common inorganic antibacterial agents. Hailer et al. demonstrated that when deposited on a porous EBM-printed Ti-6Al-4V scaffold surface, metallic silver could release silver ions over 28 days and significantly inhibit the adhesion of *Staphylococcus aureus* and biofilm formation of *Staphylococcus epidermidis* (Diez-Escudero et al. 2022). Ye et al. developed a ZnO metal oxide coating on pure titanium metal surface and achieved the local release of Zn ions and the generation of reactive oxygen species (ROS). The in vitro results revealed excellent antibacterial activity against *Staphylococcus aureus* and protected surrounding tissue cells from the toxicity of Zn ions and ROS. Metal antibacterial coatings are required to avoid cytotoxicity, and advanced surface modification techniques are needed for the establishment of antibacterial coatings (Ye et al. 2020). Metal oxides such as TiO_2, which are stable photocatalysts, can promote the production of ROS to kill bacteria under UV light radiation. In-situ chemical synthesis of TiO_2 nanostructures on titanium alloy surfaces, such as nanotubes or nanoparticles, significantly increased the local antibacterial effectiveness of the implants.

Recently, with further research on new material properties, stimulus-responsive antibacterial materials (materials that are responsive to light, magnetism, sound, electricity, etc.) have become candidates for antibacterial coatings on metal implant surfaces. Materials that are responsive to near-infrared light, such as polydopamine and graphene oxide, exhibit efficient photothermal conversion. Under near-infrared radiation, these materials can locally generate overheating effects to disrupt the structure of bacteria and biofilms in order to control infection. Wei Sun et al. developed a polydopamine-curcumin coating on the surface of titanium alloy implant that could significantly kill *Staphylococcus aureus* and *Escherichia coli* via a simultaneous combination of photothermal and photodynamic effects (Guo et al. 2023). Stimulus-responsive biomaterials can produce photothermal, magnetothermal, ultrasonic-photodynamic, and electrical effects in response to external stimuli, exerting physical antibacterial effects, rather than traditional antimicrobial effects, in disrupting biofilms and bacteria. However, the physical stimuli that are produced by the stimulus response can inevitably damage normal tissues, thus impairing the efficacy of 3D-printed customized prostheses in repairing defects. Therefore, the combination of physical and chemical antibacterial effects due to composite antibacterial coatings with multiple functional effects is an important orientation for the development of future research on new antibacterial coatings for the surfaces of 3D-printed customized prostheses.

12.2.3 Progress in the Development of New Wear-Resistant and Corrosion-Resistant Coatings

Compared to research on osteogenesis and antibacterial performance, investigations of wear-resistant and corrosion-resistant coatings on metal medical implants are relatively rare. Notably, the long-term wear and corrosion resistance requirements for customized 3D-printed implants will receive increased attention with rapid advances in their development and application. However, metal materials for medical implants can exert toxic side effects on surrounding tissues because metal fragments are produced due to wear and metal ions are released due to corrosion. Moreover, long-term corrosion can lead to a decrease in the mechanical performance of an implant. Repeated mechanical stimulation after implantation may result in implant damage, fracture, and failure along with surgical revision. Furthermore, with the emergence of magnesium-based biodegradable alloys and the development of customizable, 3D-printed, biodegradable metal prostheses, improving the degradation rate and corrosion resistance of magnesium alloys through surface treatment has become a future trend for the development of customizable, 3D-printed, biodegradable metal implants.

Developing surface coatings is the most direct strategy for improving the corrosion and wear resistance of metal implants. Among the available coating materials, bioactive ceramics such as hydroxyapatite markedly enhance the resistance of metal implants to corrosion. Amit et al. fabricated titanium alloy scaffolds containing silicon nitride (Si_3N_4), alumina (Al_2O_3), and hydroxyapatite, as well as composites of these materials, using directed energy deposition (DED) technology (Afrouzian and Bandyopadhyay 2023). The in vitro results revealed that the ceramic coatings notably improved the wear resistance (Vickers hardness) and corrosion resistance (biological friction corrosion) of the 3D-printed titanium alloy scaffolds. This further enhanced the application of 3D-printed customizable prostheses, such as artificial hip joints, in the field of orthopedic implants. Although bioceramic coatings facilitated the corrosion and wear resistance of 3D-printed metal prostheses, the hydroxyapatite coating on their surface degraded over time with protection loss. Therefore, a TiO_2 oxide layer was prepared on the surface of a 3D-printed titanium alloy prosthesis through a metal surface passivation technique, and it promoted the corrosion resistance of customized prostheses, significantly overcoming the abovementioned limitations.

In the field of surface corrosion resistance technologies, ion implantation has attracted attention in recent years because of its ease of use and definitive effectiveness. Among these methods, oxygen and nitrogen ion implantation are particularly common and can be used to directly fabricate TiO_2 or TiN thin layers on titanium metal surfaces to notably enhance the corrosion resistance of substrate materials. Microarc oxidation and hydrothermal synthesis are also frequently employed to prepare ceramic coatings or oxide layers, which have excellent corrosion resistance, on orthopedic metal implant surfaces to facilitate high service performance. However, although the increased corrosion and wear resistance of 3D-printed customized implants, which promotes their long-term in vivo safety and efficacy, has been widely achieved, systematic evaluations and comparisons of different coatings and coating preparation technologies are lacking. Rather, in vivo osseointegration and antibacterial osteogenesis are the main focus of preclinical research. Therefore, the development of corrosion-resistant coatings for implant surfaces and the establishment of related evaluation systems are crucial for the future clinical application of customized 3D-printed implants.

12.3 New Technology for Preparing Surface Coatings on Customized 3D-Printed Prostheses

12.3.1 Innovative Technology for the Physical Surface Modification of 3D-Printed Prostheses

Physical surface modification techniques involve modifying the surface of a material to achieve specific desired functionalities without altering the inherent chemical properties of the material. These techniques include mechanical surface modification, plasma injection, spray deposition, physical adsorption, and thermal treatments (such as laser melting and high-temperature annealing). Compared to chemical modifications, physical surface modifications are simpler and more efficient and do not involve the addition of extra components. However, the coatings physically bond to the substrate, resulting in weaker bonding strength (Sheng et al. 2022).

The first form of physical surface modification involves the alteration of the surface structure of the implanted substrate material, and mechanical modifications are the most direct and efficient. These modifications typically impose mechanical force on the substrate surface via high-speed particles to cause certain deformations to increase bioactivity. Sandblasting and mechanical attrition treatment, which are two common strategies for mechanical modification, can improve the surface roughness, morphology, hydrophilicity, and biocompatibility of titanium prostheses. Therefore, these approaches maximally enhance the osteoconductivity and reduce fibrotic reactions without causing significant overall mechanical variation. Sandblasting, which is a simple and low-cost technique, involves spraying materials onto a workpiece surface using a high-velocity jet in a compressed air stream. This not only enhances surface strength through plastic deformation of the subsurface layer but also removes inevitable defects (such as burrs and adhered powder) from 3D-printed prostheses, thus improving surface quality (Fig. 12.1) (Yu et. al. 2025). Mechanical attrition is commonly used for the postprocessing of customized 3D-printed prostheses and enhances strength and ductility by forming gradient nanostructures on the prosthesis surface. In addition to mechanical modification, ultrasonic nanotechnology and laser melting techniques are also utilized to modify the surface structure of implanted metal prostheses. Ultrasonic nanotechnology leverages low-frequency ultrasound vibrations on the superposition of static loads to induce severe plastic deformation on the material surface, leading to surface nanocrystallization that significantly increases the corrosion resistance and mechanical strength of the implants. Laser melting uses laser energy to remelt the topmost layer of additively manufactured parts to significantly improve the surface morphology of customized 3D-printed prostheses. However, this postprocessing behavior removes the scan layers that were produced on 3D-printed prostheses, influencing the surface chemical composition; this effect depends on the melting and solidification duration as well as the atmospheric conditions.

In the preparation of surface coatings, physical adsorption is the simplest technique for physical modification. Physically adsorbed molecules are anchored to

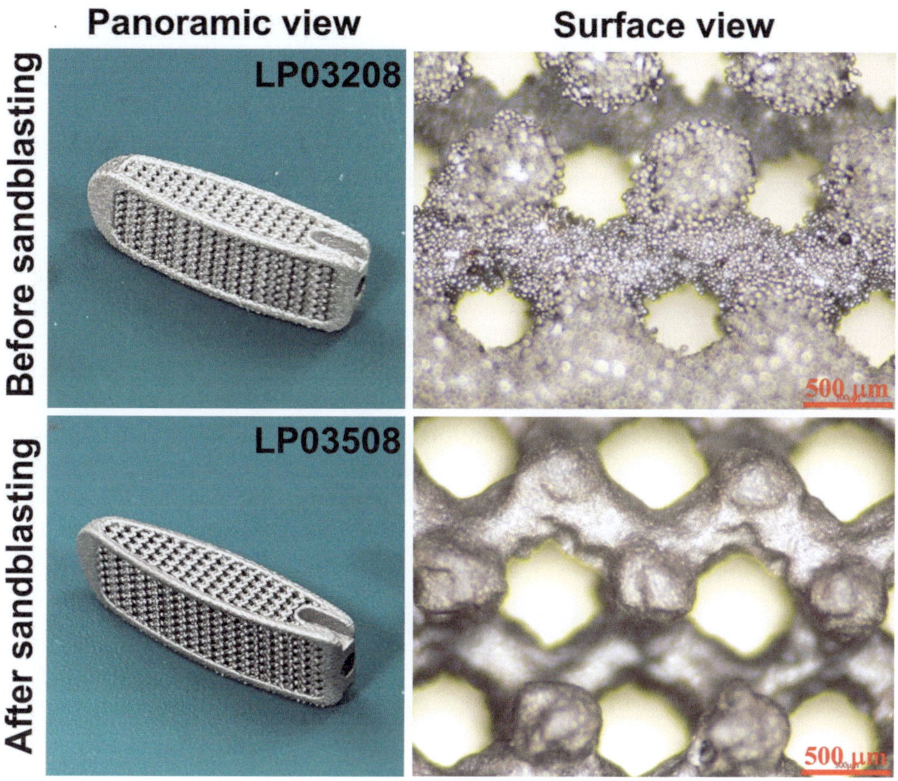

Fig. 12.1 Panoramic and surface views of 3D-printed titanium alloy cage before and after sandblasting treatment (Yu et al. 2024)

solid surfaces by mechanical interlocking and relatively weak physical binding forces. The comparatively weak nature of physical adsorption makes it appealing for drug release applications. Surface-modified adsorptive layers are made from a variety of materials, including polymers and inorganic materials such as metal ions (Wei et al. 2023).

Plasma injection and spray deposition are common techniques for the preparation of surface coatings. Plasma injection emits an ion beam of the required elements toward the solid material surface, causing variations in the surface composition, structure, and performance to increase the surface biocompatibility. Spray deposition, including cold spraying, thermal spraying, plasma spraying, and high-velocity oxy-fuel spraying, involves spraying coating materials onto a substrate surface at high pressure and velocity. For example, thermal spraying melts the spraying material through a heat source of flames or plasma and deposits it on the substrate surface via a high-speed jet to form functional coatings. This technique can deposit a wide variety of thick coatings ranging from 50 micrometers to several millimeters on customized 3D-printed prostheses made of metal materials.

With advances in physical modification technologies, progress has also been made in preparing surface coatings on 3D-printed prostheses using magnetron sputtering, atomic layer deposition, and photoradiation. Magnetron sputtering introduces an appropriate amount of argon gas into a high vacuum and creates a magnetically controlled abnormal glow discharge in the coating chamber for the ionization of argon gas. The use of non-equilibrium magnetron sputtering for the preparation of graphite-like carbon-based thin films on 3D-printed PEEK implant surfaces revealed that this technique could reduce the contact angle, indicating hydrophilicity, and enhance cell proliferation and adhesion on the surface (Jang et al. 2022). Atomic layer deposition, which is a vapor-phase thin-film deposition technique in which atoms are deposited layer by layer on a substrate, involves a deposition reaction for only one layer of atoms at a time (Fig. 12.2) (Zhang et al. 2023). This technology has significant advantages, including precise thickness control, nanoscale coatings, exceptional uniformity, strong bond strength, low growth temperatures, outstanding reproducibility, and suitability for sensitive substrates. For 3D-printed implants with complex porous structures, atomic layer deposition is well suited for the preparation of coatings on 3D-printed porous scaffolds, resulting

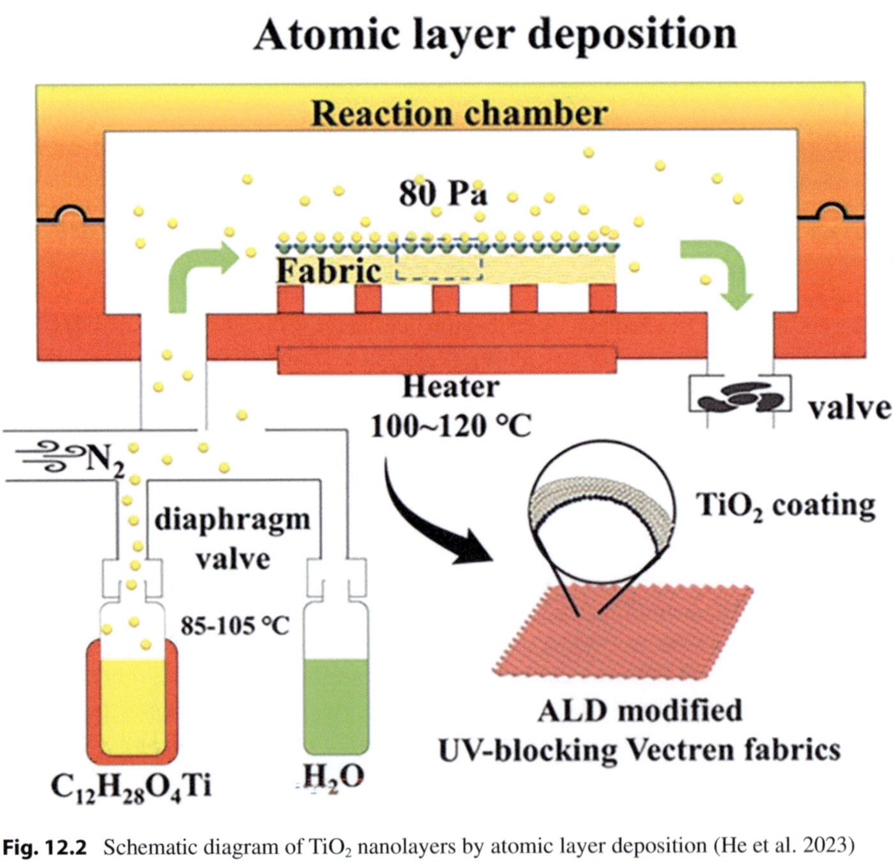

Fig. 12.2 Schematic diagram of TiO_2 nanolayers by atomic layer deposition (He et al. 2023)

in uniform, perfect films on these surfaces, but this process is expensive (Cho et al. 2020; Dorsey et al. 2019). Photonic radiation is primarily used for surface modification of customized 3D-printed biopolymer prostheses. Under UV radiation, new chemical groups can be introduced to the material surface, enhancing its chemical reactivity and laying the groundwork for subsequent modifications.

12.3.2 Innovative Technology for the Chemical Surface Modification of 3D-Printed Prostheses

Chemical surface modification alters the surface properties of raw materials via chemical reactions since the different compounds that are created or formed are chemically bonded to the raw material surface, thereby increasing the bonding strength. These techniques include chemical etching, hydrothermal treatment, electrochemical processing, chemical vapor deposition, and sol-gel methods. Moreover, chemical surface modification techniques are adaptable to implants with complex shapes, providing broad application prospects in the surface modification of 3D-printed implants.

Chemical corrosion, which includes acid and alkali corrosion, occurs when materials are exposed to acidic or alkaline environments. This process leads to the formation of corrosion pits on the sample surface, altering its surface morphology and roughness. Alkali heating, which is a cost-effective surface modification technique, is frequently used to enhance the osteoconductivity and osteoinductivity of titanium alloys. Rutile and feather-structured sodium titanate are added to surfaces treated with alkali heating, and this approach induces significant hydroxyapatite formation. Titanium metal surfaces that are exposed to alkali solution and heat treatment are negatively charged, facilitating the formation of amorphous calcium phosphate by binding with positively charged calcium ions (Ca^{2+}) (Pyka et al. 2012; Torres et al. 2018).

Hydrothermal and alkali treatments, which are straightforward processes for fabricating complex structures (especially 3D-printed porous materials), increase the bioactivity, electroactivity, and chemical activity of medical materials (Fig. 12.3). A "nanozyme-like" cerium oxide coating synthesized through hydrothermal treatment endows titanium alloys with the capability to eliminate various free radicals and regulate the immune microenvironment. Nanoceria coating accelerates early

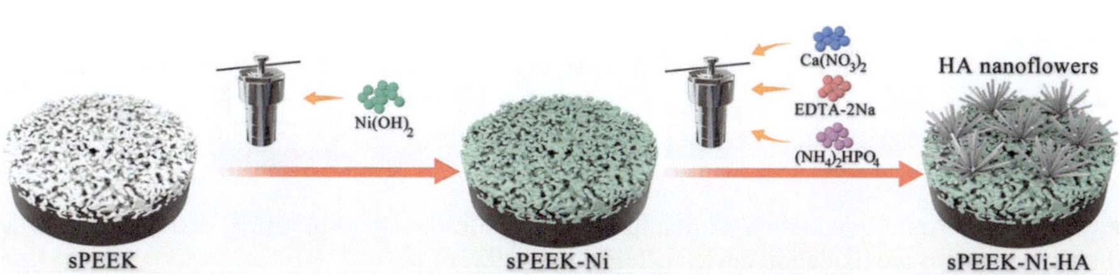

Fig. 12.3 Hydrothermal treatment of PEEK scaffold (Dong et al. 2020)

angiopoiesis and osseointegration (Bao et al. 2024). Moreover, a hydroxyapatite (HA) coating containing copper and strontium ions hydrothermally synthesized on 3D-printed porous titanium alloy surfaces not only meets the mechanical requirements of the human body but also increases the bioactivity, antibacterial properties, and bone growth of the resulting scaffold (Suchanek et al. 2015).

Electrochemical processing can be categorized into anodic oxidation, microarc oxidation, electrophoretic deposition, and electrochemical deposition according to principle and process. Anodic oxidation involves titanium alloys as anodes and lead or platinum plates as cathodes. In this process, ions in the electrolyte diffuse toward the anode under an electric field and then trigger an oxidation–reduction reaction to form a micro/nanostructure on titanium surface (Fig. 12.4a). Microarc oxidation, which is also known as plasma electrolytic oxidation, anodic spark deposition, or microarc discharge oxidation, is a technique that is used to promote the in-situ growth of porous functional oxide layers on metal surfaces using high voltages (Fig. 12.4b). Electrophoretic deposition (EPD) is a technique that is used to deposit colloidal particles on a surface in a liquid medium and an electric field, with the particles suspended in the medium between two electrodes. Electrochemical deposition is a versatile technique that is typically used to prepare coatings on metal substrates, and it can produce coatings with appropriate uniformity, thickness, and bonding strength on porous metal surfaces. This process is primarily conducted at room temperature to minimize thermal stress on implants.

Chemical vapor deposition (CVD) involves the interaction of mixed gas with the substrate surface at considerably high temperatures. This interaction causes certain components within the gas mixture to decompose and be deposited onto the substrate surface, and the resulting layer has a complex shape and provides excellent coverage (Pandey et al. 2021). Plasma-enhanced chemical vapor deposition (PECVD) frequently involves depositing active molecules onto the surfaces of biomaterials at low deposition temperatures, directly controlling the reaction parameters, and ensuring high purity. Specifically, the addition of amino groups on the surface of a carbon fiber-reinforced polyetheretherketone (CPEEK) composite

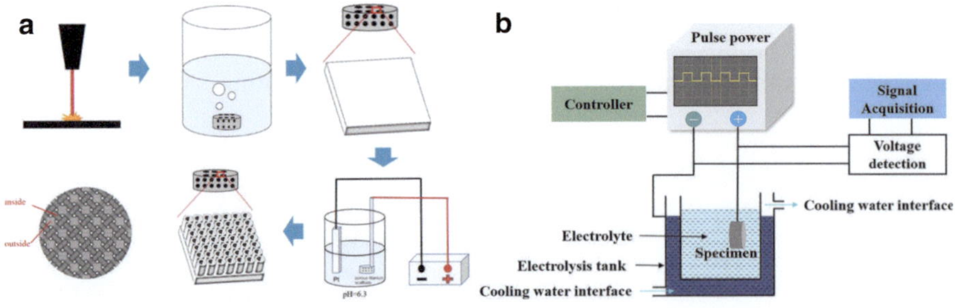

Fig. 12.4 (**a**) Anodic oxidation of titanium alloy scaffold (Fan et al. 2023) and (**b**) schematic diagram of micro-arc oxidation device (Zhang et al. 2022)

material by PECVD markedly enhances the adhesion, proliferation, and osteogenic differentiation of MG-63 cells on its surface, increasing its bioactivity and osteogenic potential (Yu et al. 2020).

The sol-gel process involves the easy hydrolysis of metal alkoxides or inorganic salts in a solvent with water, leading to sol formation through hydrolysis and polycondensation. Thereafter, this sol is coated on a metal surface, followed by drying and heat treatment to form a protective layer. This technique is suitable for 3D-printed metals and polymers. Hydrogels, which are known as excellent drug and cell carriers, can be customized to any shape and size according to specific application requirements and are capable of completely covering the microporous structures of 3D-printed implants (especially titanium implants) in current widespread applications.

12.4 Prospects for Surface Modification Technology of Customized 3D-Printed Prostheses

12.4.1 Optimization of Coating Stability on a 3D-Printed Prosthesis Surface

The two most common causes of surgical revision after joint replacement are aseptic loosening and infection (Przybilla et al. 2023), and aseptic loosening stems from the initial loss of prosthesis stability for an extended service period after implantation. Consequently, secure stability is a critical requirement for clinically implanted prostheses. For 3D-printed prostheses, long-term stability of surface modification coatings determines their service life and functionality after implantation. Coating stability involves two aspects: inherent stability (structural, physical, chemical, and biological properties), which determines coating functionality, and bonding stability of the coating and substrate, which ensures its reliability. Both effectiveness and long-term stability are vital for bone repair efficacy on surface-modified 3D-printed prostheses in vivo (Pardun et al. 2015).

12.4.1.1 Coating Property Stability

Coating properties, including physical, chemical, and mechanical properties (Gomes et al. 2021; Park et al. 2019) as well as their biomolecule-loaded bioactivity (Atefyekta et al. 2019), play a critical role in determining inherent property stability of coatings, which ensures their intended functions, such as their antibacterial, anti-inflammatory, anti-infection, and bone repair effects. However, the sensitivity of coating properties to the surrounding environment can lead to physical or chemical changes in these coatings, such as degradation, wear, reduction, oxidation, catalysis, moisture absorption, curing, deactivation, or denaturation, which in turn can result in the loss of functional properties. Therefore, for potential surface modifications of 3D-printed prostheses, a series of material structural characterizations and biological evaluations, both in vitro and in vivo, are necessary to determine the effectiveness and functionality of coating properties.

12.4.1.2 Structural Stability of Coatings

The structural stability of coatings determines the long-term biostability of implanted prostheses. Physical and chemical surface modifications can enhance the surface roughness of implants, resulting in a high degree of micromechanical interlocking that improves the primary and secondary stability of the implant (Diez-Escudero et al. 2022). Coatings that are physically bonded to the substrate surface, especially when overly thick, are prone to peeling off and forming debris, leading to structural failure of the coating. In contrast, bioceramic or bioglass coatings chemically bond to the substrate (Atefyekta et al. 2019), and biomolecular coatings are chemically immobilized on the substrate; these are important strategies for increasing structural stability (Fig. 12.5) (Rivolo et al. 2016).

12.4.2 Preparation of Composite Coatings on Surfaces of 3D-Printed Prostheses

With advances in science and technology, the demand for multifunctional composite coatings on 3D-printed prostheses has increasingly become a development trend, as single-functional coatings no longer meet the needs of clinical and scientific research. In the prevention and treatment of orthopedic surgical infections, systemic prophylactic antibiotics are commonly used to prevent infection. However, the doses of systemic antibiotics that are used, are quite limited and liable to cause bacterial resistance. Compared to systemic administration, the local application of antibiotics can provide high doses directly at the surgical site, reducing the risk of bacterial resistance (Miller et al. 2020). Yan et al. coated the surfaces of 3D-printed porous PEEK prostheses with silver nanoparticles (AgNPs) containing silk fibroin (SF) and gentamicin sulfate (GS) (Yan et al. 2018). The results indicated that modified PEEK prosthesis showed significant antimicrobial activity against both gram-positive and gram-negative bacteria. Moreover, compared to an uncoated PEEK prosthesis, modified PEEK prosthesis promoted the adhesion, proliferation, and differentiation of MC3T3-E1 cells. Yin's team developed a multifunctional PEEK prosthesis by coating sulfonated PEEK with MXene nanosheets, methacrylic acid gelatin (GelMA) hydrogel, and tobramycin, and this prosthesis exhibited antitumor, antibacterial, and osteogenic properties (Yin et al. 2020). This modified PEEK prosthesis demonstrated excellent osteogenic capabilities, the capability to kill

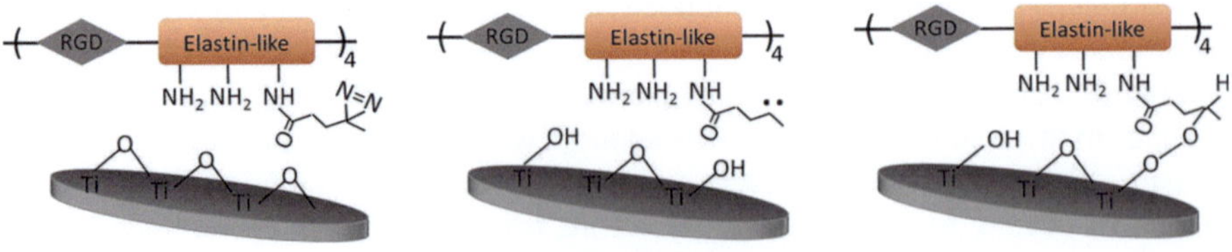

Fig. 12.5 Chemical bonding diagram of coating and substrate (Atefyekta et al. 2019)

osteosarcoma cells under near-infrared irradiation, and strong in vitro antibacterial properties due to the tobramycin coating.

The combination of antimicrobial and osteogenic coatings could be an effective strategy for treating infectious bone defects. Amin et al. developed a vancomycin and BMP-2 hydrogel coating on a porous titanium alloy surface (Yavari et al. 2020). The results indicated that biomimetic implants could effectively inhibit bacteria within 2–3 weeks and enhance ALP activity and mineralization on implant surface. Nano-ZrO_2 exhibits good biocompatibility and bioactivity, as well as antibacterial properties against both gram-negative and gram-positive bacteria (Gouda 2012; Jangra et al. 2012). Li et al. introduced bioactive ZrO_2 onto a CFR-PEEK surface through zirconium plasma immersion ion implantation (Zr-PIII). Cell culture experiments demonstrated that after PIII treatment, CFR-PEEK significantly improved the adhesion, proliferation, and differentiation of rBMSCs. The treated CFR-PEEK showed notable antibacterial activity against *Staphylococcus aureus* (Li et al. 2016).

The development of composite functionalized biocoatings on 3D-printed prosthesis surfaces is crucial for the advancement of 3D printing in biomedical applications. Numerous experiments related to the construction and biological evaluation of coatings on 3D-printed prosthesis surfaces have been conducted, and satisfactory in vitro and in vivo outcomes have been achieved. However, most research remains at the laboratory stage, and translating basic experimental data into clinical trials still poses a significant challenge. In the future, there will be many opportunities to expand this research field by filling knowledge gaps and extending capabilities, aiming to provide more effective strategies for preparing biocoatings on 3D-printed prosthesis surfaces.

References

Afrouzian A, Bandyopadhyay A. 3D printed silicon nitride, alumina, and hydroxyapatite ceramic reinforced Ti6Al4V composites – tailored microstructures to enhance bio-tribo-corrosion and antibacterial properties. J Mech Behav Biomed Mater. 2023;144:105973.

Ahn TK, Lee DH, Kim TS, et al. Modification of titanium implant and titanium dioxide for bone tissue engineering. Adv Exp Med Biol. 2018;1077:355–68.

Atefyekta S, Pihl M, Lindsay C, et al. Antibiofilm elastin-like polypeptide coatings: functionality, stability, and selectivity. Acta Biomater. 2019;83:245–56.

Bao S, Yu D, Tang Z, et al. Conformationally regulated “nanozyme-like” cerium oxide with multiple free radical scavenging activities for osteoimmunology modulation and vascularized osseointegration. Bioact Mater. 2024;34:64–79.

Chen J, Hu G, Li T, et al. Fusion peptide engineered “statically-versatile” titanium implant simultaneously enhancing anti-infection, vascularization and osseointegration. Biomaterials. 2021;264:120446.

Cho TH, Farjam N, Allemang CR, et al. Area-selective atomic layer deposition patterned by electrohydrodynamic jet printing for additive manufacturing of functional materials and devices. ACS Nano. 2020;14(12):17262–72.

Diez-Escudero A, Andersson B, Carlsson E, et al. 3D-printed porous Ti6Al4V alloys with silver coating combine osteocompatibility and antimicrobial properties. Biomater Adv. 2022;133:112629.

Dong T, Duan C, Wang S, et al. Multifunctional surface with enhanced angiogenesis for improving long-term osteogenic fixation of poly(ether ether ketone) implants. ACS Appl Mater Interfaces. 2020;12(13):14971–82.

Dorsey KJ, Pearson TG, Esposito E, et al. Atomic layer deposition for membranes, metamaterials, and mechanisms. Adv Mater. 2019;31(29):e1901944.

Ehrensberger MT, Clark CM, Canty MK, et al. Electrochemical methods to enhance osseointegrated prostheses. Biomed Eng Lett. 2020;10(1):17–41.

Fan S, Talha M, Yu X, et al. 3D printing of porous Ti6Al4V bone tissue engineering scaffold and surface anodization preparation of nanotubes to enhance its biological property. Nanotechnol Rev. 2023;12(1):0572.

Gomes OP, Batagin-Neto A, Lisboa-Filho PN. The evaluation of anchoring processes and chemical stability of zwitterionic molecules via local reactivity indexes. Comput Mater Sci. 2021;193:110418.

Gouda M. Nano-zirconium oxide and nano-silver oxide/cotton gauze fabrics for antimicrobial and wound healing acceleration. J Ind Text. 2012;41(3):222–40.

Guo Q, Li P, Zhang Y, et al. Polydopamine-curcumin coating of titanium for remarkable antibacterial activity via synergistic photodynamic and photothermal properties. Photochem Photobiol. 2023;

He J, Liu Z, Zhang W, et al. Atomic layer deposition of TiO2 nanolayer coated Vectran fabrics with enhanced UV-blocking performance and structural colors. Surf Interfaces. 2023;42(Part B):103477.

Jang TS, Park SJ, Lee JE, et al. Topography-supported nanoarchitectonics of hybrid scaffold for systematically modulated bone regeneration and remodeling. Adv Funct Mater. 2022;32(51):2206863.

Jangra SL, Stalin K, Dilbaghi N, et al. Antimicrobial activity of zirconia (ZrO2) nanoparticles and zirconium complexes. J Nanosci Nanotechnol. 2012;12(9):7105–12.

Kodama J, Chen H, Zhou T, et al. Antibacterial efficacy of quaternized chitosan coating on 3D printed titanium cage in rat intervertebral disc space. Spine J. 2021;21(7):1217–28.

Lal H, Patralekh MK. 3D printing and its applications in orthopaedic trauma: a technological marvel. J Clin Orthop Trauma. 2018;9(3):260–8.

Li J, Qian S, Ning C, et al. rBMSC and bacterial responses to isoelastic carbon fiber-reinforced poly(ether-ether-ketone) modified by zirconium implantation. J Mater Chem B. 2016;4(1):96–104.

Li Y, Li L, Ma Y, et al. 3D-printed titanium cage with PVA-vancomycin coating prevents surgical site infections (SSIs). Macromol Biosci. 2020;20(3):e1900394.

Lim HK, Ryu M, Woo SH, et al. Bone conduction capacity of highly porous 3D-printed titanium scaffolds based on different pore designs. Materials (Basel). 2021;14(14)

Miller R, Higuera CA, Wu J, et al. Periprosthetic joint infection: a review of antibiotic treatment. JBJS Rev. 2020;8(7):e1900224.

Overmann AL, Aparicio C, Richards JT, et al. Orthopaedic osseointegration: implantology and future directions. J Orthop Res. 2020;38(7):1445–54.

Overmann AL, Forsberg JA. The state of the art of osseointegration for limb prosthesis. Biomed Eng Lett. 2020;10(1):5–16.

Pandey PC, Shukla S, Pandey G, et al. Nanostructured diamond for biomedical applications. Nanotechnology. 2021;32(13):132001.

Pardun K, Treccani L, Volkmann E, et al. Mixed zirconia calcium phosphate coatings for dental implants: tailoring coating stability and bioactivity potential. Mater Sci Eng C Mater Biol Appl. 2015;48:337–46.

Park JH, Ferhan AR, Jackman JA, et al. Modulating conformational stability of human serum albumin and implications for surface passivation applications. Colloids Surf B Biointerfaces. 2019;180:306–12.

Przybilla P, Subkov E, Latorre SH, et al. Effect of 20 mum thin ceramic coatings of hydroxyapatite, bioglass, GB14 and Beta-Tricalciumphosphate with copper on the biomechanical stability of femoral implants. J Mech Behav Biomed Mater. 2023;144:105951.

Pyka G, Burakowski A, Kerckhofs G, et al. Surface modification of Ti6Al4V open porous structures produced by additive manufacturing. Adv Eng Mater. 2012;14(6):363–70.
Rivolo P, Nistico R, Barone F, et al. Study of the adhesive properties versus stability/aging of hernia repair meshes after deposition of RF activated plasma polymerized acrylic acid coating. Mater Sci Eng C Mater Biol Appl. 2016;65:287–94.
Sheng X, Wang A, Wang Z, et al. Advanced surface modification for 3D-printed titanium alloy implant interface functionalization. Front Bioeng Biotechnol. 2022;10:850110.
Suchanek K, Bartkowiak A, Gdowik A, et al. Crystalline hydroxyapatite coatings synthesized under hydrothermal conditions on modified titanium substrates. Mater Sci Eng C Mater Biol Appl. 2015;51:57–63.
Torres Y, Sarria P, Gotor FJ, et al. Surface modification of Ti-6Al-4V alloys manufactured by selective laser melting: microstructural and tribo-mechanical characterization. Surf Coat Technol. 2018;348:31–40.
Wei X, Zhou W, Tang Z, et al. Magnesium surface-activated 3D printed porous PEEK scaffolds for in vivo osseointegration by promoting angiogenesis and osteogenesis. Bioact Mater. 2023;20:16–28.
Yan J, Zhou W, Jia Z, et al. Endowing polyetheretherketone with synergistic bactericidal effects and improved osteogenic ability. Acta Biomater. 2018;79:216–29.
Yavari SA, Croes M, Akhavan B, et al. Layer by layer coating for bio-functionalization of additively manufactured meta-biomaterials. Addit Manuf. 2020;32:100991.
Ye J, Li B, Li M, et al. ROS induced bactericidal activity of amorphous Zn-doped titanium oxide coatings and enhanced osseointegration in bacteria-infected rat tibias. Acta Biomater. 2020;107:313–24.
Yin J, Han Q, Zhang J, et al. MXene-based hydrogels endow polyetheretherketone with effective osteogenicity and combined treatment of osteosarcoma and bacterial infection. ACS Appl Mater Interfaces. 2020;12(41):45891–903.
Yu D, Wu S, Zhao T, et al. Nanograin enhanced surface layer strengthening of 3D printed intervertebral cage induced by sandblasting. Biomed Mater. 2025;20:025003.
Yu W, Zhang HAL, et al. Enhanced bioactivity and osteogenic property of carbon fiber reinforced polyetheretherketone composites modified with amino groups. Colloids Surf B Biointerfaces. 2020;193:111098.
Zhang X, Guan S, Qiu J, et al. Atomic layer deposition of tantalum oxide films on 3D-printed Ti6Al4V scaffolds with enhanced osteogenic property for orthopedic implants. ACS Biomater Sci Eng. 2023;9(7):4197–207.
Zhang Z-Y, Huang T-Y, Zhai D-J, et al. Study on strontium doped bioactive coatings on titanium alloys surfaces by micro-arc oxidation. Surf Coat Technol. 2022;451:129045.
Zheng Y, Han Q, Wang J, et al. Promotion of osseointegration between implant and bone interface by titanium alloy porous scaffolds prepared by 3D printing. ACS Biomater Sci Eng. 2020;6(9):5181–90.
Yu D, Wu S, Zhao T, et al. Nanograin enhanced surface layer strengthening of 3D printed intervertebral cage induced by sandblasting. Biomed Mater. 2024; https://doi.org/10.1088/1748-605X/ad9fc5. Accessed 16 Dec 2024

MIX
Papier aus verantwortungsvollen Quellen
Paper from responsible sources
FSC® C105338

If you have any concerns about our products,
you can contact us on
ProductSafety@springernature.com

In case Publisher is established outside the EU,
the EU authorized representative is:
Springer Nature Customer Service Center GmbH
Europaplatz 3, 69115 Heidelberg, Germany

Printed by Libri Plureos GmbH
in Hamburg, Germany